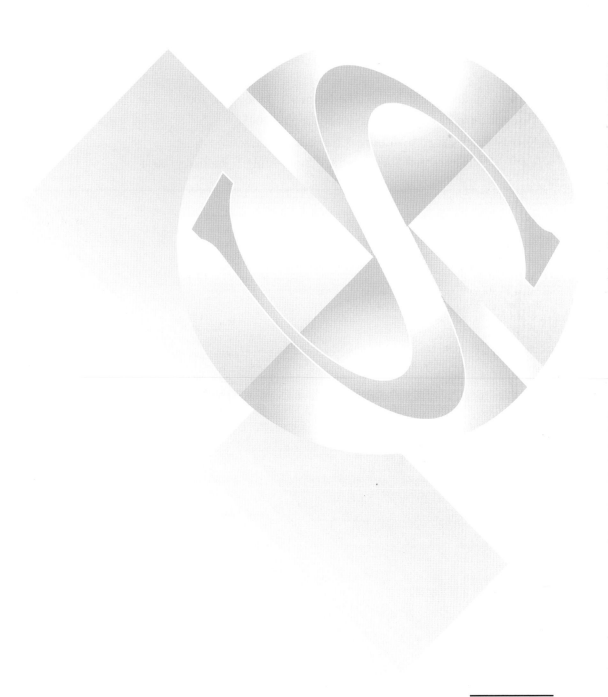

Springer
Specialist
Surgery
Series

*Other titles in this grouping include:*

Transplantation Surgery edited by Hakim & Danovitch, 2001
Vascular Surgery edited by Davies & Brophy, 2005
Neurosurgery edited by Moore & Newell, 2004
Upper Gastrointestinal Surgery edited by Fielding & Hallissey, 2004

Anne J. Moore and David W. Newell (Eds)

# Tumor Neurosurgery

## Principles and Practice

Series Editor: John Lumley

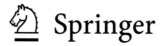 Springer

Anne J. Moore, MB BS, BSc, FRCS
South West Neurosurgery Centre
Derriford Hospital
Plymouth, UK

David W. Newell
The Seattle Neuroscience Institute
Seattle, WA, USA

British Library Cataloguing in Publication Data
A catalogue record for this book is available from the British Library

Library of Congress Control Number: 2006921750

ISBN-10: 1-84628-291-8
ISBN-13: 978-1-84628-291-1
e-ISBN: 1-84628-294-2

Printed on acid-free paper

Typeset by Florence Production, Stoodleigh, Devon, England
Printed in Singapore (FP/KYO)

9 8 7 6 5 4 3 2 1

Springer Science+Business Media, LLC
springer.com

# Preface

This book provides coverage of relevant topics in the field of tumor neurosurgery, for residents and registrars in training, and for recent graduates of training programs. As neurosurgical training incorporates expertise from centers worldwide, there is a need to have input from specialists in neurosurgery from various countries. This text is a compilation by expert authors in the USA and the UK to provide information on the basic knowledge and clinical management required for optimal care of neuro-oncology patients. The text is an up-to-date synopsis of the field of tumor neurosurgery from American and British perspectives, which covers the most common sites and tumor pathologies encountered by neurosurgeons. The chapters are organized under broad topics, including investigative studies, perioperative care and the role of newer techniques. The clinical management of CNS tumors in adults and children is described, including spinal tumors, both intradural and extradural. We anticipate that trainees will find this information useful for certification examinations and recent graduates of neurosurgical training programs can utilize this text as an update.

*Anne J. Moore*
*Plymouth, UK*

*David W. Newell*
*Seattle, USA*

# Contents

# Contributors

Ellsworth C. Alvord, Jr., MD
Department of Pathology
Neuropathology Laboratory
University of Washington School of Medicine
Harborview Medical Center
Seattle, WA, USA

Sepideh Amin-Hanjani, MD
Neurosurgery Service
Massachusetts General Hospital
Harvard Medical School
Boston, MA, USA

Kristian Aquilina, FRCS
Department of Neurosurgery
Beaumont Hospital
Dublin, Ireland

Mitchell S. Berger, MD
Department of Neurological Surgery
Brain Tumor Surgery Program
University of California
San Francisco School of Medicine
San Francisco, CA, USA

Roger A. Chisholm, MA, MB BChir, MRCP,
FRCR
Salford Royal Hospitals NHS Trust
Salford, UK

Philip Edwards, PhD
Department of Radiological Sciences
Medical School of Guy's, King's and St.
Thomas' Hospitals
King's College London
London, UK

Richard G. Ellenbogen, MD
Department of Neurosurgery
Harborview Medical Center
University of Washington School of Medicine
Seattle, WA, USA

Fred J. Epstein, MD
Hyman-Newman Institute for Neurology and
Neurosurgery
Pediatric Neurosurgery
Beth Israel Medical Center, Singer Division
New York, NY, USA

James J. Evans, MD
Division of Neuro-oncologic Neurosurgery
and Stereotactic Radiosurgery
Department of Neurosurgery
Thomas Jefferson University
Philadelphia, PA, USA

J. Russell Geyer MD
Department of Pediatrics
University of Washington School of Medicine
Children's Hospital and Regional Medical
Center
Seattle, WA, USA

Mladen Golubic, MD, PhD
Brain Tumor Institute/Department of
Neurosurgery
The Cleveland Clinic Foundation
Cleveland, OH, USA

David G. Hardy, BSc, MA, MB ChB, FRCS,
Department of Neurosurgery
Addenbrookes NHS Trust,
Cambridge, UK

Griffith R. Harsh IV, MD, MA, MBA
Neurosurgical Oncology
Stanford Medical School
Stanford University
Stanford, CA, USA

David G. Hughes MBBS, MRCP, FRCR
Department of Neuroradiology
Greater Manchester Neurosciences Centre
Hope Hospital
Salford, UK

George I. Jallo, MD
Pediatric Neurosurgery
John Hopkins Hospital
Baltimore, MD, USA

G. Evren Keles, MD
Department of Neurological Surgery
University of California
San Francisco School of Medicine
San Francisco, CA, USA

Andras A. Kemeny, FRSC, MD
The National Centre for Stereotactic
Radiosurgery
Royal Hallamshire Hospital
Sheffield, UK

Richard S. C. Kerr, BSc, MS, FRCS
Oxford Skull Base Unit
Radcliffe Infirmary
Oxford, UK

Karl F. Kothbauer, MD
Division of Neurosurgery
Department of Surgery
Kantonsspital Luzern
Luzern, Switzerland

Maryke A. Kraayenbrink, MRCP, FRCA
Department of Anaesthesia
St George's Hospital
London, UK

Charlie Kuntz, MD
Department of Neurological Surgery
University of Cincinnati
Cincinnati, OH, USA

Sandeep Kunwar, MD
Brain Tumor Research Center
Department of Neurological Surgery
University of California
San Francisco School of Medicine
San Francisco, CA, USA

Arthur M. Lam, MD, FRCPC
Departments of Anesthesiology and
Neurological Surgery
Harborview Medical Center
University of Washington
Seattle, WA, USA

Joung H. Lee, MD
Section of Skull Base Surgery
Brain Tumor Institute/Department of
Neurosurgery
The Cleveland Clinic Foundation
Cleveland, OH, USA

Henry Marsh, MA, MBBS, FRCS
Department of Neurosurgery
Atkinson Morley's Hospital
London, UK

Gregory R. McAnulty, BA, FRCA
Department of Anaesthesia
St George's Hospital
London, UK

Christopher A. Milford, BA, FRCS
Oxford Skull Base Unit
Radcliffe Infirmary
Oxford, UK

Anne J. Moore, MBBS, BSc, FRCS
South West Neurosurgery Centre
Derriford Hospital
Plymouth, UK

David W. Newell, MD
The Seattle Neuroscience Institute
Seattle, WA, USA

Michael P. Powell, MA, MBBS, FRCS
Victor Horsley Department of Neurosurgery
The National Hospital for Neurology and
Neurosurgery
London, UK

Jonathan Punt, MB BS, FRCS, FRCPCH
Children's Brain Tumour Research Centre
Academic Department of Child Health
University of Nottingham
Nottingham, UK

Matthias W. R. Radatz, MD
The National Centre for Stereotactic
Radiosurgery
Royal Hallamshire Hospital
Sheffield, UK

Robert C. Rostomily, MD
Department of Neurological Surgery
University of Washington Medical Center
Seattle, WA, USA

Jeremy G. Rowe, BM BCh, FRCS
The National Centre for Stereotactic
Radiosurgery
Royal Hallamshire Hospital
Sheffield, UK

Christopher I. Shaffrey, MD
Department of Neurological Surgery and
Orthopedic Surgery
University of Washington Medical Center
Seattle, WA, USA

CONTRIBUTORS

Cheng-Mei Shaw, MD
Department of Pathology
Neuropathology Laboratory
University of Washington School of Medicine
Harborview Medical Center
Seattle, WA, USA

Daniel L. Silbergeld, MD
University of Washington Medical Center
Department of Neurological Surgery
Seattle, WA, USA

Alexander M. Spence, MD
Department of Neurology
University of Washington Medical Center
Seattle, WA, USA

Richard J. Stacey, MBBS
Department of Neurosurgery
Radcliffe Infirmary
Oxford, UK

Kevin L. Stevenson, MD
Pediatric Neurosurgery Associates
Children's Healthcare of Atlanta
Atlanta, GA, USA

Anthony Strong, MA, DM, FRCSEd
Department of Neurosurgery
Medical School of Guy's, King's and St.
Thomas' Hospitals
King's College London
London, UK

John Suh, MD
Department of Radiation Oncology
The Cleveland Clinic Foundation
Cleveland, OH, USA

Derek A. Taggard, MD
Department of Neurosurgery
University of Iowa
Iowa City, IA, USA

Vincent C. Traynelis, MD
Department of Neurosurgery
University of Iowa Hospital
Iowa City, IA, USA

Allen E. Waziri, MD
Neurological Surgery
Columbia University
New York, NY, USA

Peter C Whitfield, BM, PhD, FRCS
Department of Neurosurgery
Aberdeen Royal Infirmary
Aberdeen, UK

Tessa L. Whitton, BM, FRCA
Department of Anesthesiology
Harborview Medical Center
University of Washington
Seattle, WA, USA

# Investigations

# 1

# Neurophysiology

Allen E. Waziri, Derek A. Taggard and
Vincent C. Traynelis

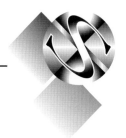

## Summary

The goal of this chapter is to provide a brief
description and critical review of the various
intraoperative monitoring techniques available to the modern neurosurgeon.

## Introduction

Since the mid-1960s, neurosurgeons have been
increasingly dedicated to utilizing technology
that allows for the monitoring of neurological
integrity and assessment of progress towards
operative goals while a procedure is under way.
Most neurosurgical procedures bear the risk
of permanent neurological injury and, in the
worst cases, devastation. In an attempt to
reduce such morbidity, numerous methods of
intraoperative monitoring have been created to
guide the neurosurgeon in altering operative
activity in a way that will prevent or minimize
neurological damage. Ideally, these monitoring
techniques involve minimal additional risks to
the patient. There are a number of methods that
have been in use for several decades and are well
described. In addition, experimental techniques
are being developed to provide further insight
into the neurophysiological changes associated
with surgical manipulation of the nervous
system.

The ideal intraoperative monitoring tool sat-
isfies several technical criteria. First is the ability
to detect neurological damage at an early and
reversible stage. Second, any modifications of
the operative technique to allow for monitoring
must not interfere with the surgeon's ability to
achieve the operative goal. Components of the
monitoring system should be easy to use and
provide consistent, reliable data. The information obtained should be resistant to variables
of the operative environment, such as depth of
anesthesia, choice of anesthetic agents, temperature, or electrical artifact. Last, the neurological function or region being monitored must
be that which is placed at risk by the operative
procedure. The goal of intraoperative monitoring is to provide the surgeon with information
that will guide or improve the current procedure
as well as subsequent procedures. All currently
available techniques fulfill these ideals to variable degrees.

In addition to the theoretical goals of intraoperative monitoring, there are a number of
practical issues that must be taken into consideration if such techniques are to be used
efficiently and successfully. Appropriate technical and analytical assistance is required from
individuals who are thoroughly familiar with
the particular technique to be used. The positioning of the patient and the monitoring
equipment must be optimized to allow for the
gathering of useful data without disruption of
the surgical field or approach. The equipment to
be used should be in excellent working order
and calibrated for the particular needs of each
case. Finally, potential sources of interference

that could mask or prohibit data acquisition, such as operating lights or other emitters of radiated electrical activity, should be minimized pre-operatively.

This chapter attempts to provide a brief description and discussion of intraoperative monitoring techniques that are currently used by neurosurgeons, some of which have been utilized with great success over the years, and others which remain in an experimental phase. Intraoperative imaging and image-guidance will be covered in Chapter 7.

# Electroencephalography

Electroencephalography (EEG) monitors and records spontaneously generated electrical potentials originating from the various surface cortical regions of the brain. EEG was first utilized as an intraoperative monitoring technique in 1965. It has subsequently grown in popularity owing to readily available equipment, familiar and consistent technique, relative simplicity of pre-operative set-up, and well- characterized patterns of response to various states of neurological function.

Traditional EEG relies on the application of a standard grid of scalp electrodes that are posi-tioned using the International 10–20 Scalp Electrode Placement System (Fig. 1.1). Data are typically gathered from both cerebral hemispheres. Appropriate personnel, including an individual trained in interpretation of the ongoing recordings, are required to apply the electrodes and maintain the system throughout the surgical procedure. Conventional EEG recording generates a great deal of data and requires continuous monitoring by a trained individual; therefore, there has been some interest in developing computer-based methods of real-time EEG analysis. Several methods of digitally processing EEG signals with subsequent computer analysis have been described, which utilize Fourier transforms to provide spectral power representations that are easier to interpret than the raw EEG data (known as compressed spectral array, or CSA). However, there has been concern over the failure of CSA to detect mild changes that could be detected with analog EEG monitoring, and the simplified data provided by CSA are more likely to be complicated by artifacts introduced by the operative environment. This may be alleviated by comparison of selected segments of raw data with the histograms generated by the computer.

The primary utility of intraoperative EEG is in monitoring for the presence of prolonged and

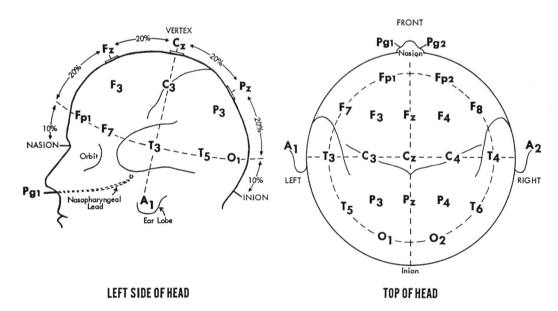

LEFT SIDE OF HEAD        TOP OF HEAD

**Fig. 1.1.** The International 10–20 Scalp Electrode Placement System used to obtain electroencephalographic recordings, as viewed from the left side and top of the head.

significant ischemia of the brain related to various surgical manipulations. Numerous studies have demonstrated that synaptic transmission is abolished when cerebral blood flow (CBF) decreases below 15 ml/100 g/min, and the ability of the neuron to maintain its membrane potential fails when flow drops below 10 ml/100 g/min. At this level, permanent neurological damage may ensue within minutes if blood flow remains reduced. Unilateral hemispheric ischemia will abrogate EEG activity within about 20 seconds. However, permanent neuronal damage, which can be detected by potassium efflux, does not begin to occur until 5 minutes post ischemia. Surgical trials in humans have demonstrated that major EEG changes occur with drops in CBF below 10 ml/100 g/min, while more minor changes occur with flows of 10–18 ml/100 g/min. The EEG pattern generally remains stable at flows of 25 ml/100 g/min or greater. Zampella et al. demonstrated that only 5% of patients will have demonstrable EEG changes at flows of 20 ml/100 g/min, while 31% of patients showed these changes at flows of less than 13 ml/100 g/min [1]. The crucial role of EEG lies in identifying the "ischemic penumbra", which is the pathophysiological state of acute ischemia in which neurons are nonfunctional but still alive and salvageable by reperfusion. As EEG is capable of detecting this state of cerebral ischemia prior to the development of permanent damage, it can be an extremely valuable technique in monitoring procedures that may result in reduced blood flow. In general, EEG has been shown to be more sensitive and to show more rapid changes than the recording of somatosensory-evoked potentials for alerting the surgeon to potentially harmful manipulations, although the rate of false-positives is higher.

Importantly, EEG is particularly sensitive to anesthesia. Most anesthetic agents, including the halogenated gases, thiopental, midazolam, etomidate and propofol, cause similar EEG changes. At doses below the minimum alveolar concentration (MAC), widespread, frontally predominant, fast rhythms appear. Increasing doses are generally characterized by a disappearance of these alpha rhythms with concurrent appearance of a beta rhythm, followed by a progressive slowing towards theta and delta rhythms. Deep anesthesia is associated with a burst–suppression pattern, and at the deepest levels measurable potentials may disappear altogether. Although the effects of different anesthetics differ slightly at lower doses in terms of the particular patterns seen, slowing with burst–suppression is the common feature of all of these drugs. Anesthetic-induced EEG changes should be seen bilaterally and symmetrically over both cerebral cortices.

Intraoperative use of EEG during neurosurgery has primarily been used in the monitoring of ischemic changes associated with carotid endarterectomy (CEA). Recordings are typically obtained pre-operatively, at induction, intermittently during dissection, and continuously during cross-clamp occlusion of the internal carotid artery (ICA). Indications of significant ischemia may potentially mandate use of of a shunt during the period of cross-clamping. Considering that the use of a shunt increases operative risk, related to either the potential for embolism or prolongation of operative time, the surgeon is required to balance these concerns with the benefits of shunting. A retrospective study by Salvian et al. compared a large cohort of patients who had undergone CEA either with routine shunting ($n = 92$) or with selective shunting using EEG changes as the indicator ($n = 213$). Of the selectively shunted group, only 16% had EEG changes that led to shunting. Postoperatively, 4 of the 92 patients who were routinely shunted had major stroke. In contrast, the selectively shunted group had only one case of post-operative stroke, suggesting that the use of EEG in determining the need for shunting may significantly reduce the risk of post-operative neurological deficit [2].

The two major EEG changes predictive of cerebral ischemia are: (1) slowing with decreased amplitude in the ischemic hemisphere, and (2) attenuation of the anesthetic-induced fast rhythms. EEG changes may be classified as major or moderate, with total or near-complete attenuation of 8–15 Hz activity and/or at least a doubling of delta activity of 1 Hz or less representing major changes. These alterations typically involve the ipsilateral hemisphere but can also be seen bilaterally or exclusively in the contralateral hemisphere. Moderate changes include amplitude attenuation of at least 50% or an increase in delta activity of 1 Hz or greater. When alterations of the recorded activity occur, whether major or moderate, they generally begin within minutes of cross-clamping the ICA. Nearly all of the major EEG changes that occur upon cross-clamping will reverse with placement of a shunt.

It has been suggested that EEG monitoring has a high false- positive rate in predicting stroke during CEA, thus unnecessarily subjecting many patients to the risks of shunt placement. However, the sum of the data on EEG monitoring in the setting of CEA indicates that it can identify the subset of patients at risk of clamp-induced ischemic insult. Redekop and Ferguson described a cohort of 293 patients who underwent routine CEA without shunting. Eight percent of these individuals demonstrated major EEG changes following clamping of the ICA; of this subset, 18% had immediate post-operative deficits, compared with only 1% of the individuals who did not have clamp-related EEG changes [3]. Another large retrospective analysis demonstrated similar success with the use of intraoperative EEG during CEA; stroke occurred in only 0.3% of patients who had been monitored with EEG during their procedure (and who had shunts placed upon the appearance of significant EEG changes), compared with a stroke incidence of 2.3% in the non-monitored group [4].

It has been pointed out that the predictive value of EEG monitoring, as measured by the actual number of strokes associated with major alterations of EEG patterns, is relatively low. There are a number of factors that are relevant to this issue. The threshold between tolerable ischemia and irreversible infarction does not clearly correlate with changes in the EEG patterns. Time is also a significant variable. A patient may well tolerate relative ischemia for the short time in which the ICA is cross-clamped during endarterectomy; however, if such ischemia were to persist for a greater length of time, permanent injury could result.

Obviously, the utility of standard methods of EEG, which require the placement of a grid of scalp electrodes, is limited by specific requirements of the operative approach, so these methods are of very little practical utility for a large proportion of intracranial cases. In addition, EEG monitoring loses efficacy in cases performed under deep hypothermic circulatory arrest (e.g. complex intracranial aneurysm); in fact, EEG activity ceases at brain temperatures of 19–26°C. Conversely, the disappearance of EEG activity has been used as a method to assess the adequacy of cooling in cases where deep hypothermic circulatory arrest is required. It has been proposed that a total of 3 minutes of electrocerebral silence (ECS) is an adequate endpoint for the assessment of therapeutic hypothermia.

# Electrocorticography

Electrocorticography (ECoG) has been used as a tool to identify loci of epileptiform activity or to delineate regions of eloquent cortex. As with EEG, ECoG records electrical potentials that are generated by the changing oscillatory activity of cortical neuronal groups. Unlike EEG, however, ECoG uses depth electrodes or surface electrode "grids" that are placed in direct contact with the cortical tissue, allowing for much finer spatial resolution of cortical electrical activity. Synchronous neuronal activity must be within approximately 6 cm$^2$ of the cortical surface in order to be detectable by scalp electrodes, while ECoG is able to detect epileptiform discharges outside of this radius. As with standard EEG, the interpretation of intraoperative ECoG is complicated by the effects of anesthetic agents.

The traditional use of intraoperative ECoG has been dedicated to the identification and demarcation of the limits of resectable epileptogenic foci, primarily based on the detection of interictal epileptiform activity. There has been no agreement, however, on which interictal discharges are predictive of continued risk of epileptiform activity. A study evaluating the implications of residual epileptogenic discharges following tumor resection suggested that surgical irritation of the cortex could induce such activity; furthermore, such discharges were not predictive of post-operative clinical seizures [5]. In addition, ECoG may not be helpful in determining whether such discharges are independent of, or propagated from, another site. The most widely accepted use of ECoG in epilepsy surgery has been in cases of extratemporal partial seizures, where it has been used routinely to set the boundaries of tissue resection. The use of ECoG in temporal lobe procedures has been more dependent on individual institutional philosophy, as some centers employ standard resection strategies or depend on pre-operative delineation of the epileptogenic focus. The use of post-excisional ECoG is also variable, although the chances of seizure-free outcome are improved if there is no evidence of persistent epileptiform activity following resection. A comprehensive discussion about the use of ECoG in the management of primary epilepsy remains beyond the scope of this chapter.

# Somatosensory Evoked Potentials

Neurosurgical monitoring of sensory evoked potentials (SEPs) relies on the recognition of characteristic alterations in the excitable properties of compromised neurons. These alterations generally occur before the onset of irreversible damage and can thus theoretically guide or alter the subsequent surgical technique. Evoked potential recordings, in contrast to those obtained via EEG, can only be generated via the use of external stimuli of various means. In general, SEPs used in intraoperative monitoring are generated by applying a peripheral stimulus to the particular sensory modality that carries its signal through the neurological region at risk, with recordings being taken at standardized points along the afferent pathway that allow for the assessment of both amplitude and latency of the signal. These stimuli can take the form of peripheral nerve shocks for somatosensory evoked potentials (SSEPs), trains of auditory clicks for brainstem auditory evoked potentials (BAEPs), or flashes of light for visual evoked potentials (VEPs). Waveforms of the SEPs are amplified and undesirable background noise may be filtered out. Prolongation of signal latency or decreased amplitude suggests diminished function at some point along the sensory pathway.

For the interpretation of SSEP data, adequate analysis of the waveforms requires averaging of at least 100 responses to provide reliable and clear waveform morphology. The rate of stimulation is usually 4–5 Hz, which minimizes acquisition time without inducing attenuation of the cortical response. Therefore, feedback can be provided to the surgeon about every 30–60 seconds. It is optimal to perform bilateral recordings, which allows the contralateral hemisphere to serve as an internal control. Components of the evoked response recording are labeled as either positive or negative, relative to a reference electrode, followed numerically by their modal peak latency in milliseconds. As an example, characteristic median nerve SSEP waves should include N13, P14, N20, P20 and P25 peaks (Fig. 1.2). The clival area generates the N13 deflection and reflects activation of the caudal medial lemniscus. Thalamocortical afferent activity is represented by the P14 wave, and N20 is associated with activation of cortical neurons in the primary somatosensory cortex. The latency difference between N13 and N20 is referred to as the "central conduction time" (CCT).

There are several variables that must be taken into consideration when using SSEP during neurosurgical procedures. Factors that can alter SSEP performance intraoperatively include anesthetic depth and type, patient temperature, blood pressure, limb positioning, and specific placement of stimulator and recording electrodes. In general, anesthetics cause an attenuation of the cortical components of the SSEP, such as N20, while the subcortical components remain resistant. Wave amplitudes are reduced and latencies are prolonged in a dose-related manner, particularly with the halogenated agents. Several exceptions include etomidate and ketamine, which can enhance the amplitude of the cortical components. Baseline recordings are crucial for evaluating changes that occur as a result of the operative procedure; individuals with carotid stenosis often demonstrate prolonged baseline CCTs and decreased amplitudes of various cortical responses.

SSEP monitoring has been used as an indicator of cerebral ischemia in much the same way as EEG. However, SSEP has several advantages over EEG as an intraoperative monitoring technique, which include greater relative resistance to general anesthesia, fewer electrode sites, and comparative ease of recording and interpretation. Generally, reductions in SSEP amplitudes are initiated by decreased cerebral oxidative mechanisms rather than by permanent neuronal damage. Decreases in CBF leading to SSEP changes parallel those causing noticeable EEG changes. Fisher et al. summarized a series of seven studies that analyzed outcomes of CEA as a function of SSEP changes. Of the total of 3,028 patients in all studies, 5.6% demonstrated a significant decline of SSEP as a direct result of surgical manipulation. Among these individuals,

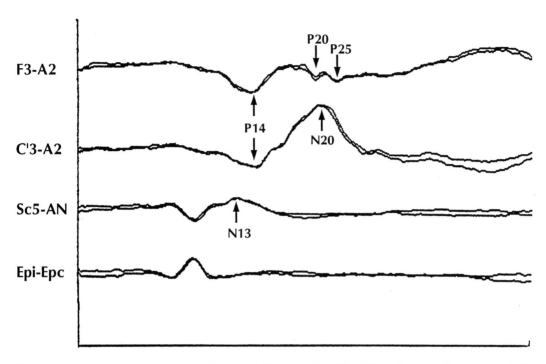

**Fig. 1.2.** Normal somatosensory evoked potentials detected after stimulation of the right median nerve. The central conduction time is calculated as the difference between the N13 and N20 peaks.

20% developed significant post-operative deficit. This number may have been larger had not a number of the patients with SSEP changes undergone shunting as a result of those changes [6]. Severe, irreversible SSEP changes appear to be a rare but ominous sign. This occurred in less than 1% of cases in a series of 994 CEAs; however, all awoke with neurological sequelae [7]. In contrast to EEG, no study has been performed with the intent to delineate the false-positive rate of SSEP monitoring – as it relates to stroke – if a shunt is not placed.

When cerebral ischemia occurs with the application of a clamp upon the ICA, character-istic changes occur in the N20, P25 and N30 components of the SSEP. A defined sequence of alterations, or stages, that occur with progres-sive ischemia has been described. Amplitude reduction combined with latency progression of N30 represents mild, or stage 1, ischemic change. Stage 2, or moderate, changes include the disappearance of N30 as well as amplitude reductions of N20 and P25 up to 50%. Severe, or stage 3, changes are defined by the loss of P25 with the concomitant progression of increasing latency and amplitude reduction of N20. Guerit

describes a similar system, which recommends shunt placement whenever moderate-to-severe SSEP alterations occur within 7 minutes after cross-clamping, and he suggests that some cases of mild-to-moderate SSEP change may be due to drops in blood pressure rather than to the ischemic effects of cross-clamping [8].

Experience of others has supported the sensi-tivity of N20 and P25 to ischemic insults, and amplitude reductions have proven to be more predictive than latency increases. Most surgeons who rely on SSEPs place a shunt when the N20-P25 complex decreases by 50% or rapidly disap-pears with clamping of the ICA. These changes typically recover when flow is re-established through the shunt. Overall, the correlation of SSEP changes to clinical outcome is quite good. Neurological dysfunction is remarkably rare in the setting of SSEP with little or no change. In the series by Haupt and Horsch, only one of the 994 patients suffered a stroke in the face of normal SSEPs. As with EEG, clamp-induced changes in SSEPs occur in about 20–30% of monitored cases. It is important to note that temporary ischemia, whether due to intended or accidental vessel occlusion, does not immediately give rise to alterations in the relevant SSEP [7].

SSEP monitoring has also been shown to be useful during intracranial procedures that directly or indirectly contribute to ischemia, including aneurysm clipping or manipulation and retraction of various brain structures. Isolated vascular territories can be assessed through judicious selection of the stimulus location to be used for SSEP. Regions of cortex subserved by the ICA and MCA can be monitored by stimulation through the median nerve; in addition, the median nerve can be used to assess flow to the thalamic segment of the somatosensory pathway, an area provided for by the PCA. Posterior tibial nerve SSEP has been used for monitoring the territory of the ACA, although concurrent monitoring of the median nerve may be necessary for adequate detection of ischemia involving the dependent regions of the recurrent artery of Huebner. In assessing the posterior circulation, isolated monitoring of either SSEP or BAEP during vertebrobasilar aneurysm clipping may be of little use, as ischemia due to basilar perforator occlusion may not affect the auditory or somatosensory pathways traversing the brainstem; however, if used in combination, SSEP and BAEP monitoring may enhance the ability to detect brainstem ischemia.

Currently, prospective data comparing EEG and SSEP monitoring for reversible ischemia and patient outcomes do not exist. On a theoretical level, EEG monitors a larger area of the cerebral cortex and does not require time averaging of signals. However, Fava et al. have suggested that SSEP monitoring, in addition to EEG, enhances the overall predictive value of monitoring during CEA. Patients ($n = 151$) with EEG changes indicating significant ischemia were shunted only if severe SSEP changes occurred within the first few minutes after vessel occlusion. Fewer shunts were placed using this protocol than if EEG were used independently. No patient with significant EEG changes in conjunction with insignificant SSEP changes had a post-operative deficit. Patients who were shunted did well, with the exception of subjects whose ischemia was felt to be embolic and who awoke with new deficit [9]. Guerit suggests that SSEP may be superior to EEG in the determination of ECS in cases using deep hypothermic circulatory arrest, as the SSEP is much less

sensitive to environmental electrical noise and is therefore better suited to identifying true ECS [8].

SSEP has also been used for functional localization in the cerebral cortex, most particularly in defining the central sulcus, via the use of phase reversal. SSEPs recorded simultaneously from the precentral and postcentral gyri exhibit typical responses of reversed polarity (Fig. 1.3). The evoked potential from the precentral gyrus is a biphasic positive-negative waveform, compared with the mirror image of the postcentral gyrus, which is negative-positive. The typically recorded response in the postcentral gyrus following median nerve stimulation is a negative deflection with a latency period of 20 ms (N20) followed by a positive deflection at 30 ms (P30). Precentral recordings reveal somewhat lower amplitude deflections that mirror the sensory strip recordings (characteristically, a P22 component followed by an N33 deflection). The precise etiology of these potentials and phase reversal is not fully understood. Brodman's area 3b, located on the primary sensory cortex along

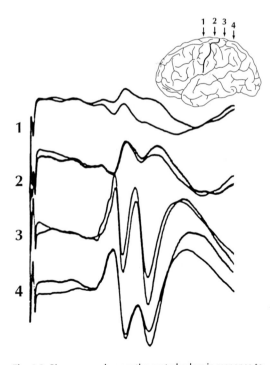

**Fig. 1.3.** Phase reversal across the central sulcus in response to contralateral median nerve stimulation. The reversal in polarity is evident when comparing leads 2 and 3, positions that bridge the central sulcus (darkened for emphasis).

the posterior wall of the central sulcus, receives sensory impulses from the thalamus. This region at least partially contributes to the generation of the N20 wave. Neurons within the precentral gyrus are thought to be responsible for generating the P22 deflection, as ablation of the postcentral gyrus does not eliminate this component of the SSEP. The P22 wave probably results from direct projections from the thalamus to the motor strip, but may be influenced by association fibers from area 3b.

SSEPs may also be recorded at the spinal level to monitor for insult to neurological tissues during spinal surgery, assuming that the location of peripheral stimulation is optimized to assess the level of cord at risk during a particular procedure (Fig. 1.4). SSEP monitoring is commonly used during a number of spinal procedures, including correction of scoliosis, resection of spinal AVM or tumor, therapeutic embolization of spinal AVMs, correction of spinal instability, and therapy for syringomyelia. Changes in spinal SSEP after the placement of hardware can suggest a need for changes in positioning of the hardware. Electrodes may be placed in the subarachnoid or epidural space, on the interspinous ligament, or attached to a spinous process. With the exception of subarachnoid leads, these leads may be placed percutaneously or at the site of surgical exposure. Recording evoked potentials at the spinal level has some advantages over cortically recorded SSEPs. Spinal evoked potentials have larger amplitudes, and repetition rates may be increased (which can reduce acquisition time). In addition, SSEPs recorded from the spinal cord are more resistant to the effects of anesthetic agents than are cortically detected SSEPs.

While median nerve stimulation has been commonly used for monitoring SSEP during cervical spine procedures, caudal portions of the cervical cord may not receive appropriate coverage with this modality. The ulnar nerve may offer more complete representation of lower cervical levels. For procedures placing the thoracic or lumbar cord at risk, SSEPs generated through the posterior tibial or common peroneal nerves can be used. Recordings taken simultaneously from both the upper and lower limb may allow for an internal control in certain procedures; specifically, evoked potentials that are lost from both the upper and lower extremity during a procedure which places the thoracic cord at risk suggest a technical error in stimu-

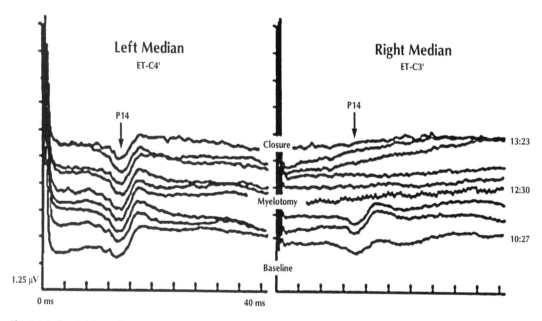

**Fig. 1.4.** Left and right median nerve somatosensory evoked potentials in a patient who underwent laminectomy and exposure of an intradural, intramedullary tumor of the cervical spine. The right P14 waveform is initially diminished at baseline and then is permanently lost during the midline myelotomy. Left-sided tracings are unaffected. The patient awoke with a permanent right hemi-proprioceptive loss.

lation or recording. However, if only lower extremity responses were lost in this case, the surgeon would be more suspicious of injury to the thoracic cord.

A large ($n = 51{,}263$), multicenter retrospective survey examining the role of SSEP monitoring in scoliosis surgery suggested a 50% reduction in the rate of neurological defects related to the procedure in patients who had intraoperative SSEP monitoring. The rate of false-negatives was remarkably low in this survey (0.06%), and the authors concluded that spinal SSEP was effective for detecting more than 90% of intra-operative neurological deficits [10]. Others have suggested that SSEPs may be useful in the assessment of compromising mechanical fac-tors or decreases in relative blood flow to the spinal cord. A small study ($n = 13$) performed on patients with syringomyelia, treated with syringo-subarachnoid shunting, demonstrated a rapid improvement in spinal SSEPs follow-ing decompression of the syrinx. This improve-ment correlated with increased local blood flow to these regions, and the patients had post-operative improvement in their symptoms [11].

However, larger trials have not demonstrated similar consistency. Falsely positive SSEP changes are relatively common [10]. In a review of 182 cervical spine procedures, complete loss of evoked potential recordings occurred in 33 subjects and was associated with post-operative deficit in only 50% of these cases [12]. Partial loss of response was even less predictive, pro-viding an overall specificity of only 27%. Further, false-negative recordings have been described. A large retrospective survey of nearly 190 spine surgeons who routinely used intraop-erative SSEP monitoring found that nearly 30% of combined post-operative deficits seen in their patients occurred in the absence of observed spinal SSEP changes [13]. Confound-ingly, recordings may show improvement dur-ing a case without correlation to post-operative neurological improvement. Positive changes to SSEP waveforms may reassure the surgeon intraoperatively, while several studies have demonstrated that improvement of SSEP ampli-tude or latency appears to be of little post-operative clinical significance.

It has been suggested that the use of SSEP monitoring in spinal surgery may be augmented with the concurrent use of another monitoring technique (such as motor evoked potentials).

However, at this time there is no consensus as to the efficacy of isolated intraoperative spinal SSEP monitoring.

Monitoring techniques for surgery of the lumbosacral spine have also been reported. In an attempt to reduce the limited morbidity associated with lumbosacral diskectomy or pedicle screw fixation of the lumbosacral spine, some surgeons monitor nerve root function in the lower extremity during the procedure. Again, no clear efficacy has been demonstrated by controlled study.

## Spinal Stimulation

Electrical stimulation of the spinal cord, both directly and indirectly, has been well described over the last decade as an additional method for monitoring the integrity of the descending tracts during surgical manipulation of the spine. The evoked motor responses, termed "neurogenic motor evoked potentials" (NMEPs), can be fol-lowed by recording from the sciatic nerve at the popliteal fossa bilaterally or by monitoring for myogenic responses in the lower limbs. The electrodes used to evoke NMEPs can be placed in several locations rostral to the region to be manipulated, including the epidural space, the spinous processes, or in a position that allows for percutaneous stimulation. Direct stimula-tion through pedicle screws has also been attempted as a means of assessing impingement upon, or damage to, nerve roots owing to misalignment of the hardware.

A recent study evaluated the efficacy of each of these electrode positions in 50 patients undergoing posterior thoracic or thoracolum-bar procedures with instrumentation. The find-ings demonstrated excellent results for each method; however, epidural placement of the stimulating electrodes was found to be most reliable in terms of the acquisition of initial NMEPs and in maintaining those NMEPs throughout the procedure [14]. The use of elec-trodes placed on the spinous processes or in the epidural space often requires enlargement of the surgical field and placement of the electrodes within the surgical field, which can result in some inconvenience.

A comparison of NMEP and SSEP was per-formed by Pereon et al. in a consecutive series of 112 patients undergoing surgical correction of spinal deformity, in which both NMEPs and SSEPs were generated and monitored. In three of the cases, surgical manipulation resulted in sudden loss of both NMEPs and SSEPs. In these cases, the electrodes used for elicitation of NMEP were moved along the spinal cord until the precise level of involvement was appreciated, with subsequent laminectomy and decompression at that level. Two of the three patients exhibiting evoked potential loss were asymptomatic following the procedure, while a third was left paraplegic. However, in two additional operations, isolated changes in NMEP were seen without a concomitant change in SSEP. In both of these cases, the surgical procedure was altered accordingly and potential neurological damage was avoided. In addition, the data from NMEP monitoring, requiring no time averaging, were acquired more quickly than data from SSEP, allowing for more timely interventions in the face of pending injury [15].

Monitoring of sacral root innervation to the anal and urethral sphincters can be performed with either evoked potential monitoring or by manometric recordings. In cases of tethered cord or tumor resection, a comprehensive strategy for monitoring has been proposed, which provides coverage from L2 to S4 [16]. This system uses a combination of SSEP monitoring from tibial nerve and nerve root stimulation with electromyographic (EMG) recordings of muscle from the sphincters and relevant leg musculature. The proposed benefit is an ability to differentiate functional neural tissue from non-functional or fibrous tissue. Despite the successful application of these various monitoring techniques, there has been no controlled study documenting improved neurological outcomes in these cases, and the circumstances in which lumbosacral spinal cord monitoring is efficacious have not been well defined.

# Motor Evoked Potentials

Identification of the primary motor cortex and the specifics of the motor homunculus can be accomplished via the use of cortical electrical or magnetic stimulation, using concomitant EMG recording to assess a response to the evoked potential in the periphery. Electrical stimulation is performed with single surface electrodes or electrode grids that are placed in direct contact with the cortex. Transcranial electrical stimulation is remarkably painful, due to current flow across the scalp. Therefore, non-anesthetized recordings are not feasible. Furthermore, transcranial electrical stimulation is contraindicated in patients with a history of seizure or an EEG suggestive of seizure tendency. Magnetically induced motor evoked potentials (MEPs) are generated by passing a changing current through a coil held perpendicular to the cortical surface, which induces a magnetic force perpendicular to the electrical field. Transcranial magnetic stimulation (TMS) of the cortex is painless, may be obtained both pre- and intraoperatively, and does not require averaging for analytical purposes. However, this method is cumbersome, expensive and non-specific with regard to the cortex it stimulates.

MEPs are exquisitely sensitive to the effects of anesthetics. It has been conclusively demonstrated that isoflurane will abolish MEPs generated by either electrical or magnetic stimulation of the cortex. Barbiturates, propofol and benzodiazepines exert a strong depressive effect on MEPs; etomidate causes a milder depression that eventually returns to baseline. Anesthetics that have been shown to have little or no effect on MEP are halothane, fentanyl and ketamine. MEPs generated by stimulation of the spinal cord avoid the cortical effects of these anesthetics and will remain intact. Cortical MEPs may be difficult to generate in young children, in whom the motor cortex is relatively inexcitable.

Enhanced patient outcome has not been clearly documented with the use of MEPs in controlled trials. A retrospective study reviewed the resections of 130 intramedullary tumors performed with the assistance of MEP recordings. The results suggested that gross total resection of these tumors was more likely when MEP monitoring was used; however, no clear reduction in morbidity or improvement in patient outcome related to monitoring was demonstrated [17].

In addition to assessing cortical elements of the motor system, MEP may prove to be a valuable technique in the assessment of intraoperative risk to the motor pathways of the brainstem and spinal cord. Considering that sensory impulses travel in the posterior tracts of the spinal cord and the lateral aspects of the brainstem, isolated monitoring of SSEP is incomplete for assessing the integrity of all spinal pathways.

The use of simultaneous MEP and SSEP monitoring has been suggested for this purpose and has been studied to a limited extent. Nagle et al. reviewed a series of 116 cases involving surgical manipulation of the spinal cord or column in which simultaneous intraoperative SSEP and MEP monitoring was utilized. Significant intraoperative changes in both SSEP and MEP patterns occurred in eight of these patients. An additional patient had isolated MEP changes. All patients with intraoperative changes awoke with post-operative deficit. Therefore, the authors support simultaneous use of both MEP and SSEP monitoring to achieve parallel, independent monitoring of spinal function [18]. Additional data from another series of patients undergoing surgical correction of spinal deformity suggested that relevant intraoperative changes are acquired in a more timely fashion with MEP than with SSEP [15].

# Cortical Mapping Techniques

Functional areas other than the primary motor cortex can be localized with electrically or magnetically driven cortical mapping techniques. Preservation of language function is a primary concern when performing dominant temporal lobe resections. Investigations that have mapped cortical regions subserving functional speech have demonstrated considerable variability in the specific location of these areas along the superior and medial temporal gyri. Resections of the dominant temporal lobe using standardized strategies have the potential to significantly damage the patient's ability to speak or, alternatively, underestimate the potential limits of resection, depending on the exact location of language areas.

The most reliable and widely used technique for identifying cortical language areas involves direct electrical stimulation of cortex that is putatively involved in functional speech. Numerous studies have shown that electrical stimulation of speech-related cortex will interfere with language tasks, generally resulting in anomia or a complete abrogation of speech. Electrical-stimulation language mapping is typically carried out in awake patients. When circumstances dictate that a resection be carried out under general anesthesia, an initial craniotomy can be performed to place indwelling surface electrode grids over the brain regions to be mapped. Following recovery from this initial procedure, detailed language-mapping protocols are carried out via the externalized electrical leads. After language mapping has been completed, with all functionally important cortical sites identified, the patient is returned to the operating room for electrode removal and an appropriately guided resection under general anesthesia.

Safe and effective language mapping is accomplished via direct electrical stimulation of the cortex at strengths that are below the after-discharge (AD) threshold. ADs are abnormal cortical discharges that are evoked by focal electrical stimulation and which persist beyond the period of stimulation. Electrocorticographic recording electrodes must be positioned immediately adjacent to the site of electrical stimulation in order to detect ADs. Stimulation strengths with the potential to evoke ADs are also capable of evoking local seizure activity. This can render stimulation mapping uninterpretable or, at worst, precipitate a generalized seizure. Typically, electrical stimuli are delivered via a hand-held probe and consist of pulse trains of charge-balanced square waves (0.2 ms duration, 50 Hz). The patient is instructed to carry out a variety of language tasks (e.g. object identification, word repetition, counting, execution of verbal commands) as disruptive electrical stimuli are delivered to various cortical surface sites. Sites that are associated with changes in speech and comprehension are identified and can be spared during the subsequent surgical resection.

# Microelectrode Recording/Stimulation

Neurosurgical treatment options for the various movement disorders have been under investigation for a number of decades. Parkinson's disease has perhaps received the greatest amount of attention, partly owing to unsatisfactory long-term outcomes with current medical therapies, improved understanding of the pathophysiological connections relevant to Parkinson's disease, and advances in monitoring techniques relevant

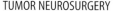
to these procedures. These cases generally involve either ablation or deep-brain stimulation of the motor thalamus, the globus pallidus or the subthalamic nucleus via stereotactic electrode placement; more recently, stem cell transplantation has emerged as a potential treatment option. Precise advancement and the final position of electrodes used for ablation or stimulation are of paramount importance in reducing post-operative morbidity as well as ensuring the best chance for therapeutic success. The primary method used over the last decade for this purpose is electrophysiological monitoring of the brain structures that are traversed by the microelectrode during the procedure.

The microelectrode mapping technique relies on the development of a "physiological map" based on the known spontaneous firing rate and pattern of particular neuronal groups and the predictable pattern changes that are related to various stimuli. The internal capsule and optic tract can be identified through the recording of firing changes related to sensory stimuli such as limb movement or flashes of light, respectively. As the recording/stimulating electrode is advanced, the physiological map that is developed can be correlated to a standardized stereotactic atlas or thin-slice high-resolution MRI images from the particular patient. Once this map is developed, lesion or stimulation electrode placement can occur with maximum precision.

The proven utility of microelectrode recording for increasing accuracy and decreasing morbidity in ablation or deep-brain stimulator placement is somewhat unclear. Although the vast majority of surgeons performing these procedures utilize microelectrode guidance, a critical review of the relevant literature compiled by Hariz and Fodstad questioned this practice. They noted that rates of severe complications and mortality appeared to be higher when microelectrodes were used, rather than MRI-based guidance, for either ablative or stimulatory purposes, while concomitant gains in accuracy and efficacy of the procedure were not seen. Their final conclusion focused on the need for a prospective, randomized trial comparing micro- and macroelectrodes in movement disorder surgery [19].

# Brainstem Auditory Evoked Potentials

The recording of cortical potentials related to auditory stimuli has proven to be difficult. In many patients, the primary auditory cortex is located deep within the Sylvian fissure. This location generates potentials whose dipole is perpendicular to the cortical surface, thereby rendering them undetectable by surface or scalp electrodes. However, detection and analysis of BAEPs have been developed for a number of neurosurgical procedures involving areas that are traversed by the ascending auditory signal, including both extra-axial (nerve) and intra-axial (brainstem) tissues. These procedures include resection of vestibular schwannomas, microvascular decompression of cranial nerves, retrolabyrinthine vestibular neurectomy, clipping of basilar artery aneurysms, treatment of posterior fossa AVMs, and resection of tumors residing in the cerebellopontine angle (CPA) or brainstem.

BAEPs are generated via the presentation of trains of clicks to one or both ears, resulting in an afferent signal that can be detected by scalp electrodes as it passes through the vestibulocochlear nerve, lower brainstem and midbrain. As with SSEP, changes in waveform amplitude or prolongation of signal latency are suggestive of impending or actual damage to the pathway, and persistent loss of the BAEP is more indicative of permanent damage than transient loss. Pre-operative assessment must be performed to obtain the baseline performance of the ascending auditory pathway for each individual prior to surgical manipulation. In most cases, hundreds or even thousands of responses to rapid (10–30 Hz) stimuli are averaged to obtain high quality waveforms. There are five major peaks, numbered I–V, which are particularly relevant in the analysis of BAEPs (Fig. 1.5). These waves are thought to be generated from the proximal eighth cranial nerve (I), the entry zone into the brainstem (II), the cochlear nuclear complex (III), the superior olive (IV), and the contralateral lemniscus or nucleus (V). These associations become important in the operating room, as brainstem ischemia may prolong the latency of peak V but leave peaks I and III essentially unaffected. Although it is possible to record directly from an exposed eighth nerve, the

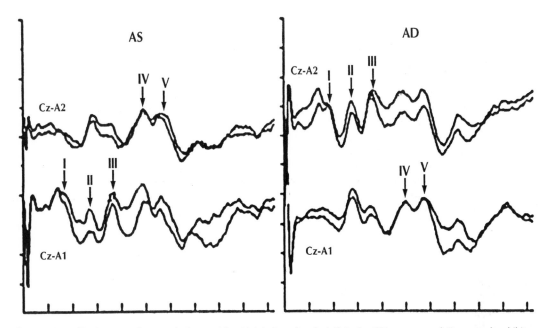

**Fig. 1.5.** Normal brainstem auditory evoked potentials with labeling of peaks I–V. During CPA surgery, peak V commonly exhibits a gradual prolongation of latency and reduction of amplitude that is not predictive of hearing loss (AS = left ear, AD = right ear).

potentials detected in this fashion are difficult to record and fail to provide insight into the functional status of ascending pathways in the brainstem.

The most frequent indication for the use of BAEP monitoring has been in the resection of vestibular schwannomas. There are a number of steps in the surgical procedure that are known to place auditory function at risk, including opening of the dura, cerebellar retraction, coagulation of tumor vessels, and removal of tumor present in the auditory canal, particularly from the most lateral portion. A series presented by Fischer et al. demonstrated that hearing was preserved in an average of 45% of patients who underwent resection of a vestibular schwannoma with concomitant recording of BAEP; this number was variable depending on the particular grade of the tumor [20]. Similar findings were described by Fahlbusch et al. in a series of 61 patients who underwent resection of large vestibular schwannomas via a lateral suboccipital approach with pre-operative and intraoperative BAEP monitoring. In this cohort, hearing was preserved in approximately 43% of patients in the early post-operative phase; however, a number of patients had subsequent decreases in hearing, resulting in a decrease in the final

number of hearing-intact individuals to 27% [21]. BAEP monitoring has also been used in cases focusing on microvascular decompression of the facial or trigeminal nerves. Both retrospective and prospective studies have suggested that post-operative hearing loss can be reduced in these cases with the use of BAEP monitoring before and during the procedure.

Changes in BAEP that have been referred to as significant indicators of post-operative hearing loss are: decreases in waveform amplitude of 50%, prolongation of waveform latency of 10% or greater, and dramatic alterations in waveform morphology. Obviously, disappearance of the waveform is most concerning and is most likely to correlate with subsequent loss of hearing. Upon exposure of the CPA, wave V may exhibit prolonged latency and amplitude reduction that gradually continues until the potential is lost. When wave V is lost, no prediction of post-operative hearing can be made. If the potential is unchanged throughout surgery, the patient's post-operative auditory function will be stable. Loss of wave I occurs more acutely over minutes and is always associated with loss of wave V; return of this potential will occur within 15 minutes or will not return at all. If it fails to reappear within this time, hearing will inevitably be lost. Hearing will be preserved if both waves remain unaffected.

# Cranial Nerve Monitoring

The most extensive experience with brainstem and cranial nerve monitoring has come from procedures involving the CPA. Various sensory and motor functions of the cranial nerves can be monitored in an attempt to preserve function or to assist intraoperative decision making. As previously, sensory nerves are typically monitored with evoked potentials and motor nerves with EMG recordings. The theoretical rationale for monitoring spontaneous EMG activity relies on the property that thermal, mechanical or metabolic irritation of the intracranial portion of a cranial motor nerve will lead to a predictable and measurable activity in the innervated muscle.

Logistically, intraoperative EMG monitoring of muscles innervated by the various cranial nerves is relatively simple. Needle insertion into the appropriate muscle is preferable to surface electrode placement for increasing the sensitivity and specificity of the system. Intramuscular electrodes increase the sensitivity of detection for spontaneous EMG activity, while surface electrodes are more appropriate for the assessment of compound muscle action potentials (CMAPs). Most systems amplify and convert the muscle action potential to audible signals that are immediately available to the surgical team. A variety of probes are available for the purposes of stimulation. Both constant current and constant voltage stimulation paradigms exist, and both have been used effectively and safely. Monopolar and bipolar stimulating electrodes are available, with the latter providing more focal stimulation. Finally, appropriate communication with the anesthesiologist is crucial, as EMG potentials will be abrogated by significant neuromuscular blockade.

The efficacy of facial nerve monitoring in reducing post-operative facial palsy during CPA tumor surgery is well established. Monitoring during vestibular schwannoma resection is particularly crucial, as up to 78% of these cases involve an impairment of the facial nerve. Facial nerve activity is usually recorded from the ipsilateral frontalis, orbicularis oculi, orbicu-

laris oris, and/or mentalis muscles. EMG responses have been classified as either spontaneous or evoked. Spontaneous activity is common with the onset of monitoring, generally characterized by low-amplitude, low-density unit potentials presenting as steady trains or small repetitive bursts. Evoked responses, which are more common, are further subdivided into three patterns. "Pulse patterns" result from purposeful stimulation of the facial nerve with the stimulating probe and have a frequency identical to that generated by the stimulator. A second response, the "burst pattern", results from mechanical, chemical or thermal stimuli. Such alterations of nerve firing occur soon after the inciting event, with the observed pattern consisting of short (<1 s) bursts of synchronous motor activity. The final type of activity, known as the train pattern, presents as groups of asynchronous discharges with durations of several minutes. These potentials may have a latency of seconds to minutes after the aggravating event occurs. Traction on the nerve is usually the causative event, but chemical or thermal irritation may also be responsible. Activity may also be seen if cold irrigation fluid is used. The train pattern is most concerning as an indicator of potential or current damage to the nerve; the effect is typically delayed and outlasts the stimulus that incited it.

Post-operative function of the facial nerve can be predicted based on stimulation studies performed prior to wound closure. Inability to produce facial motion with high current stimulation is predictive of post-operative paralysis. When stimulation of more than 3.0 mA in a constant voltage setting is required to produce facial movement, post-operative palsy of the seventh cranial nerve is expected. However, potential for recovery exists if the nerve is intact. Good movement induced by 0.05–0.2 mA at the brainstem has been correlated with normal or minimal paresis of the facial nerve. Using a constant current setting, elevation of stimulus threshold to 0.2 or 0.3 V following the procedure is usually associated with good post-operative function of the nerve. However, threshold potentials greater than 0.3 V may be indicative of post-operative loss of function.

Antidromic stimulation of the facial nerve is also possible via the use of a hand-held electrode placed in the surgical field, with nerve stimulation at the stylomastoid foramen. This technique is advantageous in cases where neuromuscular blockade is required; however, continuous monitoring of nerve function is obviously extremely difficult, and a certain amount of inconvenience is added due to the need to introduce a hand-held device into the surgical field.

EMG monitoring of the facial nerve has also been an important part of procedures performed to relieve hemifacial spasm. Abnormal muscle response to stimulation of the appropriate branch of the facial nerve, which is typically seen in this patient population, disappears when the nerve is released from the offending vessel. This finding has been associated with good postoperative outcomes, while perseverance of an abnormal response parallels residual post-operative spasm.

Intraoperative monitoring of the other cranial nerves is also possible. Needle electrodes can be placed into any of the extraocular muscles, thereby monitoring cranial nerves III, IV and VI. The masseter or temporalis serve as recording sites for the motor division of the trigeminal nerve. Electrodes placed into the soft palate or posterior pharyngeal musculature can be used to monitor the function of cranial nerve IX. However, great care must be taken when stimulating these motor fibers, as some of them innervate the carotid body and stimulation may result in bradycardia or hypotension. Similarly, vagal monitoring, using electrodes placed endoscopically into the vocal cords or cricothyroid muscle, may also result in marked bradycardia, arrythmias or alterations of blood pressure. The absence of vagal activity, as recorded in laryngeal muscles, can be used to determine whether posterior pharyngeal recordings are attributable to cranial nerve IX rather than to nerve X. EMG recordings from either the trapezeus or sternocleidomastoid muscles will indicate activity of cranial nerve XI; however, stimulus intensity should be kept low to minimize the possibility of forceful jerking of the head with resulting trauma at the pin sites. Electrodes placed in the tongue allow for recording of evoked potentials from hypoglossal stimulation.

## Visual Evoked Potentials

There has been interest in developing a reliable method of measuring and interpreting visual evoked potentials (VEPs) for use during procedures that could compromise elements of the visual pathway from the retina to the occipital cortex. Optic stimuli have been traditionally delivered through LED-emitting goggles or fitted contact lenses. There have been very few studies assessing the role of VEP monitoring in neurosurgical procedures, perhaps due to the enormous variation in observed waveform characteristics in conjunction with persistently unreliable recordings. Preliminary results have been mixed, but the overriding consensus suggests that the use of VEP monitoring is not justified as a technique owing to this extensive variability. It has been demonstrated that alterations in VEP have very poor sensitivity and specificity for the prediction of post-operative visual changes. Therefore, this technique remains primarily in the experimental arena.

## Measurement of Cerebral Blood Flow

Two major methods have been devised for the purpose of primary quantification of CBF. As opposed to EEG or SSEP monitoring, which give a secondary glimpse of CBF by detecting physiological changes that occur owing to decreases in flow, direct measurement of flow would hypothetically provide more rapid and relevant intraoperative feedback. The first of these methods relies on measuring the clearance of an injectable tracer from brain tissue. The tracer that has been used for this purpose, due to its relative insolubility in water and rapid diffusion across the blood–brain barrier, is 133Xe. Typically, clearance is detected with a hand-held sensor placed over the region of interest following injection of the tracer into the ICA. A clearance curve is generated and the area under the curve is used for calculating CBF. The use of 133Xe for CBF measurement during CEA has been well described. Sundt has reported the greatest experience with regional CBF (rCBF) measurements during CEA [22]. It is primarily his analysis of nearly 2,200 monitored patients that supports shunt placement for flows of less than 18–20 ml/100 g/min. Others have questioned the efficacy of measuring rCBF during CEA. Zampella et al. performed EEG monitoring and rCBF measurements during 431 consecutive

CEAs without shunting [1]. No correlation was found between rCBF measurements and neurological morbidity or overall complication rate.

A second method of measuring CBF relies on near-infrared spectroscopy to assess cerebral oxygenation status. Also known as "cerebral oximetry", this technique measures changes in the levels of oxygenated, deoxygenated and total hemoglobin as well as oxidized cytochrome in the local cerebral blood supply. The advantage of using the near-infrared spectrum is that this wavelength of light passes easily through the extracranial tissues, allowing for non-invasive monitoring. However, variations in anatomy or extra- to intracranial collateral blood supply can make interpretation of the results somewhat difficult. The sensor patch is placed over the forehead on the ipsilateral side and continuous measurements of regional cerebral oxygen saturation ($rSO_2$) are obtained. Several studies have assessed the utility of cerebral oximetry as a monitoring technique during CEA; results have been mixed and it is clear that significant improvements need to be made to this technique before it can be used with any consistency for intraoperative monitoring.

# Intraoperative Ultrasound

B-mode ultrasound began to be used by neurosurgeons soon after it became available in the early 1980s. It quickly proved its value for localizing lesions, delineating normal and pathological anatomy, guiding instrumentation, and identifying residual tumor following resection. It can be particularly useful for localizing intramedullary spinal cord pathology. More recently, stereotactic intraoperative ultrasound has been employed as an adjunct during surgical procedures using image guidance. As intraoperative "shift" can instill significant error into these systems, real-time ultrasound imaging can be compared with the pre-operative scans used for image guidance, and appropriate corrections can be made.

Transcranial Doppler (TCD) ultrasound has been used for the intraoperative assessment of flow velocities and detection of embolic events during CEA by insonation of the terminal ICA, MCA or ACA through a temporal window. A large study ($n = 1058$) of patients undergoing CEA with intraoperative TCD monitoring concluded that microemboli detected during dissection/wound closure, decreases of MCA velocities equal to or greater than 90%, and increases of pulsatility index of 100% or more were significantly associated with post-operative stroke [23].

Microvascular Doppler has several intraoperative uses, including evaluation of flow in the carotid artery following CEA, documentation of graft patency in cases of EC–IC bypass, and assessment of flow in an aneurysm and adjacent vessels before and after clip application.

# Intraoperative Angiography

Intraoperative angiography is used during a wide range of neurovascular procedures including aneurysm clipping, AVM resection, and EC–IC bypass. The imaging procedure itself is identical to non-operative angiography; however, patient positioning and preparation and the use of radiolucent stabilizing equipment are crucial for the successful use of this technique in the operating room. The potential complications are similar to those seen during non-operative cerebral angiography, namely groin hematoma, femoral artery thrombosis, stroke and vasospasm.

The utility of intraoperative angiography has been documented by several studies. In a series of 115 patients undergoing various neurovascular procedures with angiography, the operative procedure was altered in 19 of these cases owing to concerns raised by the intraoperative angiogram, while only 2 of the 115 patients had a post-operative complication that could potentially have been related to angiography [24].

# Peripheral Nerve Monitoring

Peripheral nerve monitoring relies primarily on EMG recordings, nerve conduction velocity (NCV), nerve action potentials (NAPs) and SSEPs, all of which are performed in the same fashion as during routine non-operative evaluation of nerve function. These techniques can be used to assess the pre-operative function of the nerve, as related to pathological changes, in addition to allowing for the monitoring of functional status of the nerve during surgical manipulation. Sources of insult to the nerve, capable of instigating changes detectable with these techniques, include compression, laceration, stretching or ischemia.

EMG recordings are particularly helpful in establishing the location, severity and extent of a peripheral nerve problem. The recording electrode is placed into the belly of the muscle innervated by the peripheral nerve that is pathologically involved or placed at risk by surgical manipulation. During the procedure, nerve integrity can be monitored by proximal application of an electrical stimulus with assessment of the resulting muscle activity through EMG recordings. This technique can also be used to demonstrate the identity of a nerve by the pattern of muscle responses seen after stimulation.

NCVs can be used to specifically localize a region of pathological change in a peripheral nerve. Measurement of NCVs requires the placement of stimulating and recording electrodes along the length of the nerve of interest. Relevant pathology can be localized by measuring the conduction time (and therefore velocity) and amplitude of an action potential passing through a particular segment of the nerve. A decrease in velocity suggests a problem with myelination (seen in entrapment syndromes) whilst a diminished amplitude is indicative of axonal loss. Sensory and motor fibers cannot be delineated by this method. Direct stimulation of a lesion may be extremely helpful in differentiating between pathological nervous tissue (e.g. neuroma) and normal nervous tissue and for guiding the appropriate limits of surgical resection.

Typically, bipolar stimulation is used for optimal focusing of the stimulus current. Hooked electrodes can be used, which allow for the nerve to be lifted free of surrounding tissue in a gentle fashion, thereby minimizing stimulus artifact due to volume conduction. Adequate stimulation can be accomplished using a setting of 50 V (constant current) or 10 mA (constant voltage) for a duration of 0.05 ms. Greater current may be necessary in cases where the nerve is fibrotic or has decreased myelination.

In general, the recording electrode must be placed at a minimum of 5 cm from the stimulation electrode; if the distance is smaller, any relevant NAP may be obscured by shock artifact. NAPs will not be affected by general anesthetics or neuromuscular blockade. However, local ischemia, as caused by application of a tourniquet, may result in obliteration of the NAP. Circulation should be restored for a minimum of 20 minutes before reliable NAPs can be recorded.

In a review of 25 years of experience, including more than 2,000 patients, Kline and Happel found that recording intraoperative NAPs was essential to surgical decision making and successful outcome. When a NAP could be successfully recorded across a lesion in continuity, 93% of patients had good recovery of function following neurolysis. If the NAP failed to cross the region of pathology, the dysfunctional tissue could be resected and repaired with satisfactory results in nearly two-thirds of cases [25].

# Conclusions

To assure the greatest possible success of any of the aforementioned intraoperative monitoring techniques, a number of factors need to be considered on a case-by-case basis. Cooperation and communication between the surgeon, anesthesiologist and physiologist or technician responsible for collection and interpretation of the monitoring data are paramount for accurate intraoperative information. The operative team must be dedicated to the proper set-up and use of the monitoring equipment, although the preparation may take a few extra moments, in order to maximize data acquisition and avoid the unlikely possibility of harm related to the monitoring process itself. Similarly, the monitoring team should maintain an unobtrusive presence in the operating room and provide no unnecessary distraction or delay to the procedure. Appropriate selection of a particular technique for a given case is crucial and the surgeon must be willing to change his operative technique if the appropriate warning signs become apparent. Finally, it is important to note that no form of intraoperative monitoring guarantees a good post-operative result, even in the absence of the relevant warning signs.

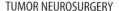

# Key Points

- *Various techniques for intraoperative neuro-physiological monitoring are available to neurosurgeons for use during procedures that involve both the central and peripheral nervous system.*

- *Some of these techniques have a proven utility and play an integral role during a number of neurosurgical cases. Other techniques are used as a matter of personal preference or remain in the experimental realm.*

- *Several of these methods, particularly EEG and SSEP monitoring, are effective at demonstrating neurophysiological changes attributable to ischemia, and therefore are of use in procedures that place the CBF at risk.*

- *Techniques such as SSEP, MEP, BAEP, EMG and NCV recording allow for monitoring of afferent or efferent activity through regions of the nervous system placed at risk by neurosurgical manipulation.*

- *Monitoring/mapping of cortical functions can be performed using techniques such as phase reversal, microelectrode recording or cortical stimulation (either electrical or magnetic).*

# References

1. Zampella E, Morawetz RB, McDowell HA, Zeiger HE, Varner PD, McKay RD et al. The importance of cerebral ischemia during carotid endarterectomy. Neurosurgery 1991;29:727–30.
2. Salvian AJ, Taylor DC, Hsiang YN et al. Selective shunting with EEG monitoring is safer than routine shunting for carotid endarterectomy. Cardiovasc Surg 1997;5:481–5.
3. Redekop G, Ferguson G. Correlation of contralateral stenosis and intraoperative electroencephalogram change with risk of stroke during carotid endarterectomy. Neurosurgery 1992;30:191–4.
4. Plestis KA, Loubser P, Mizrahi EM, Kantis G, Jiang ZD, Howell JF. Continuous electroencephalographic monitoring and selective shunting reduces neurologic morbidity rates in carotid endarterectomy. J Vasc Surg 1997;25:620–8.
5. Schwartz TH, Bazil CW, Forgione M, Bruce JN, Goodman RR. Do reactive post-resection "injury" spikes exist? Epilepsia 2000;41:1463–8.
6. Fisher RS, Raudzens P, Nunemacher M. Efficacy of intraoperative neurophysiological monitoring. J Clin Neurophysiol 1995;12:97–109.
7. Haupt WF, Horsch S. Evoked potential monitoring in carotid surgery: a review of 994 cases. Neurology 1992;42:835–8.
8. Guerit JM. Neuromonitoring in the operating room: why, when, and how to monitor? Electroencephalogr Clin Neurophysiol 1998;106:1–21.
9. Fava E, Bortolani E, Ducati A, Schieppati M. Role of SEP in identifying patients requiring temporary shunt during carotid endarterectomy. Electroencephalogr Clin Neurophysiol 1992;84:426–32.
10. Nuwer MR, Dawson EG, Carlson LG, Kanim LE, Sherman JE. Somatosensory evoked potential spinal cord monitoring reduces neurologic deficits after scoliosis surgery: results of a large multicenter survey. Electroencephalogr Clin Neurophysiol 1995;96:6–11.
11. Milhorat TH, Kotzen RM, Capocelli AL Jr, Bolognese P, Bendo AA, Cottrell JE. Intraoperative improvement of somatosensory evoked potentials and local spinal cord blood flow in patients with syringomyelia. J Neurosurg Anesthesiol 1996;8:208–15.
12. May DM, Jones SJ, Crockard HA. Somatosensory evoked potential monitoring in cervical surgery: identification of pre- and intraoperative risk factors associated with neurological deterioration. J Neurosurg 1996;85:566–73.
13. Dawson EG, Sherman JE, Kanim LE, Nuwer MR. Spinal cord monitoring. Results of the Scoliosis Research Society and the European Spinal Deformity Society survey. Spine 1991;16:S361–4.
14. Wilson-Holden TJ, Padberg AM, Parkinson JD, Bridwell KH, Lenke LG, Bassett GS. A prospective comparison of neurogenic mixed evoked potential stimulation methods: utility of epidural elicitation during posterior spinal surgery. Spine 2000;25:2364–71.
15. Pereon Y, Bernard JM, Fayet G, Delecrin J, Passuti N, Guiheneuc P. Usefulness of neurogenic motor evoked potentials for spinal cord monitoring: findings in 112 consecutive patients undergoing surgery for spinal deformity. Electroencephalogr Clin Neurophysiol 1998;108:17–23.
16. Kothbauer K, Schmid UD, Seiler RW, Eisner W. Intraoperative motor and sensory monitoring of the cauda equina. Neurosurgery 1994;34:702–7.
17. Kothbauer K, Deletis V, Epstein FJ. Intraoperative spinal cord monitoring for intramedullary surgery: an essential adjunct. Pediatr Neurosurg 1997;26:247–54.
18. Nagle KJ, Emerson RG, Adams DC et al. Intraoperative monitoring of motor evoked potentials: a review of 116 cases. Neurology 1996;47:999–1004.
19. Hariz MI, Fodstad H. Do microelectrode techniques increase accuracy or decrease risks in pallidotomy and deep brain stimulation? A critical review of the literature. Stereotact Funct Neurosurg 1999;72:157–69.
20. Fischer G, Fischer C, Remond J. Hearing preservation in acoustic neurinoma surgery. J Neurosurg 1992;76:910–17.
21. Fahlbusch R, Neu M, Strauss C. Preservation of hearing in large acoustic neurinomas following removal via suboccipito-lateral approach. Acta Neurochir (Wien) 1998;140:771–7.
22. Sundt TM. The ischemic tolerance of neural tissue and the need for monitoring and selective shunting during carotid endarterectomy. Stroke 1983;14:93–8.
23. Ackerstaff RG, Moons KG, van de Vlasakker CJ et al. Association of intraoperative transcranial doppler monitoring variables with stroke from carotid endarterectomy. Stroke 2000;31:1817–23.

24. Barrow DL, Boyer KL, Joseph GJ. Intraoperative angiography in the management of neurovascular disorders. Neurosurgery 1992;30:153–9.

25. Kline DG, Happel LT. A quarter century's experience with intraoperative nerve action potential recording. Can J Neurol Sci 1993;20:3–10.

# 2

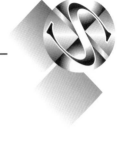

# Neuroradiology and Ultrasound

David G. Hughes

With a contribution on Ultrasound by

Roger Chisholm

## Summary

Neuroradiology utilises a wide range of imaging modalities in the diagnosis and treatment of CNS pathologies. MRI is the investigation of choice for most neuro-radiological imaging. CT remains the foremost modality in the emergency situation, and is superior to MRI in the visualisation of calcification, bone detail and acute hemorrhage. Angiography should be considered for all patients without a clear cause of hemorrhage and who are surgical candidates. Digital subtraction angiography is currently the gold standard in the investigation of subarachnoid hemorrhage, but in the future MRA and CTA will replace it. Technological advances are moving towards less invasive imaging modalities, supported by functional and physiological data. Ultrasound is the primary investigation in a neonate with an enlarging head and will reliably diagnose ventriculomegaly. It is accurate in the assessment of internal carotid artery stenosis for potential carotid endarterectomy patients.

## Introduction

Neuroradiology has evolved as a subspecialty of radiology by the application of different radiological techniques to the investigation of clinical problems related to the central nervous system (CNS) and spine. Initially limited to radiographs, a number of techniques became available that required skill in performance and interpretation, demanding the establishment of "neuroradiology". We now have a core of imaging modalities that allow ever more accurate diagnosis, and increasingly treatment, of CNS pathologies. These modalities include radiographs, computed tomography (CT), magnetic resonance imaging (MRI), angiography, ultrasound, nuclear medicine, myelography and interventional neuroradiology. These present a complex permutation of possible investigation of given clinical conditions that may be further influenced by local availability and expertise.

This chapter will review these imaging modalities and discuss the basic principles, indications, weaknesses and complications illustrated by clinical examples. A comprehensive imaging review of neurological disease is not possible in the length of this chapter and the reader is referred to recent neuroradiological textbooks for further reading [1, 2].

# Radiographs

Radiographs, once the only investigation available, are nearly redundant in modern neuroradiology. The use of skull radiographs has been greatly reduced even in trauma, and are now used in the UK as part of a triage exercise in minor head injury cases to decide on the safe discharge of a patient.

A person who has sustained a mild head injury, has no skull fracture, is Glasgow Coma Scale 15 and has adequate support at home can be discharged with a head injury advice chart. Even in this situation there is a case for CT scanning, the limiting factors being radiation dosage (ten times that of skull radiographs) and extensive workload to the CT scanner. There may be a role for skull radiographs in mild trauma to exclude a depressed skull fracture that is suspected from the mechanism of injury. The skull radiograph is still requested in myeloma and renal bone disease "screens".

Radiographs of the spine can be more helpful. They still form the basis of trauma cervical spine imaging "clearing the spine", although there are advocates of CT in this role if the patient is already undergoing CT of another part of the body.

A vast number of radiographs are still used in the assessment of neck and back pain. The yield of significant abnormalities is generally very low; in low back pain it is more productive if the use of radiographs is limited to the young patient (under 20 years) for the detection of spondylolisthesis (Fig. 2.1) and to older patients (over 55 years) where metastasis is more likely. Degenerative disease seen on a radiograph correlates poorly with clinical signs and symptoms. Where surgical management of degenerative disease is considered, then there is a case for MRI only [3].

# Computed Tomography

The first patient to be scanned using CT was at Atkinson Morley's Hospital in London in 1972. The technology invented by Sir Godfrey Hounsfield [4] (an engineer at the Central Research Laboratories, EMI, England) was the single most important development in neuroradiology.

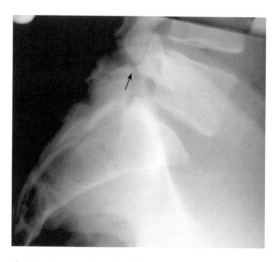

**Fig. 2.1.** Lateral radiograph of the lumbosacral junction. Defect in the pars interarticularis of L5 is clearly shown (arrow).

There have been great improvements since the early machines, with excellent resolution and very fast scanning times, making it possible to scan a head in a few seconds. Although MRI is superior in the investigation of most neurological and spinal diseases, CT scanners are both readily available in virtually all hospitals and very cost effective, so they are widely used as the workhorse of neuroimaging. CT remains the foremost imaging modality in the emergency situation. This applies particularly to trauma, where intracranial hematoma can be rapidly assessed in the unstable patient and where, in the case of polytrauma, other areas such as the cervical spine or abdomen can be scanned. CT is superior to MRI in the visualization of calcification, bone detail and acute hemorrhage.

The CT appearances of hematoma are well recognized in the acute phase, being of higher attenuation than the adjacent brain. In hyperacute hematoma, areas of low density may be seen consistent with active bleeding before a clot has formed. The appearance of the hematoma changes to become the same density as brain and eventually lower (Table 2.1). This typical evolution of hematoma can be altered by clotting disorder, anticoagulation, low haemocrit and anemia, when the acute hematoma can be isodense with brain in 50% of cases [5].

The presence of fluid–fluid levels within an extra-axial hematoma often represents acute hemorrhage with a chronic bleed. Fluid levels within a parenchymal hematoma are not only

NEURORADIOLOGY AND ULTRASOUND

**Table 2.1.** CT appearances of hematoma (relative to brain)

| Phase | Time | Attenuation |
| --- | --- | --- |
| Hyperacute | Minutes to hours | Hyperdense with hypodense areas |
| Acute | Hours to 1 week | Hyperdense |
| Subacute | 1–6 weeks | Isodense |
| Chronic | >6 weeks | Hypodense |

seen in hemorrhagic tumors but also in any of the many causes of cerebral hemorrhage.

Low-density extra-axial collections are not necessarily hematomas. Empyemas are low density with mass effect and, when subdural, may expand the interhemispheric fissure (Fig. 2.2). Often the patient is more clinically unwell than would be suggested by the size of the collection. Intravenous contrast typically causes enhancement of a surrounding membrane, which may aid diagnosis. Contrast medium is used routinely in CT scanning, particularly if there is a possibility of infection, tumor or vascular lesion. Unnecessary use should be avoided, e.g. in acute trauma or hydrocephalus, as there is a risk of serious reaction in 1 in 2,500 injections [6].

When subarachnoid hemorrhage (SAH) mixes with CSF, the attenuation of the hema-

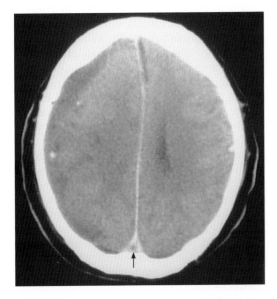

**Fig. 2.2.** CT scan post i.v. contrast. Low-density subdural collection with mass effect. Note fluid in the interhemispheric fissure, which suggests a subdural empyema. This is complicated by a sagittal sinus thrombosis (arrow points to the delta sign).

toma is reduced, becoming the same as brain. Therefore smaller SAHs will be subtle with apparent effacement of sulci and cisterns – an appearance that should not be mistaken for brain swelling. CT will detect 95% of SAHs within 24 hours of the ictus. A reliable indirect sign is the presence of mild hydrocephalus. After 1 week, CT is much less reliable as the density of the hematoma is significantly reduced.

Current CT scanners use multislice techniques of acquisition, allowing greater coverage in shorter times. This reduces any movement artifact and facilitates CT angiography as a significant length of vessel can be scanned while the bolus of contrast medium passes through. Reformation of the scans can be performed in several ways, such as multi-planar reconstructions, maximum intensity projections, volume-rendered images or even "fly through" endoluminal views. CT angiography (CTA) has been used to demonstrate carotid artery disease, intracranial vascular anatomy, including arteriovenous malformations (AVMs), and aneurysms [7] and is now frequently used as a first investigation of SAH. The three-dimensional images obtained can be used to decide between an endovascular or open neurosurgical operation on an aneurysm. It is useful in the emergency situation when a large hematoma has been demonstrated and when there is a suspicion of an underlying vascular lesion. CTA in this situation may demonstrate an underlying aneurysm, enabling the patient to proceed rapidly to evacuation of the clot and clipping of the aneurysm without the delay of organizing a formal angiogram.

CTA requires the administration of iodinated contrast media and also for the patient to lie very still during the scan time of approximately 30 seconds.

A large aneurysm may be apparent on the initial CT scan as blood within the aneurysm is less dense than the surrounding hematoma (Fig. 2.3).

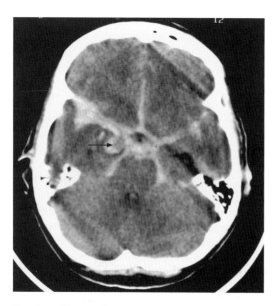

**Fig. 2.3.** CT scan demonstrating extensive subarachnoid hematoma with the lower density aneurysm lumen visible (arrow).

The ability of CT to detect subtle calcification and show excellent bone detail highlights its use as an adjunct to MRI. Detection of calcification within a tumor may aid the differential diagnosis. Subtle calcification may not be apparent on an MR scan but is obvious on a CT scan, which may lead to the diagnosis of tuberous sclerosis in the investigation of epilepsy. Skull base detail is very well shown on a CT scan and is complementary to MRI in fully defining complex lesions of this region. This ability to define bone detail is also very useful in spinal imaging, particularly in trauma, to define and classify fractures. Reconstruction of data into sagittal and coronal planes is easily achieved and adds essential information on alignment and extent of abnormality.

# Magnetic Resonance Imaging

The principles of nuclear magnetic resonance were first described in the 1930s by C.J. Gorter and used extensively as spectroscopy to study physical and chemical properties of matter. It was not until the late 1970s that images of human anatomy were produced and the technique became known as "magnetic resonance imaging". Extensive development has enabled MRI to become the investigation of choice for most neuroradiological imaging.

The quantum mechanics and mathematics that attempt to explain MRI are beyond this author and are not required for image interpretation. An understanding of the simplified principles and the various sequences produced is necessary [2, 8].

From a practical view of image interpretation, we need to know what is white, black or gray on a particular MR sequence. These are summarized in Table 2.2. Fat, very proteinaceous tissues, certain degradation products of hemorrhage, and gadolinium influence free protons to produce high signal on T1 weighting. Gray and white matter will be intermediate signal, but white will be slightly higher signal because of its increased fat content. Brain edema and most pathologies will be intermediate signal, i.e. grey, and CSF will be black.

On T2 weighting, CSF is high signal and gray matter is higher signal than white matter. Air and cortical bone are very low signal owing to the small amount of free protons in these. Arterial blood flow and certain venous flow will present no signal (flow void) on standard spin-echo sequences. Most pathologies will be high signal, as are certain hemorrhagic breakdown products. So most tumors will be high signal on T2 weighting and low on T1, although atypical patterns of signal can help to characterize certain tumors (Fig. 2.4).

Routine scanning with MRI usually involves T1- and T2-weighted sequences in at least two planes. The weighting can be gained by various scanning techniques, including conventional spin echo (CSE), fast spin echo (FSE) and gradient echo (GE). Acquisitions can be acquired in two- or three-dimensional modes. Very fast scanning is possible with techniques such as echo-planar imaging (EPI) or half-Fourier acquisition single-shot turbo spin-echo ("HASTE"), although they may be limited by artifact and poor signal-to-noise ratio. Special sequences can be used to suppress fat, such as in "STIR" (short tau inversion recovery), which is useful for skull base and orbital imaging, and to suppress CSF, as in "FLAIR" (fluid-attenuated inversion recovery), which increases the conspicuity of lesions at brain–CSF interfaces. More recently, specialized applications of MR scan-

inner membrane, and one must also recognize the much more rapid organization of an epidural hemorrhage with its immediate access to the surrounding connective tissue and blood vessels.

## Neoplasms

This category is obviously the largest – neurosurgeons' biases historically shaped this direction! – and consists of 70–80% of all neurosurgical specimens, but the distribution depends on the populations served and the strengths of subspecialties of neurosurgeons in any one institute. The magnet effect of individuals – so obvious in Cushing's pituitary tumors, but also involving public, private, academic, large and small institutions – is still in play! There are already many books describing gross and microscopic findings for each type of tumor and there are already too many revisions of classifications of tumors [4,5,6,7,8], so we will not be repetitive in describing each tumor. Books that not only describe the findings of each tumor but also discuss the differential diagnoses more extensively are more helpful [6]. The authors would caution, however, that the types of tumors have changed dramatically, from "wait until the tumor is large enough to be seen by pneumoencephalography" to " biopsy after the MRI after the first fit". They would also suggest that the character of a tumor can be defined biologically (i.e. only the ranges of growth and invasive characteristics can be inferred, not measured histologically, and these ranges are notoriously wide: fast, slow, diffuse, etc.). But this may be a subject for discussion in its own right!

Having reached a tentative conclusion that a given specimen probably represents a neoplasm, one should be able to say whether it is: (1) primary or secondary (metastatic), (2) intrinsic (neural) or extrinsic (non-neural), and (3) its type and grade.

The nature of the edge is very helpful since primary intrinsic neoplasms tend to be infiltrative of the CNS whereas metastatic or extrinsic neoplasms tend to be sharply demarcated from the CNS. Of course, truly extrinsic neoplasms are rarely excised with any CNS but there may be a capsule of fibrous tissue that helps. One must always be aware that rapidly growing primary gliomas may break through the pia, infiltrate the arachnoid and dura and grossly resemble meningiomas. The reverse is also true

– that even benign meningiomas and craniopharyngiomas may break through the pia and infiltrate the CNS, craniopharyngiomas especially evoking a remarkable gliosis with many Rosenthal fibers.

In determining the type and grade of neoplasms, one usually relies on the cell morphology, frequently assisted by the pattern of cellular arrangement as well as by stromal and vascular changes. Let us consider each of these below.

*Cell Morphology* The authors assume familiarity with the neurohistology of normal neurons, astrocytes, oligodendroglia, ependymal cells and microglia, as well as that of blood vessels and meninges. In general, touch or smear preparations of freshly removed specimens stained with H&E generally reveal the structure of individual cells better than frozen or even subsequently prepared paraffin sections, provided, of course, that enough cells stick to the slide. Touch or smear preparations are especially useful with pituitary adenomas as the normal pituitary cells do not come out of their enclosure in small pockets or capsules of connective tissue. In adenomatous tissue, the connective tissue septa diminish and large nodules of adenoma cells are easily squeezed out. Cells with abundant processes that are tightly woven together, as in schwannomas and astrocytomas, come out only as thick chunks. Patterns of cellular arrangement and vascular changes are usually not discerned in touch preparations. Necrotic coagula are easily seen but may be missed as an artifact.

To make a diagnosis of the cell type, one looks for resemblance of tumor cells to normal cells. Sometimes our concept of "normal" may seem a little strange; witness the "fried egg" or " honeycomb" (Fig. 3.5) pattern of oligodendrogliomas. This pattern is really an autolytic artifact that most pathologists find diagnostic, even though the normal oligodendrocyte usually shows much less of this artifact.

Cells showing more deviation away from the norm are said to be less differentiated or more anaplastic. At its maximal end, the cells appear so undifferentiated and uncharacteristic – consisting only of nuclei with little or no cytoplasm or processes – that their identity is lost and they can only be designated as primitive neuroectodermal cells. However, whether they are truly

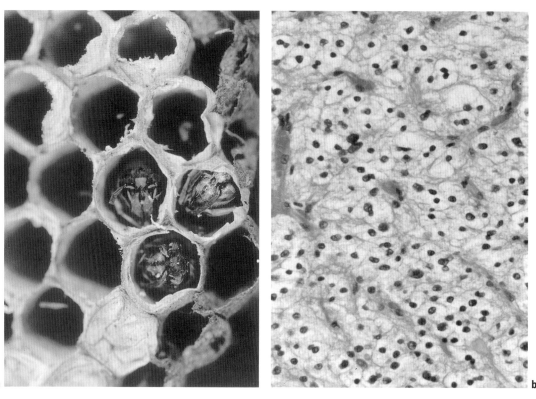

a                                                                                        b

**Fig. 3.5. a** A honeycomb, some still filled with baby bees, corresponding to the nuclei of an oligodendroglioma. **b** "Honeycomb" pattern of an oligodendroglioma. S-4362-81, H&E.

neuroectodermal or not needs to be proven by other studies.

Many well differentiated tumors frequently consist of more than one type of cell, just as a family contains old and young persons, male and female, tall and short, even skinny and obese. This is especially true in gliomas, as astrocytes (fibrillary, gemistocytic or protoplasmic), oligodendroglia and even ependymocytes share the same progenitor. When a diagnosis of a particular type of glioma is made, it does not necessarily imply a pure culture of that particular type of glia cell, only a majority of that type of cell. When the proportion of other types becomes significant, a diagnosis of mixed glioma can be made, although a determination of the necessary proportion is quite arbitrary and subjective – usually at least 25%. This is another area where controversies arise.

## Patterns of Cellular Arrangement

Each tumor appears to be different. In order to classify tumors into groups, one has to find some common denominator for each group. As we mentioned above, we first use the morphology of the tumor cells to estimate the lineage of the cell and tumor. However, although the histological variations on normal cells are very limited, those of tumor cells are quite marked. No matter how we combine the shape, size and degree of staining of the nucleus and cytoplasm and the shape, size and number of cell processes, we can make only a limited number of normal cell types, which can resemble the tumor cells to various degrees. Not all tumors are diffusely infiltrating or consist of randomly arranged or packed cell masses. Tumors belonging to a similar lineage have a tendency to show a particular pattern formed by groups of cells. These patterns are not specific and frequently overlap among different groups but are helpful when combined with cell morphology. The patterns are not necessarily present in the whole tumor but are often found only in small foci, which one has to search for.

*Diffusely Infiltrating with No Significant Pattern*
This type of pattern can be seen in all types of gliomas: gangliogliomas, lymphomas, primitive neuroectodermal tumors (PNETs), germinomas, melanomas, sarcomas and some types of carcinoma. Some show relatively subtle patterns: germinomas can be identified because of the mixture of two distinct cell types: large epithelioid cells and small lymphocytes. Islands of nuclei in a sea of glial fibers are seen in the adult spinal cord (Fig. 3.6a) and are typical of subependymomas (Fig. 3.6b). Lymphoma cells tend to be densely packed around blood vessels, even laminated. Homer Wright pseudorosettes, described below, may be found in PNETs with neuroblastic differentiation but frequently require careful search.

*Perineuronal Satellitosis* Oligodendrogliomas have a tendency to proliferate close to the cell bodies of neurons in the gray matter, a phenomenon known as "perineuronal satellitosis". Astrocytes and microglia also occur normally and abnormally in a satellite position but oligodendrogliomas seem to be the most common neoplasm to produce this pattern. Two or three glial cells around a neuron are common, indeed normal, but more than that is abnormal. In tumors, there are an increased number of satellite cells, which usually show some nuclear pleomorphism (Fig. 3.7). Often the presence of a neuron in the center is obscure and one sees only a regular scattering of clumps of tumor cells in the gray matter, suggesting the distribution of neurons previously present. Satellitosis is not specific for a neoplasm, but can be seen in reactions to various non-specific infections and intoxications.

*Streams and Bundles* Most frequently seen in schwannomas, streams of interlacing bundles of elongated spindle-shaped cells are present in Antoni Type A regions (Fig. 3.8); cut in cross-section, the spindle-shaped nuclei become small and round. Meningiomas, especially of the fibrous variant, can also show this pattern, but

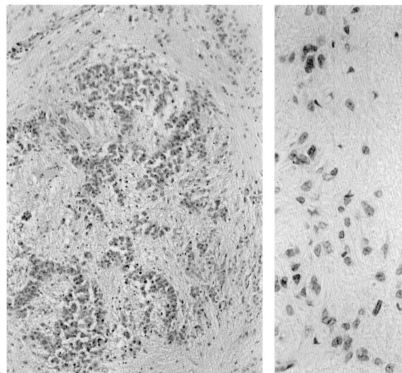

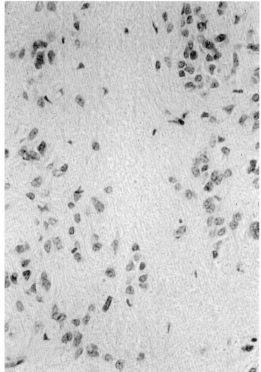

a                                                                                          b

**Fig. 3.6. a** Islands of nuclei in a sea of glial fibers in a normal adult spinal cord. NP282, H&E. **b** Similar islands in a subependymoma. NP171, H&E.

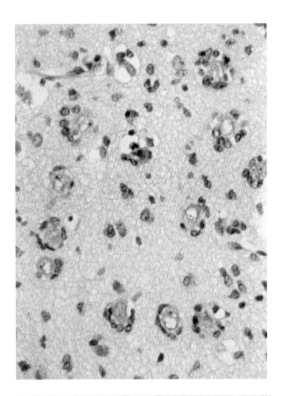

**Fig. 3.7.** Perineuronal satellitosis in an oligodendroglioma. NP7146, H&E.

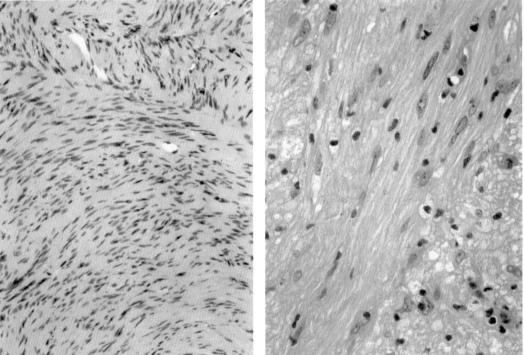

a

b

**Fig. 3.8. a–b** Streams or bundles of spindle cells typical of a schwannoma. NP16042, H&E. **a** Low magnification. **b** High magnification.

the nuclei of meningioma cells tend to be less spindle-shaped. In addition, streaming cells forming parallel rows with little interlacing can be seen in pilocytic astrocytomas, fibrillary astrocytomas and oligodendrogliomas.

*Whorls, Loops, Onion-skin Pattern and Psammoma Bodies* These patterns are characteristic of meningiomas in which there are concentric layers of tumor cells around a center, which may contain no structure or which may show a small blood vessel, a hyaline body or even a calcified granule. Psammoma bodies are calcified granules that are usually laminated and non-specific, unless one can see the whorling meningioma cells around them (Fig. 3.9a, b). Whorls can also be seen in schwannomas but they are not as distinctly outlined by a thin fibrous membrane as in meningiomas and tend to be larger with an indistinct border (Fig. 3.9c). Larger whorls may look more like oval loops. Cross-sections of neurofibromas may show a somewhat similar pattern, known as an "onion skin" or "onion bulb". These structures are more numerous and loosely spaced, typically with a demonstrable axon in the center of the onion bulb.

*Nodular, Lobular and Alveolar Patterns* Tumors consisting of nodules and lobules of various sizes are numerous. Small nodules and large lobules separated by thin fibrous membranes are typical of meningiomas, separated by capillaries or hypocellular gliotic tissue frequently in oligodendrogliomas and separated by connective tissue septa in pituitary adenomas. Similar lobular patterns are also seen in chordomas, chemodectomas, metastatic carcinomas and alveolar soft-part sarcomas. Alveolar and follicular patterns are more or less synonymous with a lobular pattern (Fig. 3.10).

*Palisades and Pseudo-palisades* Nuclei that form parallel rows are known as "nuclear palisades". Anuclear eosinophilic cytoplasmic bands between nuclear rows in a schwannoma are known as "Verocay bodies" (Fig. 3.11). The combination of nuclear palisades, Verocay's bodies and interlacing bundles of spindle-shaped cells (see Fig. 3.8) is relatively specific for schwannoma, although an almost identical pattern can be seen in occasional astrocytomas (bipolar spongioblastomas or "central schwannoma"). Palisading of nuclei can also occur in PNET, again as a clone of the rare primitive spongioblastoma. An area of coagulative necrosis surrounded by rows of nuclei is often called "pseudopalisading", more accurately called "perinecrotic palisading", and is often seen in glioblastoma multiforme. Adjacent areas of dense (Antoni A) and loose (Antoni B) tissue is typical of schwannoma (Fig. 3.11).

*Rosettes and Pseudo-rosettes* There are four types of these patterns: two types of true rosettes and two types of pseudo-rosettes. All show cells radiating around a center. One true rosette is an ependymal rosette that has a small or large lumen in the center, resembling the central canal of the spinal cord with cilia or blephaloplasts around the lumen (Fig. 3.12a). Such rosettes are found in some ependymomas (Fig. 3.12b). Another true rosette is composed of rods and cones and is seen in some retinoblastomas. One type of pseudo-rosette includes a blood vessel in the center, a perivascular pseudo-rosette (Fig. 3.13a, b), the cell processes from the surrounding cells tapering toward the vascular wall. These can be seen with H&E stain but more easily seen with van Gieson (VG) stain (Fig. 3.13c). Perivascular pseudo-rosettes are very common in ependymomas, and are much more common than true rosettes. When the center consists of anuclear eosinophilic cytoplasm (on H&E stain), it is known as a "Homer Wright pseudo-rosette", a pattern typical of neuroblasts growing in culture. They are found in some PNETs but more frequently in neuroblastomas (Fig. 3.14), central neurocytomas and pineocytomas. The eosinophilic amorphous areas tend to be larger and more irregular in pineocytomas and neuroblastomas.

*Cartwheels and Perivascular Crowns* Difficult to distinguish from perivascular pseudorosettes, a cartwheel formation has been described as characteristic of astroblastomas in which radially arranged tumor cells show cell feet attached to the vascular wall, whereas only tapering cytoplasmic processes are demonstrable in ependymomas. When no cellular processes are present around the blood vessel, the pattern is simply called a "perivascular crown", as seen in numerous types of tumors, including astrocytomas (Fig. 3.15), adenomas and carcinomas .

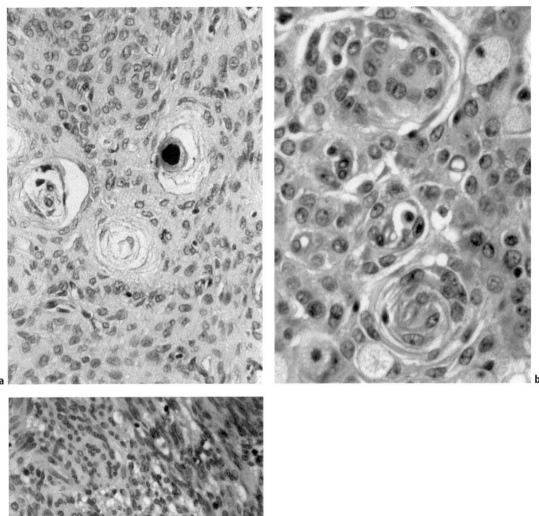

**Fig. 3.9. a** Whorls of plump viable meningioma cells progressively condensing into small, tight whorls of thin cells and then into psammoma bodies. NP7807, H&E. **b** Transitional forms of whorls typical of meningiomas. NP17354, H&E. **c** Looser whorls of cells seen occasionally in schwannomas. S-67-787, H&E.

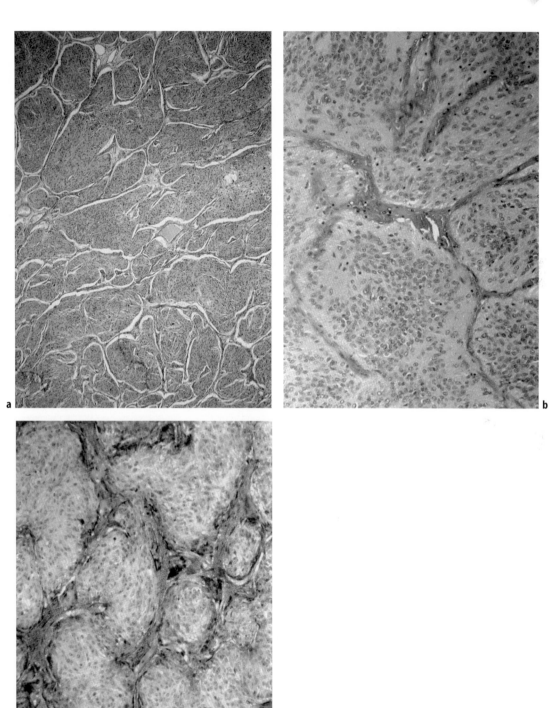

**Fig. 3.10. a** Lobular pattern in a meningioma. N90, H&E. **b** Lobular pattern in an oligodendroglioma produced by "chicken wire" pattern of thick capillaries. Note absence of the autolytic honeycomb pattern shown in Fig. 3.5b. NP10891, H&E. **c** Lobular pattern in a prolactinoma. NP7275, H&E.

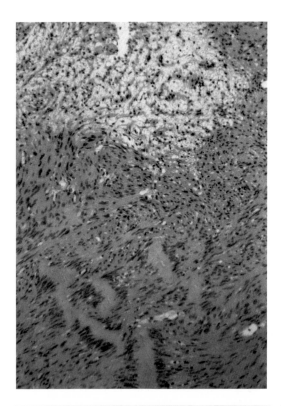

**Fig. 3.11.** Schwannoma showing nuclear palisades forming Verocay bodies in Antoni A (dense) region next to Antoni B (loose, foamy) region. NP15094, H&E.

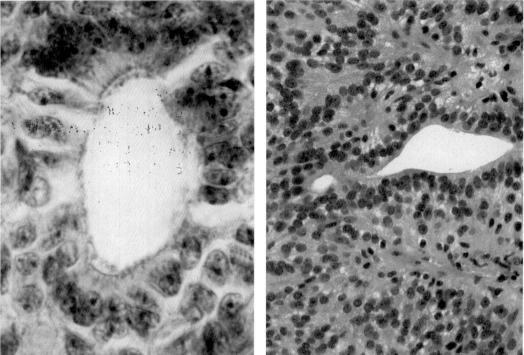

a

b

**Fig. 3.12. a–b** True rosettes. **a** Normal ependymal canal and **b** ependymal rosette in an ependymoma. NP27902, H&E.

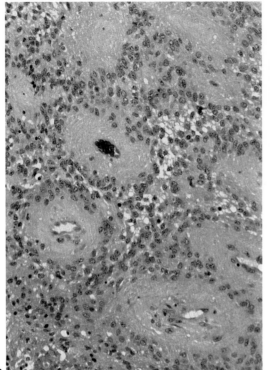

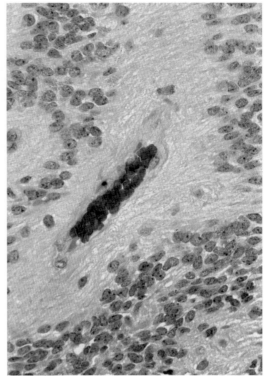

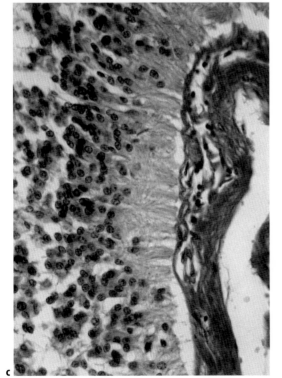

**Fig. 3.13. a–c** Perivascular pseudo-rosettes in an ependymoma. NP20617, H&E. **a** Low magnification. **b** High magnification. **c** Special stains such as this Verhoeff–van Gieson stain can differentiate the perivascular collagen (red in the original) from the glial fibers (yellow in the original), the latter tapering to a point in ependymomas rather than expanding into a footplate, as in astroblastomas. NP709.

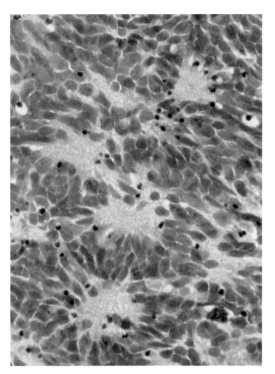

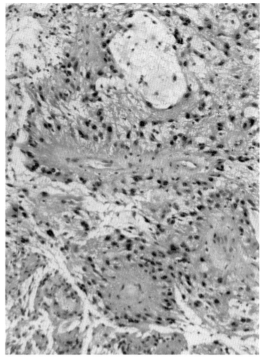

**Fig. 3.14.** Homer Wright neuroblastic pseudo-rosette in a medulloblastoma (cerebellar PNET). NP25458, H&E.

**Fig. 3.15.** Perivascular crowns in an astrocytoma. NP13936, H&E.

*Papillae* Papillae are finger-like processes of hyperplastic tumors, each process with a connective tissue stroma, usually with accompanying blood vessels, covered by epithelial cells. The best example is, of course, a choroid plexus papilloma but papillae can also be seen in ependymomas, pituitary adenomas, metastatic adenocarcinomas (Fig. 3.16) and in a rare form of meningiomas known as "papillary meningiomas".

*Checkerboard and Lattice Formations* This mosaic pattern with alternating dense fibrillary and loose hypocellular areas is typically found in pilocytic astrocytomas (Fig. 3.17a, b). The loose areas represent areas of mucinous degeneration and the beginning of cyst formation. Rosenthal fibers are usually found in the dense part. A similar pattern with tumor nodules partitioned by connective tissue septa is found in optic gliomas (Fig. 3.17c).

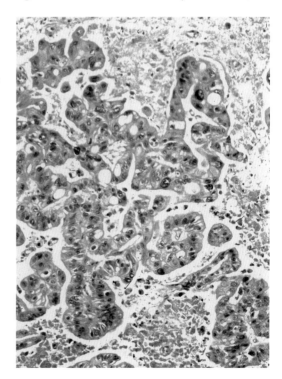

**Fig. 3.16.** Papillary adenocarcinoma. NP16375, H&E.

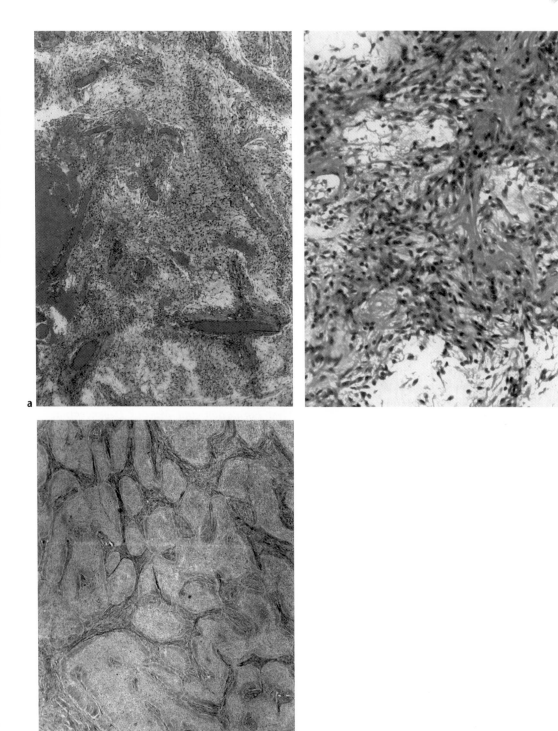

**Fig. 3.17. a–c** Lattice pattern in a pilocytic astrocytoma. NP14609, H&E. **a** Low magnification. **b** High magnification. **c** Septate pattern in an optic glioma. NP4260, H&E.

The various patterns described above are not necessarily specific for any one type of tumor but are useful in beginning to formulate a histological differential diagnosis. When combined with other findings, such as the morphology of the tumor cells and stromal and vascular changes, the particular pattern is very helpful.

### Stromal Changes

In addition to the appearance of the principal cells, there are many ancillary changes that occur in tumor tissue. These changes again are not specific and diagnostic by themselves but are helpful in making a diagnosis, especially in determining the degree of anaplasia of the tumors.

*Necrosis with or without Palisading* Necrosis represents death of tissue. There are two types, liquefactive and coagulative, but most of the latter become liquefactive in time as macrophages digest it. Liquefactive necrosis from the beginning is typical of an abscess with pus, but the later stage of any other necrosis can be progressively soft and eventually liquid. Tumor necrosis and radiation necrosis tend to be coagulative with very little phagocytic activity. Necrosis due to infarction is initially coagulative, although grossly soft, but slowly becomes liquefactive with extensive phagocytosis to digest the dead tissue. Even when tumor necrosis is considered to be due to vascular occlusion within the tumor, the dead tumor tissue does not appear to attract many phagocytic cells. The presence of tumor necrosis with surrounding palisading is indicative of cellular proliferation without concomitant vascular and/or nutrient support and is, therefore, a sign of a rapidly growing tumor. The presence of necrosis is one of critical importance in the diagnosis of glioblastoma. The clinical correlate of necrosis in ependymomas and oligodendrogliomas is not as clear as in astrocytomas [9].

Radiation also induces coagulative necrosis, predominantly in the white matter, frequently almost identical to that of untreated glioblastomas. In cases of a re-operated tumor with a history of previous radiotherapy, it is practically impossible to distinguish the necrosis as being an inherent part of the tumor or secondary to radiation. Some emphasize the presence of pseudo-palisading around the necrosis as specific to tumor necrosis, but the absence is ambiguous since there may not be sufficient numbers of remaining tumor cells necessary to form palisades or their growth rate may have been slowed by the radiotherapy.

*Mineralizations (Calcification, Ferrugination and Ossification)* Calcification is found in relatively slow growing tumors, including meningiomas, oligodendrogliomas, gangliogliomas, craniopharyngiomas and astrocytomas, but it can also follow irradiation. It can be found in the parenchyma and adjacent cerebral tissue and in the blood vessel walls in oligodendrogliomas. In meningiomas, calcification may be present in the form of psammoma bodies, which may show concentric lamination, and in the form of more amorphous larger calcified masses. In craniopharyngiomas, teratomas, chordomas and dermoid cysts, the calcification appears as masses of various sizes. Scattered calcified granules within coagulative necrosis are typically seen in radiation necrosis.

*Cyst Formation and Mucoid Degeneration* A cyst is simply a fluid-filled closed cavity and tends to be found in slow-growing tumors. The fluid may be dark brown (so-called "motor oil"), watery (like CSF), xanthochromic of various degrees or hues, milky or mucinous depending on the amount of hemosiderin and protein present, and with or without cholesterol crystals in craniopharyngiomas. The cyst usually arises from liquefactive necrosis or mucoid degeneration of the tumor tissue. In oligodendrogliomas, pilocytic astrocytomas and chordomas, both mucoid degeneration and cyst formation may be present. A large, more or less solitary, cyst is typically found in hemangioblastomas and pilocytic astrocytomas that appear as a mural nodule. Numerous microcysts are common in oligodendrogliomas (Fig. 3.18) and astroblastomas as well as in pilocytic astrocytomas. Cysts in craniopharyngiomas or chordomas are variable in size. Cysts are uncommon in meningiomas and schwannomas and rare in PNETs and germinomas. Glioblastoma has been defined as a multiform glioma, so it should not be surprising to find foci of low-grade glioma with cysts and calcifications, not to forget cysts due to necrosis.

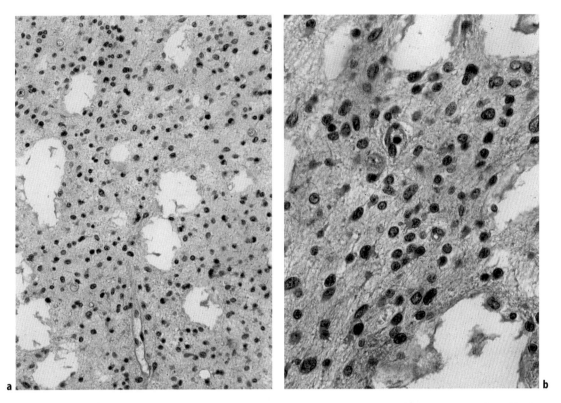

**Fig. 3.18. a–b** Microcysts are frequently seen in oligodendrogliomas, usually owing to mucinous degeneration, as evidenced by the faintly stained contents. NP19529, H&E. **a** Low magnification. **b** High magnification.

*Rosenthal Fibers, Cytoid Bodies and Eosinophilic Hyaline Bodies* Eosinophilic hyaline bodies of variable shapes and thicknesses (commas, sausages or just thick bands) are known as "Rosenthal fibers". These structures are usually densely red with a mild purplish tinge and sometimes resemble columns of red blood cells. They are found typically in pilocytic astrocytomas and gliotic white matter surrounding craniopharyngiomas. The origin of Rosenthal fibers has been debated but they probably represent a degenerated form of glial fibers on which crystalline is deposited. They stain variably with GFAP but not so intensely as do the usual astrocytic fibers. Eosinophilic hyaline bodies, cytoid bodies and eosinophilic granular bodies are found in low-grade gliomas, such as pilocytic astrocytomas and oligodendrogliomas, but their origin has not been clarified.

*Keratin (Dry Keratin) and Parakeratin (Wet Keratin)* Multilaminated desquamated epithe-lial membranes appear as thin parallel lines to hexagonal plates, depending on the plane of section. They are known as "keratin" or "dry keratin" ("dandruff") and are typically seen in epidermoid and dermoid cysts (Fig. 3.19a), where the dehydrating pattern of maturation is to be expected on exposure to air. By contrast, dead, swollen, mucosal epithelium ("wet keratin", where the swelling represents maturation of cells exposed to moisture) appears as eosinophilic masses with pale membranous septa representing cell walls and ghosts of nuclei (Fig. 3.19b). Wet keratin is characteristic of craniopharyngiomas, which develop from Rathke's duct and nasopharyngeal mucosa.

*Desmoplasia and Fibrosis* Excessive fibrous connective tissue sometimes forms the stroma of tumors and at times divides tumors into numerous small nodules or cords. This phenomenon is seen especially when a tumor invades and infiltrates the leptomeninges, even

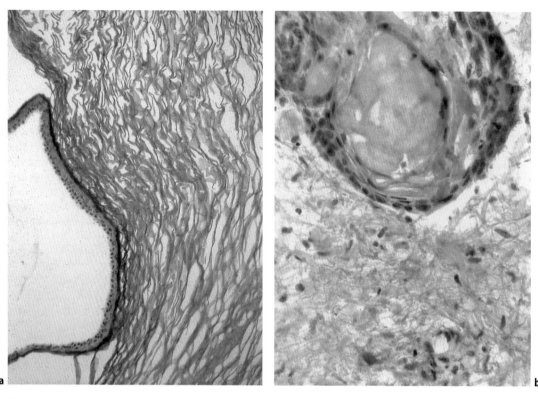

**Fig. 3.19. a** Dry keratin appears as parallel lines expanding into hexagonal plates depending on the plane of section. NP3880, H&E. **b** Wet keratin appears as swollen cells with ghosts of nuclei in a craniopharyngioma. NP-02-286, H&E.

more when it invades the dura, or when there is an excessive reaction in the connective tissue portion of the vascular components. Fibrous scar formation is almost always found in cases with previous surgical intervention. Irradiation also induces excessive proliferation of connective tissue. The differentiation from a sarcoma or a mixed glio-sarcoma is difficult unless one can demonstrate neoplastic features in the connective tissue, i.e. mitoses and numerous cycling nuclei in addition to the pleomorphism frequently seen in actively reacting fibrous tissue.

Terminology may be deleted with experience, and the "cerebellar sarcoma" – so diagnosed decades ago because of its rich fibrous connective tissue dividing the tumor into nodules (Fig. 3.20a) – is now known to be a desmoplastic medulloblastoma, but the prognosis remains the same with CSF metastases (Fig. 3.20b, c), just as in other medulloblastomas. Terminology also increases, of course, and both desmoplastic

infantile ganglioglioma (DIG) and desmoplastic cerebral astrocytoma of infancy (DCAI) occur in the superficial cerebrum of infants, are rich in collagenous tissue, and tend to have a relatively favorable prognosis.

*Inflammation* Mild focal perivascular lymphocytic cuffs are common but non-specific in many gliomas and other tumors. Pre-operative diagnostic procedures such as angiography may contribute to a mild inflammation. Foci of neutrophilic reaction are occasionally seen in glioblastomas, causing differential diagnostic problems with other causes of necrosis or inflammation, especially when the specimen is inadequate. Lymphocytes of various types constitute the small cells of germinomas and become of diagnostic importance.

*Hemorrhages, Old and Recent* Evidences of recent and old hemorrhages may follow various treatments but also occur spontaneously in

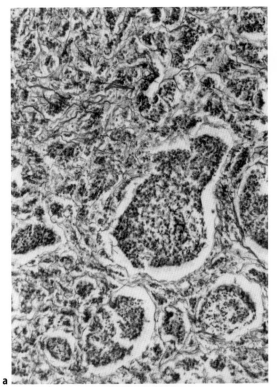

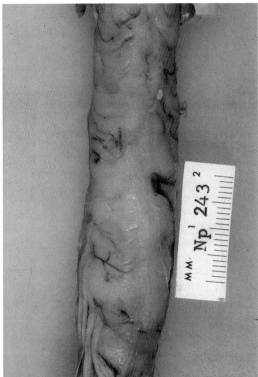

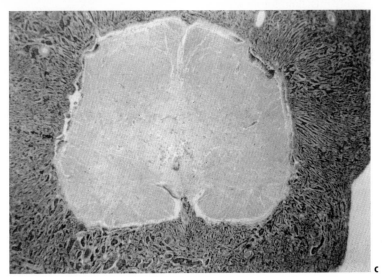

**Fig. 3.20. a** Medulloblastomas sometimes evoke so much connective tissue reaction as to suggest sarcoma (NP243, reticulin). **b** Although the posterior fossa was irradiated, the failure to appreciate that the tumor was really a medulloblastoma led to the patient's death by metastases through the CSF, surrounding the spinal cord. **c** gross. H&E.

many tumors characterized by hypervascularity: hemangioblastomas, meningiomas, schwannomas, oligodendrogliomas and ependymomas. Melanomas often bleed and the cells may contain both melanin and hemosiderin pigments.

*Vascular Changes*

In general, high-grade neoplasms are more vascular than low- grade ones, but there are many exceptions. Obviously, tumors of vascular origin, such as capillary hemangioblastomas, hemangioendotheliomas and hemangiopericytomas, are vascular by definition regardless of their degree of anaplasia. Meningiomas have long been known to be vascular, fed both intra- and extra-cranially, and their surgical resection was sometimes disastrous in the old days, but they are easily handled today with pre-operative selective embolization. Among metastatic neoplasms, melanomas, hepatomas and choriocarcinomas are well known to be vascular and to bleed easily. Ependymomas are inherently vascular as part of their perivascular pseudo-rosettes, but an avascular cellular ependymoma without perivascular pseudo-rosettes can be readily mistaken for an astrocytoma. Oligodendrogliomas can also be very vascular and have spontaneous intracerebral hemorrhages. Pilocytic astrocytomas and schwannomas often show focal areas of hypervascularity, usually markedly hyalinized, but occasionally even with capillary endothelial proliferation.

*Capillary Endothelial Proliferation* Excessive proliferation of capillary endothelium filling the lumen and/or extending externally to form glomerulus-like masses (Fig. 3.21) or chains is one of the common ancillary "proofs of malignancy" in glioblastomas. However, it is also common in oligodendrogliomas and the walls of cysts of any nature, and is occasionally found in pilocytic astrocytomas and schwannomas without affecting the grading or prognosis.

*Telangiectasia and Angioma Formations* Foci of telangiectasia and angioma formations are frequently found in high-grade glioblastomas and low-grade oligodendrogliomas, but are not useful as criteria for grading the neoplasm. Spontaneous hemorrhages most frequently occur in these tumors.

*Capillary Networks Intersecting the Tumor into Lobules* So-called "chicken-wire capillary networks" that intersect the tumor into multiple lobules are one of the characteristic architectural patterns of oligodendrogliomas (see Figs. 3.5b and 3.10b).

*Sinusoidal Networks Intersecting the Tumor into Lobules* The normal pituitary gland consists of small acini of cells of different types separated by connective tissue septa with sinusoidal vessels. The acini expand in adenomas to destroy the connective tissue septa but the basic pattern may remain, only with enlargement of the acini (see Fig. 3.10c).

*Hyalinized Necrosis and Thrombosis of Blood Vessels* Hyalinized necrosis of blood vessel walls and recent thrombosis, together with marked proliferation of abnormal blood vessels, including thin-walled and dilated veins and thick-walled fibrous blood vessels of indeterminate nature, may be at least as diagnostic of

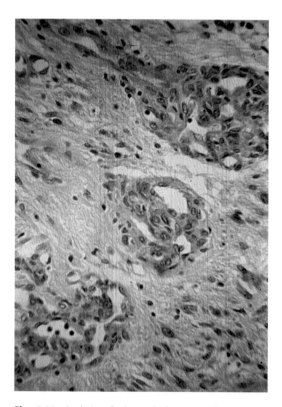

**Fig. 3.21.** A chain of glomeruloid masses of endothelial proliferation is typical of glioblastoma. NIH-575, H&E.

glioblastoma as the presence of necrosis. Tumor necrosis is most likely the result of these abnormal vascular channels with neovascularization, which inappropriately slows or shunts the blood flow away from the tumor.

*Perivascular Fibrosis* Perivascular fibrosis is very common and non-diagnostic. With multiple capillary channels it is characteristic of radiation, but it can be found in untreated glioblastomas as a "radio-mimetic effect".

## If It Belongs to One of the Above Processes, Can You Narrow Your Diagnosis More Specifically as to the Type of Process?

In narrowing one's list of differential diagnoses, it is frequently necessary to consult textbooks and journals [4,5,6,7,8,10]. Pathology is largely a visual science, so that picture-matching becomes important!

## Does Your Tentatively Final Pathological Diagnosis Make Sense Clinically and Anatomically?

There is rarely anything so satisfying as reaching the same diagnosis as did the clinician, both independently using different techniques inherent in each specialty. Even more satisfying is suggesting a better diagnosis that each can then independently confirm by further studies!

## 2. How Can One Understand the Changing Diagnostic Terminologies?

Time and space do not permit us to answer this question! The only safe method is to ask the other persons what terminology they are using and try to work out a mutually satisfactory translation! One may refer to books already in print on tumors [4,5,6,7,8] and other diseases [10], but one must remember that these were probably out of date before they were published! The classifications and terminologies on tumors are especially numerous, complicated and controversial, particularly when considering gliomas. The logical difficulties are circular: without knowing the histological variations, one cannot tabulate the biological variables. Even though there are some strange compromises that provoke continuing criticisms, the current World Health Organization's classification should be supported as an heroic attempt to standardize terminologies internationally – with all the inherent biases of international relations considered – since this approach is likely to be far more advantageous in the long run. In the mean time, a comment comparing other terminologies is frequently necessary.

As for the future, at least one of us believes that the ultimate resolution lies in actually measuring the growth rates and degree of infiltration to truly define high, intermediate or low grades and to suggest the probable degree of resection that should be attempted. The past behavior should predict the future at least sufficiently accurately to suggest when the next follow-up scans should be obtained and how frequently thereafter, thus providing some estimate of how effective the therapy has been in that particular patient [11,12]. Figure 3.22 illustrates the growth of the average diameter linearly with time, a pattern typical of infiltrating gliomas of low and high grade, the velocities differing by a factor of 10, each extreme being an average of +50%, as estimated by Woodward et al. [13]. By contrast, constant volume-doubling times are typical of the exponential growth of solid tumors (Fig. 3.23). Over short periods of time the proof of one mathematical formula or the other may be difficult clinically, but the difference over long periods of time is really quite striking (Fig. 3.23). The biological difference relates to the subclinical and more or less submicroscopic, invisible, infiltrating cells that convert the "edge" of the detectable tumor into a "travelling wave" that expands linearly with time rather than exponentially, as occurs if there is no external diffusion of cells.

When all is said and done, there are only a few gliomas that are susceptible to total resection: cerebellar astrocytomas and PXAs. In these cases, frozen section studies of the "margins" should be useful, and the surgeon should be tempted into resecting more than the gross may suggest, without, of course, increasing the patient's disability.

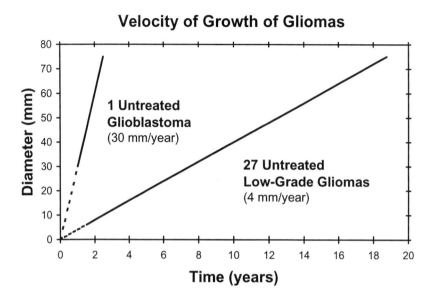

**Fig. 3.22.** Linear increase in diameter with time: about 4 mm/year as the average of 27 untreated low-grade gliomas (data from Mandonnet et al. [11]) and about 30 mm/year in an untreated glioblastoma (data from Swanson et al. [12]).

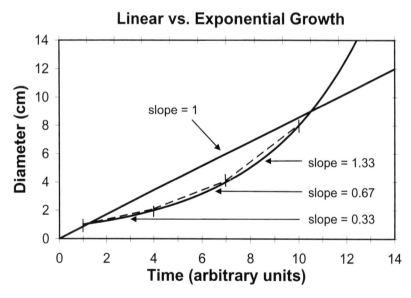

**Fig. 3.23.** Comparison of linear diametrical growth of infiltrating gliomas and constant volume-doubling time (exponential) growth of solid tumors over the clinically visible portion of most tumors. Time in arbitrary units: years for low-grade and months for high-grade tumors.

# 3. What are the Limitations of the Histopathological Diagnosis of Surgical Specimens?

The classification and definition of diseases can be purely academic but they also serve two practical purposes: namely interpersonal communication and prediction of a patient's outcome. If the terminologies of all diseases were standard and unified, a patient could carry that diagnosis to any physician anywhere in the world and all physicians would understand the significance of the condition and know the types of treatment that particular patient should receive. Obviously this is only the ideal. The reality is not that simple, as we all know. There are some common diseases that are familiar to most physicians. For instance, most physicians are familiar with meningiomas, which are common adult tumors, and know roughly what types of treatment are useful, even though they may not know that there are double digits of variants that may be descriptively added to the histological diagnosis. By contrast, there are many uncommon or relatively newly described conditions in which the diagnostic terms are not always precise, well established or standardized. Indeed, they are still being modified and changed from time to time as more is learned about their variations in appearance and behavior.

It is always interesting and usually helpful to know the historical transition of the concepts and changes in the terms of particular diseases but it is cumbersome and potentially confusing for neophytes. Thus, it is not uncommon to find many different or similar names given to the same condition. A new disease is usually found and defined by its discoverer. But with time, more cases are described with some variations, resulting in the modification of the definition and expansion of the diagnostic criteria until they overlap with other conditions. The borderlines between these different conditions become obscure. Consequently, arguments start as to whether they should be lumped together under one term or kept as separate entities based on some findings obtained by special diagnostic techniques. Under these conditions the diagnostic terms become ambiguous, even subjective, depending on the different training and experiences of various pathologists.

In addition, some classifications or divisions may be rather artificial, resulting in continuous debates. The best example is seen in the grading of gliomas. The line drawn between grades II and III is still controversial and one first needs to know whether the highest possible grade is grade III or IV! A similar argument concerns the reporting of the degree of cycling activity: Should one report the average (such as might be most accurately measured by flow-cytometry) or the highest percentage of cycling cells that one can find in a high-dry field? What degree of staining should one regard as "positive"? Should one actually count or just "eye-ball" it as a rough approximation? Satisfactory comments explaining the problems are required when reporting these types of results.

Another important role of diagnostic terms is to predict the outcome of a patient, so that both the physician and the patient know what to expect and what treatment would be best for the patient. The long-term outcome and the life expectancy of the average patient with a brain tumor are frequently compared with the pre-scan days, but these are not even a baseline for comparison with today's results since the clinical diagnostic criteria have changed so much. If there is advancement in the timing of diagnosis, say 4 years in the case of the usual oligodendroglioma [14], then there had better be an increase in survival of those same 4 years before improvement in treatment can be claimed! The Will Rogers' effect all over again!

Furthermore, we are making a diagnosis from the specimen that has been removed from the patient, but the outcome of the patient really depends on what remains in the patient's CNS. That variable, plus the variety of individualized treatments, makes it difficult to evaluate the results that are currently being continuously updated. How can one begin to define the histological features that characterize the malignancy of a particular type of neoplasm when one starts with subtotally resected tumors, the residual volumes not measured even if solid and not measurable if infiltrating? Even the most benign such tumor will "recur", i.e. continue to grow!

Contrary to the layman's belief that all answers are there on the slides when neuropathologists look through the powerful microscope with or without special stains and even

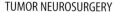
with electron microscopy, there are many limitations to the histological diagnosis. Another problem is probably fixable: an accurate diagnosis depends on a good specimen. This problem is an everyday affair. A representative site, an adequate quantity and no artifact are three essential requisites from the supplier's side. Good technical and staining techniques are crucial from the preparer's side, to which inquisitive eyes and a brain connected to an effective searching machine containing an appropriate list of differential diagnoses is the final key!

# References

1. Fulton J. Harvey Cushing. A biography. Springfield, Ill., Charles C. Thomas, 1946.
2. Bailey P, Cushing H. A classification of the tumors of the glioma group on a histogenetic basis with a correlation study of prognosis. Philadelphia, Lippincott, 1926.
3. Shaw CM, Alvord EC Jr. Congenital arachnoid cysts and their differential diagnosis. In: Vinken PJ, Bruyn GW, editors. Handbook of clinical neurology, vol 31: congenital malformations of the brain and skull, part II. Amsterdam: North-Holland Publishing Co, 1977; 75–135.
4. Zulch KJ. Brain tumors, their biology and pathology. Berlin Heidelberg New York: Springer, 1986.
5. Bigner DD, McLendon RE, Bruner JM. Russell & Rubinstein's pathology of tumors of the nervous system, 6th edn. London Sydney Auckland: Arnold; 1998.
6. Berger PC, Scheithauer BW. Atlas of tumor pathology (vol 10, Tumors of the central nervous system). Washington DC: AFIP, 1994.
7. Asa SL. Atlas of tumor pathology, vol 22: tumors of the pituitary gland. Washington DC: AFIP, 1998.
8. Scheithauer BW, Woodruff JM, Erlandson RA. Atlas of tumor pathology, vol 24: tumors of the peripheral nervous system. Washington DC: AFIP, 1999.
9. Alvord, EC Jr. Is necrosis helpful in the grading of gliomas? Editorial. J Neuropathol Exp Neurol 1992;51: 127–32.
10. Graham DI, Lantos PL (editors). Greenfield's neuropathology, 6th edn. London Sydney Auckland: Arnold, 2002.
11. Mandonnet E, Delattre JY, Tanguy ML, Swanson KR, Carpenter AF, Duffau H et al. Continuous growth of mean tumor diameter in a subset of WHO Grade II gliomas. Ann Neurol 2003;53:524–8.
12. Swanson KR, Alvord EC Jr, Murray JD. Virtual brain tumors (gliomas) enhance the reality of medical imaging and highlight inadequacies of current therapy. Br J Cancer 2002;86:14–18.
13. Woodward DE, Cook J, Tracqui P, Cruywagen GC, Murray JD, Alvord EC Jr. A mathematical model of glioma growth: the effect of extent of surgical resection. Cell Prolif 1996;29:269–88.
14. Mork SJ, Lindegaard K-F, Halvorsen TB, Lehmann EH, Solgaard T, Hatlevoli R et al. Oligodendroglioma: incidence and biological behavior in a defined population. J Neurosurg 1985;63:881–9.

# II

# Perioperative Care

# 4

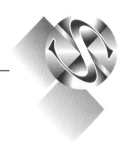

# Neuroanesthesia

Maryke Kraayenbrink and Gregory McAnulty

## Summary

The basis of general anesthesia is to establish the "triad" of hypnosis, muscle relaxation and suppression of sympathetic reflexes. This, together with manipulation of mechanical ventilation, fluid therapy, temperature and the circulation by the use of anesthetic and vasoactive drugs, can produce the required operating conditions for complex neurosurgery.

Most intravenous anesthetics decrease cerebral metabolism and blood flow and tend to have a cerebral protective effect and decrease intracranial pressure. The inhalational agents are all cerebral vasodilators that can be offset by the induction of hypocapnia through to hyperventilation. The overall effect on cerebral blood flow (CBF) depends on a balance between the concentration of the inhalational agent and the degree of hyperventilation.

Moderate hyperventilation reduces CBF and brain volume. Extreme hyperventilation may be associated with critical reduction in flow to compromised areas and focal ischemia. It is likely that barbiturates offer some protection for the brain against ischemia, but there is evidence that mild hypothermia has a cerebral protective effect that exceeds that of the barbiturates and which is out of proportion to the degree to which the cerebral metabolic rate is lowered.

The induction of general anesthesia depresses normal protective reflexes, and patients are at risk of aspiration of gastric contents. Those with raised intracranial pressure or who have suffered recent trauma causing vomiting are at particular risk.

Manipulation of the blood pressure may facilitate some procedures (e.g. the induction of hypotension during aneurysm surgery). Patients must be appropriately monitored and the risks of the failure of normal autoregulation of the cerebral circulation in patients with cerebral vasospasm must be considered. Careful monitoring control of the arterial pressure is also required where there is potential for cord ischemia.

A significant number of patients suffer moderate or severe pain after craniotomy. Morphine appears to be a safe analgesic and is more effective than codeine in postcraniotomy patients.

Management of the multiply injured patient must initially focus upon the ABC (airway, breathing and circulation) of basic life support.

## Introduction

Modern anesthetic drugs, improvements in monitoring, a better understanding of cardiovascular, respiratory and neurological physiology, and advances in intensive care medicine have all contributed to safer neuroanesthesia. It is probably true to say that the development of modern neurosurgery would not have been possible without the advances that have taken place in anesthesia.

# Drugs in Neuroanesthesia (see Table 4.1)

The complex interplay between the effects of drugs and physiological variables, such as arterial carbon dioxide ($CO_2$) tension, body temperature and arterial blood pressure, during clinical neuroanesthesia makes the interpretation of experimental data from the use of particular drugs in isolation difficult. However, in most cases, the administration of a combination of agents, together with manipulation of mechanical ventilation, fluid therapy and temperature, will allow the anesthesiologist to produce the physiological conditions required for optimal surgery. The basis of general anesthesia is to establish the 'triad' of hypnosis (or amnesia), muscle relaxation and suppression of sympathetic reflexes (or analgesia). Each aspect of this triad may be achieved with a variety of drugs and, in order to minimize dose-dependent adverse effects, combinations of agents are generally used. Neuroanesthetic agents will therefore be discussed here under the headings of "sedatives/hypnotics" (including volatile anesthetics), "neuromuscular blocking drugs" (muscle relaxants) and "opioids" (analgesics).

## Sedatives/Hypnotics

A diverse group of agents produce sedation at lower doses and hypnosis at higher doses. There is generally also a dose-related suppression of protective reflexes and automatic functions such as respiration and cardiovascular control. The drugs are usually grouped into intravenous and volatile agents. The volatile (or inhalational) agents are administered from a vaporizer via an anesthetic breathing circuit.

Intravenous agents include the barbiturates, propofol, benzodiazepines, etomidate and ketamine. With the exception of ketamine, all intravenous anesthetics decrease cerebral metabolism and blood flow and tend to have a cerebral protective effect and decrease intracra-

nial pressure (ICP). Ketamine, in the spontaneously breathing patient, produces increased cerebral blood flow (CBF) and ICP, but may also have cerebral protective effects as an N-methyl-D-aspartate (NMDA) receptor inhibitor [1].

Unlike the intravenous agents, inhalational agents are all cerebral vasodilators that can be offset by hyperventilation to hypocarbia. They also decrease cerebral metabolism, leading to a coupled decrease in CBF. The overall effect on CBF depends on a balance between the concentration of the inhalational agent and the degree of hyperventilation [2,3]. In addition, nitrous oxide is frequently used in anesthesia of all types as an adjunct to other agents, allowing them to be used in lower doses. Its use in neuroanesthesia is controversial because it increases CBF and may increase ICP in susceptible patients [4]. This effect can also be offset by hyperventilation. Thus, while nitrous oxide has been extensively used in neuroanesthesia without apparent detrimental effect, it is probably prudent to avoid its use in the presence of decreased intracranial compliance.

## Neuromuscular Blocking Drugs

Neuromuscular blocking drugs, or muscle relaxants, facilitate intubation of the trachea and mechanical ventilation of the lungs, and prevent movement during surgery. They are charged molecules that do not cross the blood–brain barrier, and so have no direct cerebral effects. However, they may indirectly influence the central nervous system via cardiovascular side-effects, histamine release and active metabolites. These drugs may be depolarizers or non-depolarizers, depending on their mechanism of action at the neuromuscular junction.

Depolarizing drugs (of which succinylcholine – Anectine – is now the only commonly used example) act very rapidly, have a short duration of action and produce excellent intubating conditions. Succinylcholine remains the drug of choice for rapid-sequence intubation to protect at-risk patients against aspiration of stomach contents. It produces initial muscle fasciculation and, frequently, post-anesthetic myalgia. A non-depolarizing-type block may be produced with repeated doses. Vagal stimulation may occur, inducing bradycardia and asystole. Serum potassium concentrations increase

NEUROANESTHESIA

**Table 4.1.** Drugs used in neuroanesthesia

| Drug class | Examples | Beneficial effects | Adverse effects |
|---|---|---|---|
| Barbiturates | Pentobarbitone Methohexitone | Cerebral vasoconstriction (in normo- or hypocapnia) Decrease in $CMRO_2$ **Decrease in CBF** Decrease in ICP Isoelectric EEG with high doses of anticonvulsant | Respiratory depression Myocardial depression (potential for circulatory collapse in hypovolemia or with high doses) Enhanced seizure focus activity (methohexitone) |
| Isopropyl phenol | Propofol | Rapid recovery Appropriate for total intravenous anesthesia (TIVA) and prolonged sedation Decrease in $CMRO_2$ **Decrease in CBF** Decrease in ICP | Hypotension due to vasodilatation and cardiac depression (may compromise CPP) |
| Benzodiazepines | Diazepam Midazolam | Anxiolysis Anterograde amnesia Anticonvulsants Decrease in $CMRO_2$ Decrease in CBF Antagonist (flumazenil) available | Active metabolites (prolonged action in renal failure) Respiratory depression |
| Carboxylated imidazoles | **Etomidate** | Rapid recovery Hemodynamic stability Decrease in $CMRO_2$ Decrease in CBF | Suppression of adrenocortical axis |
| Phencyclidine derivatives | Ketamine | Analgesic at subhypnotic doses NMDA antagonist Respiratory and cardiovascular stimulation | Increase in CBF and ICP in non-ventilated patients Emergence of delirium and hallucinations |
| Volatile liquids | | | |
| Alkanes | Halothane | Non-irritant | Myocardial depression Cardiac arrhythmias Rare hepatotoxicity |
| Ethers | Enflurane | Non-irritant | Epileptiform paroxysmal spike EEG activity in high concentrations, accentuated by hypercapnia |
| | Isoflurane | Minimal metabolism Least cerebral vasodilatation Rapid induction and recovery | Irritant |
| | Desflurane | Very rapid induction and recovery | Irritant Hypotension Cerebral vasodilatation |
| | Sevoflurane | Non-irritant, ideal for inhalational induction Very rapid induction and recovery Cerebral pressure autoregulation maintained | |
| Muscle relaxants | | | |
| Depolarizers | Succinylcholine | Rapid onset and recovery Excellent relaxation | Occasional prolonged action May cause increase in ICP in patients with low intracranial compliance Potassium release, especially in burns patients and following denervation Arrhythmias |

**Table 4.1.** continued

| Drug class | Examples | Beneficial effects | Adverse effects |
|---|---|---|---|
| Non-depolarizers | Tubocurarine Gallamine Alcuronium Pancuronium Atracurium Vecuronium Doxacurium Mivacurium Pipecuronium Rocuronium | Flaccid paralysis without fasciculation Atracurium, vecuronium, doxacurium, mivacurium, pipecuronium, rocuronium with minimal cardiovascular side-effects Atracurium and mivacurium do not accumulate in renal failure Reversible with neostigmine | Tubocurarine: histamine release, ganglion blockade (hypotension) Gallamine: muscarinic blockade Pancuronium: sympathetic action, muscarinic blockade Atracurium: histamine release |
| Opioids | | | |
| Ultra-short-acting | Remifentanyl | Rapidly metabolized by plasma esterases, rapid termination of effect (minutes) | Depressant effect on blood pressure No residual analgesia |
| Short-acting | Alfentanil | Short duration (redistributed) | Hypotension ? Increases ICP |
| | Fentanyl | Short duration (redistributed) | Cardiovascular stability |
| | Sufentanil | Short duration (redistributed) | Cardiovascular stability (less than fentanyl) |
| Long-acting | Morphine | Lasting analgesia | Histamine release (hypotension) Active metabolites |
| | Codeine | Limited analgesic and respiratory effects | Wide variation in efficacy (genetic variation in demethylation ability) |

$CMRO_2$, cerebral metabolic rate for oxygen; CBF, cerebral blood flow;
ICP, intracranial pressure; CPP, cerebral perfusion pressure

owing to leakage of intracellular potassium. Where sodium–potassium channel populations increase (following burns, denervation, crush injury or tetanus), potassium release may be catastrophic. Approximately 1 : 3,000 of patients given succinylcholine fail to metabolize the drug normally. This may lead to prolonged (several hours) paralysis, the so-called "Anectine apnea". The effect of succinylcholine on ICP and CBF is controversial. There is evidence that succinylcholine can cause an increase in ICP in individuals with compromised intracranial compliance [5]. This may be because the increased muscle spindle activity resulting from fasciculation causes increased cerebral afferent input and increases CBF. Many different stimuli that affect CBF and ICP occur at the time of induction of anesthesia when succinylcholine is given, and it is likely that the effect of succinylcholine on ICP is relatively unimportant in the clinical setting. It can be abolished by pretreatment with a non-depolarizing neuromuscular blocker [6].

Non-depolarizing muscle relaxants competitively block the action of acetylcholine at the neuromuscular junction. They lead to a flaccid paralysis and can be displaced from the acetyl choline receptor by increasing the concentration of acetylcholine by the use of an anticholinesterase (neostigmine). Earlier introduced agents of this group have side-effects such as histamine release or sympathetic stimulation. Atracurium, cisatracurium and mivacurium are broken down to inactive metabolites in the plasma and can be used without prolonged effect in patients with renal failure [7].

## Opioids

Drugs of this group are extensively used during neurosurgical anesthesia and for post-operative analgesia. If given in sufficiently large doses, all will cause unconsciousness; however, awareness and recall may occur in the absence of other anesthetics. All are respiratory depressants and, therefore, in the absence of artificial ventilation, can cause $CO_2$ retention leading to cerebral vasodilatation. All can cause muscle rigidity and some release histamine. The evidence concerning the effects of these drugs on cerebral hemodynamics and ICP is conflicting and depends on their cardiovascular effects as well as the background anesthetic.

The drugs act on specific opioid receptors and their effects can be reversed by specific antagonists. The drugs in this group differ in their onset and duration of action.

Shorter acting drugs fentanyl, alfentanil and sufentanil will allow rapid awakening at the end of the procedure. Remifentanil is an ultra-short-acting opioid. It is broken down in the plasma and can be given as an intravenous infusion [8]. Morphine and codeine are used for postoperative analgesia after neurosurgery.

Naloxone is a specific competitive antagonist that reverses the analgesia and respiratory depression caused by morphine and other opioids. It has no agonist activity. Its duration of action may be shorter than that of the opioid it is intended to reverse, and therefore repeated dosing may be necessary. Naloxone may have deleterious effects in neurosurgical patients, including increased CBF and cerebral metabolic rate (CMR), hypertension and rupture of intracranial aneurysms [9]. Naloxone has been shown to dramatically reverse the lateralizing deficits in patients with cerebral ischemia [10].

# Clinical Neuroanesthesia

The selection of anesthetic drugs and techniques is planned so as to provide an optimal environment for the brain and good conditions for surgery, and will vary according to the patient's condition and the planned operation. There is no single correct "recipe" for neuroanesthesia and attention to detail is as important as the choice of drugs.

## Pre-operative Assessment and Medication

In all cases, anesthetic care starts with a pre-operative visit and assessment by the anesthesiologist, who will be interested in the patient's general health, comorbidities, current medications and known allergies. For emergency cases, the time of last oral intake of food and fluids is important. The neurological status will be evaluated with particular regard to specific deficits, evidence of raised ICP, brainstem dysfunction and, in the case of cervical spine surgery, stability of the cervical spine.

Investigations will depend on the patient's age, medical condition and the proposed surgery, and institutions will have their own guidelines for investigations as well as for the amount of blood to be cross-matched before specific procedures. The perioperative management of coexisting diseases such as diabetes mellitus and ischemic heart disease is part of the anesthesiologist's responsibility, in consultation with other specialists.

Pre-operative medication is sometimes prescribed in order to provide anxiolysis and sedation, and a drying and vagolytic agent may also be given. Other drugs, such as beta-blockers, may be prescribed for specific indications. Sedative pre-medication is commonly a benzodiazepine or opioid, but sedatives should be used with caution in patients with evidence of raised ICP. Vagolytic drugs, such as atropine, glycopyrrolate and hyoscine, are given to dry oral secretions and to block undesirable vagal reflexes such as bradycardia. A drying agent is particularly important in patients who are to undergo fiberoptic intubation. Glycopyrrolate is preferable to atropine in neurosurgical patients, as it does not cause the same degree of tachycardia. Hyoscine causes sedation and can be associated with delayed recovery, making it unsuitable for craniotomy patients. It can be used before spinal surgery but is best avoided in older patients in whom it can cause post-operative confusion. In general, it is best for patients to take their usual medications, apart, perhaps, from diuretics, on the morning of surgery.

Guidelines for fasting before surgery aim to prevent pulmonary aspiration of gastric contents whilst avoiding dehydration from prolonged fasting. Fasting times of 2 hours for clear fluids, 4 hours for milk and 6 hours for solids have been shown to be safe in patients with normal gastric emptying. Those with raised ICP causing vomiting are at risk of dehydration and may require pre-operative intravenous fluids.

## Induction of Anesthesia

Induction of anesthesia is a time when the patient is subjected to the action of several drugs and stimuli that have profound cardio-vascular and respiratory effects. These need to be managed carefully in order to avoid adverse effects on intracranial dynamics; therefore good monitoring and venous access must be present from the outset. The aim is to prevent large swings in blood pressure and heart rate, to maintain good oxygenation at all times and to avoid hypercapnia.

The airway must be secured with an endotra-cheal tube for all intracranial and major spinal surgery. For some non-invasive investigations performed under anesthesia or for minor pro-cedures, a laryngeal mask airway may be used. The endotracheal tube must be carefully posi-tioned and very well secured, as access is diffi-cult once surgery has started. Intubation is carried out after induction of anesthesia when relaxation has been achieved by muscle relax-ants, except where there is an indication for awake intubation.

While the induction agents are generally car-diovascular depressants, and the blood pressure often falls on induction, laryngoscopy and intu-bation are stimulating and cause a rise in heart rate and blood pressure. It is essential to monitor the blood pressure closely throughout the whole period of induction and for the anes-thesiologist to be prepared to intervene to treat hyper- or hypotension. A number of drugs have been recommended to obtund the hypertensive response. Commonly used drugs include a small increment of the induction agent, a short-acting opioid such as alfentanil or sufentanil, a short-acting beta-blocker, or lignocaine. There should be no attempts to intubate until muscle relax-ation has been achieved in order to avoid coughing, with its attendant effect on ICP.

Some patients are difficult to intubate for anatomical or pathological reasons and special techniques may be needed. Awake fiberoptic intubation may be the preferred approach in such patients as well as for those with an unsta-ble cervical spine.

## Monitoring

Monitoring requirements will depend on the nature and extent of the planned surgery and the patient's condition. In all cases, there should be continuous monitoring of the electrocardio-gram (ECG), blood pressure, pulse oximetry, inspired oxygen, expired $CO_2$ and anesthetic gas concentrations. Invasive blood pressure monitoring via an intra-arterial line is required for major intracranial and spinal surgery, but non-invasive blood pressure monitoring may be adequate for less extensive operations such as shunts, burr-hole biopsies and more minor spinal surgery where there is no risk of cord ischemia. The central venous pressure (CVP) should be monitored for vascular cases and where major blood loss is anticipated. More extensive cardiovascular monitoring, such as of pulmonary artery pressures, may be indicated by the patient's condition (e.g. severe ischemic heart disease), but is not routinely nec-essary. The core temperature should be moni-tored except in the shortest cases and can be recorded at several sites including the esopha-gus, where the temperature probe can be combined with an esophageal stethoscope. A peripheral nerve stimulator is mandatory in order to monitor the effects of the neuro-muscular blocking drugs, as patient movement or coughing could be disastrous during neuro-surgical operations.

For patients in the sitting position, precordial Doppler ultrasonography, transesophageal echocardiography and pulmonary artery pres-sure monitoring may be used to detect venous air embolism.

## Positioning

The position of the patient depends on the site and nature of the surgery and the preference of the surgeon. Serious complications can occur as a result of careless positioning and, because neurosurgical operations may last for many hours, it is particularly important that patients are correctly positioned and pressure or trac-tion on nerves and venous or arterial obstruc-tion are avoided. Spinal cord damage can result from poor positioning and great care must be taken when moving the anesthetized patient with an unstable spine. Pressure on the eye can result in blindness.

Specific problems are associated with the use of the sitting position for operations in the posterior fossa and craniocervical region, including venous air embolism and postural hypotension [11]. Resuscitation may be difficult if cardiac arrest occurs in a patient in an unusual position, but a successful outcome is still possible [12].

## Maintenance of Anesthesia

Anesthesia is maintained by inhalational agents or by an infusion of an intravenous agent such as propofol. Rapid awakening is desirable after neurosurgery to allow neurological assessment of the patient, and is best achieved with short-acting drugs. Opioid analgesics and muscle relaxants are given as needed and the patient's lungs are ventilated. Moderate hyperventilation is used for craniotomies in order to reduce CBF and brain volume, thereby providing good operating conditions. However, extreme hyperventilation may be associated with critical reduction in flow to compromised areas and focal ischemia, and is best avoided [13].

Mannitol, frusemide, steroids and CSF drainage can all be used to decrease brain swelling. In patients at risk of cerebral ischemia, mild hypothermia may be achieved by passive cooling. A core temperature of 34°C provides some degree of cerebral protection without exposing the patient to the risks of more severe hypothermia. Patients should be actively warmed to 36°C by the end of surgery if they are to be wakened and extubated.

Cardiovascular parameters are kept as near as possible to physiological in order to ensure good cerebral perfusion. Normovolemia is the ideal, with a hematocrit of about 30%. Normal saline is the intravenous fluid of choice and 5% dextrose should be avoided [14]. Occasionally, deliberate hypotension is indicated for surgical reasons.

In a number of centers, surgery that requires total circulatory arrest is undertaken. In order to minimize ischemic cerebral damage, this is accomplished after the establishment of profound hypothermia by femoral–femoral cardiopulmonary bypass. Barbiturates or propofol are administered beforehand.

## Perioperative Brain Protection

The means by which it may be possible to protect the brain from ischemia are pharmacological or physical. Direct pharmacological interventions have focused on drugs that reduce the cerebral metabolic rate (and therefore reduce the demand for oxygen and energy substrate) and on agents that block the cellular mediators of ischemic injury (including calcium influx and the production of destructive protein kinases and free radicals). Physical means include the maintenance of an adequate cerebral perfusion pressure and arterial oxygen carriage and the optimizing of blood viscosity and temperature control.

With the exception of barbiturates [15], direct pharmacological brain protection has been, so far, disappointing. Traditionally, the dose of barbiturate is titrated to achieve burst suppression of the electroencephalogram (EEG). However, this has been questioned and there is evidence from animal studies that lower doses may be equally effective [16]. Barbiturates depress the myocardium, dilate arterioles and interfere with normal baroreflexes and sympathetic tone, and may induce cardiovascular collapse in patients who are hypovolemic or have already impaired cardiovascular systems. Careful monitoring is essential and circulatory support may be required particularly in patients receiving higher doses. The intravenous anesthetic agent propofol may achieve a similar degree of protection with better cardiovascular stability [17].

There is evidence that mild hypothermia has a cerebral protective effect that exceeds that of the barbiturates and which is out of proportion to the degree to which the cerebral metabolic rate is lowered [18]. Profound hypothermia during total circulatory arrest has been shown to be remarkably protective on gross measurement of outcome [19]. Animal studies suggest that prolonged periods of arrest (>70 min) may be associated with damage to Purkinje's cells of the cerebellum [20]; however, the technique may allow procedures to be performed that would be otherwise impossible.

Hypothermia has a number of adverse effects, including poor wound healing, increased susceptibility to infection, alterations in platelet function, changes in drug metabolism and increased oxygen consumption during rewarming. However, with mild hypothermia (brain temperature of 34°C) the benefits seem to outweigh the risks.

Action to increase the mean arterial pressure whilst temporary vascular clips are in place during clipping of cerebral aneurysms is advocated by many authors. Some evidence exists for a beneficial effect of judiciously timed application of hyperbaric oxygen in focal and global ischemia, but the treatment may itself induce oxygen-free radical formation [21].

Despite the many possible avenues for intervention in the face of impending, established or relieved cerebral ischemia, in clinical anesthetic practice, only barbiturates given in anticipation of focal ischemia, and hypothermia before and after focal or global cerebral ischemia, have been shown to be useful in humans [21].

Attention to cerebral perfusion pressure, avoidance of hyperthermia, appropriate levels of anesthesia and maintenance of normoglycemia are probably of greater overall importance.

## Emergence

Towards the end of surgery, anesthetic agents are reduced and then discontinued. The residual neuromuscular block is reversed when the operation is finished and, when the patient is able to breathe and protect his airway; the tracheal tube is removed. As with induction, emergence from anesthesia is a time when hemodynamic instability can occur, and the awakening patient may cough on the tracheal tube. Specific medications may be needed to control the blood pressure at this time.

On occasion, immediate extubation is not desirable, for example when there have been serious intraoperative difficulties and the brain is swollen at the end of surgery, or if problems with the airway are anticipated. In such cases a decision may be made to keep the patient sedated and ventilated post-operatively for a period. Decisions of this kind should be made jointly by the anesthesiologist and surgeon. Patients who have had surgery in the posterior fossa or craniocervical region may have inadequate airway protective reflexes post-operatively and should not be extubated until airway reflexes have returned.

## Recovery

Patients who have had major intracranial or spinal surgery should be cared for in a high-dependency area where they can receive intensive nursing care post-operatively. Frequent observations of cardiac and respiratory variables as well as neurological observations are mandatory for the early detection and treatment of complications such as bleeding. Post-operative nausea and vomiting are common after anesthesia and surgery, particularly posterior fossa surgery, and are multifactorial in

origin [22]. Post-anesthetic shivering may occur, particularly after long operations, and is associated with a number of undesirable effects. Oxygen consumption, $CO_2$ production and metabolic rate may increase by up to 500% and it is not well tolerated by patients with cardiac or pulmonary disease. Patients should be actively warmed to a core temperature of 36°C. Surface warming with a hot-air mattress is very effective.

## Post-operative Analgesia

It is now recognized that a significant number of patients suffer moderate or severe pain after craniotomy. There is a tendency to avoid morphine for post-operative analgesia in craniotomy patients for fear of respiratory depression leading to hypercapnia and excessive sedation and because it may interfere with the assessment of the size and reactivity of the pupils. However, morphine appears to be safe and provides more effective analgesia than codeine in post-craniotomy patients [23]. Patient-controlled analgesia (PCA) with morphine may be better for patients with normal levels of consciousness.

Non-steroidal anti-inflammatory drugs (NSAIDs) can be a useful adjunct for post-operative pain control. However, NSAIDs have some well-known adverse effects, including effects on platelet function and renal function, and may increase CBF [24]. Further studies comparing the efficacy and safety of different analgesic regimens in craniotomy patients are needed.

# Neuroanesthesia for Specific Circumstances

## Pediatric Neuroanesthesia

Induction of anesthesia in children can be intravenous or inhalational, depending on the child's preference. A smooth, calm induction with avoidance of crying and struggling is more important than which drug is used. Gaining venous access can be made more acceptable to the child by the prior application of local anesthetic preparations to the skin, such as eutectic mixture of local anesthetic ("Emla") cream or amethocaine gel. Maintenance of anesthesia is with controlled moderate hyperventilation, and many pediatric neuroanesthesiologists use nitrous oxide despite evidence that it is a significant cerebral vasodilator in children [25]. Muscle relaxants and analgesics are given as indicated. Good positioning is essential to avoid venous congestion, but positioning can be more difficult in small children as their relatively large heads and short necks can easily give rise to venous obstruction if the head is rotated.

Because of the relatively large size of the head in a child, significant blood loss is to be expected in craniotomies and excellent venous access is essential. Accurate estimation of blood loss can be difficult and the anesthesiologist may be aided by cardiovascular parameters such as heart rate, blood pressure, capillary refill time and core-peripheral temperature difference in maintaining normovolemia. Small children can become hypoglycemic during long procedures and blood glucose levels should be monitored during surgery.

Children, because they have a larger surface-area-to-weight ratio and less subcutaneous fat, can become significantly hypothermic during long operations unless active steps are taken to maintain body temperature. As with adults, the aim is for normo- or mild hypothermia. Hyperthermia is highly detrimental.

Midline posterior fossa tumors account for a significant proportion of brain tumors in children, and some pediatric neurosurgeons prefer to operate on them with the patient in a sitting position. This provides excellent operating conditions and is associated with decreased blood loss [11]. Venous air embolism (VAE) is a serious complication that must be detected and treated immediately. Nitrous oxide will equilibrate rapidly with the air bubbles and, being 30 times more soluble than nitrogen, will cause them to increase in size. If an air embolus is suspected, immediate attempts should be made to aspirate the air via a right atrial catheter. The surgeon should flood the wound with saline and the anesthesiologist should apply digital pressure to the jugular veins. This allows the site of the open vein or sinus to be identified and controlled.

Surgery for tumors in the floor of the fourth ventricle can be associated with cardiovascular instability, usually bradycardia and hypertension, owing to surgical interference with vital areas in the brainstem. This may also lead to

bulbar problems post-operatively and such children may need prolonged intubation.

Craniofacial surgery often involves children who have difficult airways, and special techniques and expertise may be needed to gain control of the airway. These operations are frequently prolonged and major blood loss is likely. Post-operatively the airway may be in jeopardy from local edema and it may be safer to keep the child intubated and ventilated until the swelling has abated.

Children who are awake, warm and breathing well with no airway problems can be extubated at the end of surgery.

## Sedation

Children may require sedation for procedures that adults are able to tolerate without sedation. Proper supervision and monitoring are essential for the safe provision of sedation to children whether they are under the care of anesthesiologists or other medical personnel.

The aim should be for conscious sedation. However, it is important to realize that the child may lapse into deep sedation once the stimulus of the procedure stops or if drug absorption is delayed. Because of the possibility of respiratory and cardiovascular depression with deeper levels of sedation, it is essential that the attending personnel are trained in life-support techniques and that full resuscitation equipment is immediately available. Pulse oximetry should be monitored as the minimum and should be continued until the child has recovered completely.

Children must be adequately assessed before receiving sedation and the fasting guidelines used for general anesthesia apply equally to patients undergoing sedation. The presence of a parent or carer can often give great comfort to a child undergoing medical procedures. Where procedures are expected to be painful, local anesthetics or analgesics, used as adjuncts, may reduce the necessity for increasing the level of sedation. Drugs commonly used in pediatric sedation include benzodiazepines, opioids, chloral hydrate, ketamine and trimeprazine.

## Anesthesia for Neuroradiology and Magnetic Resonance Imaging (MRI)

Absolute patient immobility is often necessary for high-quality images to be obtained in neuroradiology and, as these procedures are often prolonged and uncomfortable, general anesthesia or sedation may be needed. Additional factors reducing patient acceptability of the MRI scanner are claustrophobia and the loud noise during scanning. Patients who need anesthesia or sedation include infants and children and confused or mentally ill adults. Unconscious or critically ill patients will need airway protection and ventilatory and cardiovascular support.

Procedures for which anesthesia may be required include computerized axial tomography (CAT scan), myelography, angiography and interventional radiology. The X-ray department is sometimes considered to be a hostile environment for anesthesia, and patient access may be limited, but exactly the same standards of monitoring and patient care are needed as in the operating room.

The requirements for anesthesia are similar to those for neurosurgery and include avoidance of fluctuations in heart rate and blood pressure, prevention of hypoxia, hypercapnia and raised venous pressure, and rapid recovery to allow for early neurological assessment. In many cases the laryngeal mask airway can be used to maintain the airway and avoid the need for intubation. Angiography in adults under local anesthesia with sedation may provide greater cardiovascular stability than with general anesthesia [26].

Many conditions are now treated by interventional neuroradiology, including arteriovenous malformations (AVMs), vascular tumors and aneurysms. Sometimes frequent neurological assessment is needed during the procedure, e.g. during embolization of AVMs. The patient needs to be awake and able to cooperate with testing but can be sedated for comfort between assessments. Propofol, with its rapid onset and offset of action, is ideal for this purpose. Sedation of this kind should be administered by an anesthesiologist as respiratory depression and even apnea can easily ensue. Adequate monitoring must be used, including pulse oximetry, ECG and blood pressure monitoring, and supplemental oxygen should be available. Equipment and drugs to support the airway, breathing and cardiovascular system must be readily available.

Endovascular obliteration of aneurysm sacs through superselective catheters placed during angiography is an increasingly popular alternative method of treatment to surgical clipping. The procedure can be prolonged in particular with large aneurysms and, as there is less need for patient assessment during the procedure, general anesthesia is often used for patient comfort.

The strong magnetic field of an MRI scanner can interfere with monitoring and anesthetic equipment. At the same time the equipment can cause degradation of the nuclear magnetic signals, leading to poor-quality images. Because of the strength of the magnetic field, ferromagnetic objects can become dangerous missiles in close proximity to the scanner and must be excluded or adequately secured. Special non-ferromagnetic equipment is available but adds significantly to the cost. Metal objects distort the field and result in poor image quality, and can also heat up and cause burns when subjected to radiofrequency electromagnetic fields. Reliable and accurate monitoring is essential in the MRI scanner as the patient cannot be easily seen and is remote from the anesthesiologist. Artifacts can be induced in the ECG by the radiofrequency currents but can be minimized by the use of shielded cables, telemetry or fiberoptics. ECG electrodes must be non-magnetic and should be place carefully to reduce artifacts. Shielded MRI-compatible oximeters are available. Good airway control is important, as the anesthesiologist is not easily able to intervene if airway obstruction develops during the scan. The laryngeal mask airway is ideal for this purpose.

## Anesthesia for Posterior Fossa Surgery

Interference with the cardiorespiratory centers in the brainstem can result in cardiovascular instability during surgery and in airway and breathing problems post-operatively. Pressure on the nucleus of the vagus results in profound bradycardia, even cardiac standstill, and other cardiac arrhythmias and hypertension can be caused by brainstem manipulation. Vigilance by the anesthesiologist and close cooperation between surgeon and anesthesiologist are essential.

Respiratory complications can occasionally result from interference with the respiratory centers, giving rise to impaired respiratory drive post-operatively. More commonly, edema around the lower cranial nerve nuclei results in inadequate airway protection with respiratory obstruction, difficulty in swallowing and pulmonary aspiration. As a result, patients occasionally need to remain intubated post-operatively and a few need prolonged respiratory support.

## Anesthesia for Aneurysm Surgery

During induction of anesthesia, intubation and the placement of the pin head rest, meticulous attention to the patient's hemodynamics is essential. Mean arterial pressure is the critical determinant of cerebral perfusion but systolic arterial pressure is probably more important in determining the wall stress and tendency to rupture in a cerebral aneurysm [27].

Induced hypotension may be used during aneurysm surgery to reduce aneurysm wall tension and operative bleeding. However, it must be used with caution as autoregulation is disrupted in patients with cerebral vasospasm. Measurement of jugular bulb oxygen saturation can help to determine the minimum level of mean arterial pressure that should be allowed [28]. Vasodilating drugs are used to induce hypotension (isoflurane, sodium nitroprusside, phentolamine), frequently in combination with a beta-adrenergic receptor blocker. Careful monitoring is required and drugs that have a relatively short half-life are preferred to allow restoration of normal perfusion pressures as soon as possible once control has been gained. The advent of temporary aneurysm clips has lessened the requirement for hypotension during clipping of cerebral aneurysms and may result in better patient outcomes. Cerebral vasospasm is less of a problem when AVM is the cause of subarachnoid hemorrhage; therefore induced hypotension can more safely be used during excision of AVM where it may reduce bleeding and the need for blood transfusion.

The surgical exposure of the vessels at the base of the brain by retraction of brain tissue can be aided by positioning of the patient, withdrawal of CSF and dehydration with diuretics. The use of induced hypocapnia by hyperventilation is controversial in aneurysm patients as it may enhance vasoconstriction in those with cerebral vasospasm. It is probably safe to use mild hyperventilation, but in the presence of induced hypotension, normocapnia should be maintained.

## Anesthesia and the Cervical Spine

Several anesthetic problems may occur during cervical spine surgery. The pathology for which the patient is receiving surgical treatment may, in itself, render normal techniques for securing the airway difficult or hazardous to the patient. For the anesthesiologist, access to the airway and the tracheal tube is difficult once surgery has started, so the possibility of tube dislodgment or disconnection from the breathing circuit is a real hazard. Trauma to, or ischemia of, the cervical cord or damage to the phrenic nerves may lead to respiratory paralysis or severe compromise post-operatively. Partial or complete airway obstruction may occur post-operatively as a result of edema of the tissues of the airway, recurrent laryngeal nerve palsy, or hemorrhage into the neck.

Many conditions are associated with restricted movement or instability of the cervical spine. The list includes: degenerative osteoarthritis and spinal canal stenosis, ankylosing spondylosis, Down's syndrome, Klippel–Feil syndrome, Arnold–Chiari malformation, other congenital malformations such as dwarfism, type IV Ehlers–Danlos syndrome, metastatic lesions, osteomyelitis and rheumatoid arthritis, as well as trauma with demonstrated or suspected cervical spine injury.

Induction of anesthesia and intubation results in the loss of protective muscle tone as well as the potential for flexion and extension greater than that which would be tolerated by the awake patient. The cervical cord may be at risk if there is a tight stenosis or potential for subluxation from either movement or a fall in the perfusion pressure of the neural tissue owing to hypotension. Potential for cord injury dictates careful immobilization during manipulations to secure the airway and will frequently require special techniques and monitoring. Fixed cervical vertebrae may make conventional intubation very difficult or impossible because conventional laryngoscopy requires a certain amount of flexion of the neck and extension of the head. Awake intubation (most usually with a flexible fiberoptic bronchoscope) may be the safest option in many cases where there is potential risk to the cord or where a secure airway cannot be obtained conventionally. This is carried out with intravenous sedation and local anesthesia of the airway.

Careful control of the arterial pressure during induction and maintenance of anesthesia is clearly critical when there is potential for cord ischemia in order to ensure maintenance of an adequate cord perfusion pressure. Good communication and cooperation between the anesthesiologist and the surgical team is essential during patient transfer and positioning, particularly if the patient is to be turned prone.

At completion of surgery, patients are usually extubated upon return of protective reflexes. However, if there is a risk of upper airway obstruction, for example after transoral procedures, the safest option is elective ventilation with sedation in the intensive care unit until the danger of post-extubation obstruction is past. Emergency re-intubation of patients who have developed upper airway obstruction after cervical spine fixation may be extremely difficult, particularly if the neck has been immobilized in a device that interferes with access and vision. Efforts to maintain oxygenation may result in undesired movement of the unstable neck and damage to the cord. It is therefore imperative that the patient is able to maintain a safe airway before extubation, and in some cases an elective tracheostomy performed at the time of surgery may be advisable.

Post-operative hematoma formation in the neck, although fortunately rare, can severely compromise the airway. Not only does the hematoma compress and distort the airway; it may interfere with venous and lymphatic drainage, resulting in edema of the airway. Decompression of the hematoma may not relieve the obstruction if there is significant airway edema, and re-intubation may be required but may be very difficult due to distortion and swelling of the tissues. A high morbidity may be associated with such cases [29]. Because of the danger of airway obstruction, all patients who have had cervical surgery should be cared for in a high-dependency environment with close nursing supervision and frequent monitoring. Those who have had extensive procedures will need full intensive care.

## Emergency Neuroanesthesia

Neurosurgical patients who require emergency anesthetic intervention fall into two groups. There are those who present with, or who have suffered an acute deterioration of, a condition of the brain or spinal cord. These patients may have compromised ventilation or other system failure as a consequence of their primary disease. They have the potential for aspiration of stomach contents if they have lost protective airway reflexes or if they are anesthetized without specific measures to prevent regurgitation. They may be hemodynamically unstable because of dehydration, sepsis or interference with autonomic reflexes. They may have specific effects of a disease process that affects a number of organ systems (e.g. rheumatoid disease, metastatic carcinoma).

The other group of neurosurgical patients are victims of trauma in whom neurological damage may be only one of a number of life- or limb-threatening conditions. In these patients there may be several injuries that compete for intervention, but appropriate management of one may be detrimental to the management of others. A methodical and coordinated approach will minimize the risk of missing serious injuries and will treat life-threatening injuries in appropriate order of priority. Management of the multiply injured patient must initially focus upon the ABC (airway, breathing and circulation) of basic life support. Implicit in management of the airway is avoidance of unnecessary movement of a potentially unstable cervical spine. However, hypoxia and aspiration of gastric contents into the lungs are more certain killers than theoretical cervical instability. Aggressive management to maintain cerebral perfusion pressure in these patients appears to be associated with improved outcome [30]. Novel therapies that may decrease secondary injury may have a place in the future.

## Anesthesia for Awake Craniotomy

In these procedures the patient is required to be responsive and cooperative so that immediate assessment of the function of areas such as the motor cortex or speech areas can be made during resection of tissue close to, or involving, these areas. However, until the brain tissue is exposed and after the intended resection is completed, sedation or anesthesia can be administered to improve patient acceptability during such phases of the procedure as scalp incision, drilling of the skull, fashioning of the bone flap and closure. In the past, neurolept techniques (using fentanyl, alfentanil or sufentanil) were generally used, but short-acting opioid and propofol combinations are now the norm. The airway may be secured with the laryngeal mask airway, which is removed for the awake part of the procedure. Additional local anesthetic infiltration is given to reduce the stimulation of insertion of cranial pins and scalp incision. Monitoring must be of the same intensity as for conventional craniotomy as complications such as venous air embolism, airway obstruction and convulsions can occur. The anesthesiologist must have a full understanding of surgical intentions in order to anticipate the need to alter the depth of sedation appropriately. Very close cooperation between the surgeon and the anesthesiologist is absolutely essential to the success of this procedure.

# Key Points

- *The complex interplay between the effects of drugs and physiological variables during clinical neuroanesthesia makes the interpretation of experimental data from the use of particular anesthetic drugs in isolation difficult.*

- *Moderate hyperventilation reduces CBF and brain volume. Extreme hyperventilation may be associated with critical reduction in flow to compromised areas and focal ischemia. Intravenous anesthetics generally decrease cerebral metabolism, CBF and ICP. Inhalational agents are all cerebral vasodilators. The overall effect on CBF depends on a balance between the concentration of the inhalational agent and the degree of hyperventilation.*

- *Pharmacological brain protection has been, so far, disappointing.*

- *Adequate monitoring must be used when patients are sedated. Supplemental oxygen, equipment and drugs to support the airway, breathing and cardiovascular system must be readily available.*

- *Close cooperation between the surgeon and the anesthesiologist is absolutely essential.*

# Self-assessment

☐ What are the three components of general anesthesia? Which of these is most important for neuroanesthesia?

☐ How might rapid awakening at the end of surgery be best achieved?

☐ Which patients may require post-operative ventilation?

☐ How may anesthetic agents and techniques contribute to neuroprotection?

☐ Discuss the implications of the use of induced hypotension in aneurysmal surgery.

☐ What is the rationale for pre-operative starvation? What precautions are needed for emergency anesthesia?

# References

1. Mayberg TS, Lam AM, Matta BF, Domino KB, Winn HR. Ketamine does not increase cerebral blood flow velocity or intracranial pressure during isoflurane/nitrous oxide anesthesia in patients undergoing craniotomy. Anesth Analg 1995;81:84–9.
2. Reinstrup P, Ryding E, Algotsson L, Messeter K, Asgeirsson B, Uski T. Distribution of cerebral blood flow during anesthesia with isoflurane or halothane in humans. Anesthesiology 1995;82:359–66.
3. Cho S, Fujigaki T, Uchiyama Y, Fukusaki M, Shibata O, Sumikawa K. Effects of sevoflurane with and without nitrous oxide on human cerebral circulation. Transcranial Doppler study. Anesthesiology 1996;85:755–60.
4. Algotsson L, Messeter K, Rosen I, Holmin T. Effects of nitrous oxide on cerebral haemodynamics and metabolism during isoflurane anesthesia in man. Acta Anaesthesiol Scand 1992;36:46–52.
5. Marsh ML, Dunlop BJ, Shapiro HM. Succinylcholine: intracranial pressure effects in neurosurgical patients. Anesth Analg 1980;59:550–1.
6. Stirt J, Grosslight K, Bedford R, Vollmer D. 'Defasciculation' with metocurine prevents succinylcholine-induced increases in intracranial pressure. Anesthesiology 1987;53:50–3.
7. Boyd AH, Eastwood NB, Parker CJ, Hunter JM. Comparison of the pharmacodynamics and pharmacokinetics of a cis-atracurium (51W89) or atracurium in critically ill patients undergoing mechanical ventilation in an intensive care unit. Br J Anaesth 1996; 76:382–8.
8. Rosow C. Remifentanil: a unique opioid analgesic. Anesthesiology 1993;79:875–6.

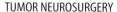

9. Estilo A, Cottrell JE. Naloxone hypertension and ruptured cerebral aneurysm. Anesthesiology 1981;54:352.

10. Baskin DS, Hosobuchi Y. Naloxone reversal of ischemic neurological deficits in man. Lancet 1981;2:272.

11. Porter JM, Pidgeon C, Cunningham AJ. The sitting position in neurosurgery: a critical appraisal. Br J Anaesth 1999;82:117–28.

12. Kelleher A, Mackersie A. Cardiac arrest and resuscitation of a six month old achondroplastic baby undergoing neurosurgery in the prone position. Anesth Analg 1995;50:348–50.

13. Tung A. Indications for mechanical ventilation. Int Anesthesiol Clin 1997;35:1–17.

14. Ravussin P, de Tribolet N, Boulard G. Neuroanésthesie. Quelques aspects nouveaux. Neurochirurgie 1993;39: 145–8.

15. Cheng MA, Theard MA, Tempelhof R. Intravenous agents and intraoperative neuroprotection. Beyond barbiturates. Crit Care Clin 1997;13:185–99.

16. Warner DS, Zhou JG, Ramani R, Todd MM. Reversible focal ischemia in the rat: effects of halothane, isoflurane, and methohexital anesthesia. J Cereb Blood Flow Metab 1991;11:794–802.

17. Stone JG, Young WL, Marans ZS, Solomon RA, Smith CR, Jamdar SC et al. Consequences of electroencephalographic-suppressive doses of propofol in conjunction with deep hypothermic circulatory arrest. Anesthesiology 1996;85:497–501.

18. Nemoto EM, Klementavicius R, Melick JA, Yonas H. Suppression of cerebral metabolic rate for oxygen (CMRO2) by mild hypothermia compared with thiopental. J Neurosurg Anesthesiol 1996;8:52–9.

19. Kouchoukos NT, Daily BB, Wareing TH, Murphy SF. Hypothermic circulatory arrest for cerebral protection during combined carotid and cardiac surgery in patients with bilateral carotid artery disease. Ann Surg 1994;21:699–705.

20. Fessatidis IT, Thomas VL, Shore DF, Sedgwick ME, Hunt RH, Weller RO. Brain damage after profoundly hypothermic circulatory arrest: correlations between neurophysiological and neuropathological findings. An experimental study in vertebrates. J Thorac Cardiovasc Surg 1993;106:32–41.

21. Stamford J. Beyond NMDA antagonists: looking to the future of neuroprotection. In: Stamford J, Strunin L, editors. Neuroprotection. London: Baillière Tindall, 1996; 581–98.

22. Rowbotham DJ. Current management of postoperative nausea and vomiting. Br J Anaesth 1992;69:46S–59S.

23. Goldsack C, Scuplak SM, Smith M. A double-blind comparison of codeine and morphine for postoperative analgesia following intracranial surgery. Anesthesia 51:1996;1029–32.

24. Cashman J, McAnulty G. Nonsteroidal anti-inflammatory drugs in perisurgical pain management. Mechanisms of action and rationale for optimum use. Drugs 1995;49:51–70.

25. Leon JE, Bissonnette B. Transcranial Doppler sonography: nitrous oxide and cerebral blood flow velocity in children. Can J Anaesth 1991;38:974–9.

26. Clayton DG, O'Donoghue BM, Stevens JE, Savage PE. Cardiovascular response during cerebral angiography under general and local anesthesia. Anesthesia 1989; 44:599–602.

27. Ferguson GG. The rationale for controlled hypotension. Int Anesthesiol Clin 1982;28:89–93.

28. Moss E, Dearden NM, Berridge JC. Effects of changes in mean arterial pressure on SjO2 during cerebral aneurysm surgery. Br J Anaesth 1995;75:527–30.

29. Bukht D, Lanford R. Airway obstruction after surgery in the neck. Anesthesia 1983;38(4):389-90.

30. Rosner MJ, Rosner SD, Johnson AH. Cerebral perfusion pressure: management protocol and clinical results. J Neurosurg 1995; 83:949-62.

# 5

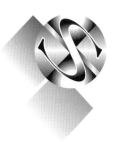

# Neurosurgical Intensive Care

Tessa L. Whitton and Arthur M. Lam

## Summary

Neurological disease frequently has multiple systemic manifestations, and management of patients with critical neurological illness requires a multidisciplinary approach with meticulous attention to organ dysfunctions. Many of these patients will suffer a poor outcome not as a result of the primary neurological disease, but as a result of medical complications. Thus, improvement of the intensive medical care of these patients will lead to an overall improvement of morbidity and mortality.

## Introduction

The prevention of secondary insults to the central nervous system and close monitoring of neurological function are mainstays in the treatment of patients requiring neurosurgical care. The neurosurgical intensive care unit provides a setting for an integrated approach to the care of these patients and an organizational framework for delivery of this care. It represents the continuum of care applied to monitoring and treatment modalities instituted prior to or during surgery, which is essential for optimal recovery. Early treatment of complications may reduce morbidity from secondary insults; the intensive care unit should provide conditions for the rapid recognition and management of such complications. This chapter will discuss the theory and practice of intensive care management of the neurosurgical patient, with reference to general principles and specific neurological conditions.

## Basic Physiological Concepts

### Intracranial Pressure

The skull and vertebral canal form a rigid covering for the brain, spinal cord, cerebrospinal fluid (CSF) and blood. All of these intracranial compartments are non-compressible, thus the intracranial volume is essentially constant (the "Monro–Kellie doctrine"). Volume expansion of any compartment can only occur at the expense of compression of other compartments. The only buffering capacity is secondary to compression of the venous sinuses and the caudal displacement of CSF to the lumbosacral axis. Once this is exhausted, any tendency to increase volume in any of the compartments (as in an expanding mass) will result in an increased intracranial pressure (ICP).

The compliance of the intracranial system is often expressed as the "compliance curve" by plotting ICP against the expanding volume, although it should more accurately be described as the "elastance curve" (Fig. 5.1). A steep curve implies increased elastance or decreased compliance, as occurring with a rapidly expanding mass, as in a subdural or intracranial

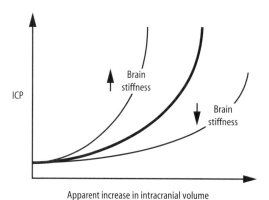

**Fig. 5.1.** Intracranial compliance curve.

hematoma. This "compliance" can be quantified by adding or withdrawing a known volume of saline to the CSF via a ventriculostomy, and noting the rise in ICP – the volume pressure response.

Elevation of ICP decreases cerebral perfusion, and may result in secondary ischemia, as the net cerebral perfusion pressure (CPP) is determined by the difference between mean arterial blood pressure (MAP) and ICP. (CPP = MAP – ICP or MAP – JVP, where JVP = jugular venous pressure. This applies when the cranium is open and ICP is zero.) In addition to its effect on CPP, an elevated ICP can also result in herniation. Although a clear-cut threshold cannot be determined, an elevated ICP >30 mmHg is associated with an increased risk of transtentorial or brainstem herniation. Thus monitoring and treatment of ICP is of paramount importance in the ICU.

In patients with spinal cord injury, the perfusion pressure to the cord is similarly determined by the difference between MAP and CSF pressure. Although most cord-injured patients present with complete lesions, anatomical disruption is rare, and maintenance of adequate perfusion is important to preserve cord function to ischemic regions proximal to the main site of injury.

## Cerebral Blood Flow, $CO_2$ Reactivity and Cerebral Autoregulation

Reduction in cerebral blood flow (CBF) is one of the major causes of secondary cerebral ischemia in the damaged or edematous brain. Under normal circumstances CBF is tightly controlled by homeostatic mechanisms. Normal CBF is approximately 50 ml/100 g/min, coupled to a cerebral metabolic oxygen consumption rate of 3.2 ml/100 g/min. In patients with brain injury, CBF of 18–20 ml/100 g/min is generally considered to be the ischemic threshold, below which secondary injury may occur, although cellular integrity is usually preserved until CBF is <8–10 ml/100 g/min. Many factors control the cerebrovascular tone, including endothelial factors (nitric oxide, endothelin), cerebral metabolism, neurotransmitter release, systemic blood pressure, blood carbon dioxide content, blood viscosity and humoral substances. In physiological terms the important considerations include flow-metabolism coupling, $CO_2$ reactivity, and pressure autoregulation. Under normal circumstances, blood flow to the brain is tightly coupled to its metabolism, globally as well as regionally. The cerebral vasculature is exquisitely sensitive to carbon dioxide, changing by 3–4% per mmHg change in $P_aCO_2$. In contrast, $P_aO_2$ has a negligible effect on CBF. Although the molecular mechanism of cerebral autoregulation remains unknown, CBF is generally maintained constant between CPP of 50–150 mmHg. Blood flow becomes pressure-dependent at blood pressures outside the normal range, and this flow–pressure curve is shifted to the right in the presence of chronic hypertension. The purported mechanisms of autoregulation control include metabolic feedback and myogenic feedback.

Intracranial pathology may impair one or more of these homeostatic mechanisms [1]. $CO_2$ reactivity appears to be more robust than autoregulation, and is frequently preserved even with severe brain injury. With the exception of arteriovenous malformation and vasospasm (see below), the loss of $CO_2$ reactivity is generally associated with a poor prognosis.

## Cushing's Response

CBF changes according to the formula:

CBF = CPP / CVR
or (MAP – ICP) / CVR

where CVR is the cerebral vascular resistance.

With elevation of ICP and compression of the brainstem, compensatory changes involving both MAP and CVR may occur. This compensatory rise in MAP, effected by increased sympathetic discharge from the vasomotor center in response to a rise in ICP causing brainstem ischemia, was first documented in 1901 by Cushing and is known as "Cushing's response". While MAP increases as a result of increased systemic vascular resistance, cerebral vasodilation occurs in response to the decrease in CPP as the autoregulatory compensatory response. However, with decreased intracranial compliance (increased intracranial elastance), this vasodilation may lead to further increase in ICP and reduction in CPP.

## Critical Closing Pressure

The CPP has traditionally been calculated as the difference between MAP and ICP or JVP and thus may easily be derived when ICP is monitored. Although not a frequent occurrence, regional compartmentalization of ICP may result in regional variation in CPP, and hence in CBF. Moreover, when venous pressure is elevated or higher than ICP, both the arterial inflow from the systemic driving force (MAP) and the venous outflow need to be considered in order to optimize CPP.

On the basis of studies of other organs and the peripheral circulation, it can be demonstrated that the critical closing pressure (CCP), located at the arteriolar level, determines the downstream pressure in the vasculature of that organ. The cerebral CCP is defined as the arterial pressure threshold below which arterial vessels collapse, and is determined by both the ICP and the cerebral arterial tone. Thus CCP is the minimum perfusion pressure necessary to keep the cerebral vessels open. This is influenced by the surrounding extrinsic pressure (ICP) as well as by any distal resistance (e.g. jugular venous obstruction). This is not an easily quantifiable variable, but it represents the overall downstream resistance of the cerebral vasculature, and may be a more important determinant of CPP than ICP (i.e. CPP = MAP – CCP) [2]. Complex relationships therefore exist between ICP, systemic blood pressure, cerebral metabolism and CBF, all of which must be taken into consideration in the intensive care management of neurosurgical patients. These principles apply whether the patients had suffered traumatic brain injury, subarachnoid hemorrhage

or ischemic stroke. Recent advances in monitoring modalities, which will be discussed later in the chapter, have made it theoretically possible to manipulate 'real-time' information to optimize treatment of these patients.

# Management of Elevated Intracranial Pressure

Intracranial hypertension is defined as an ICP >15 mmHg. A progressive rise from this level, or sustained ICP >20 mmHg, should prompt investigation and treatment. A progressive rise in ICP may indicate the development of hemorrhage/hematoma, edema, hydrocephalus or a combination of these causes, and an immediate CT scan is indicated. A sustained elevated ICP increases the risk of secondary injury from ischemia and/or herniation.

In patients with surgically correctable pathology, such as subdural/epidural/intracerebral hematoma, or hydrocephalus, prompt surgical treatment is indicated. In other patients ICP can be effectively controlled by manipulating the different compartments of the intracranial contents. In patients refractory to medical management, decompressive craniectomy is indicated. These approaches are discussed below and summarized in Table 5.1.

## Reduction of Cerebral Blood Volume

### Head Elevation

Elevation of the head of the bed to an angle of 20–30° reduces ICP by optimizing cerebral venous return. However, in hypovolemic patients, head elevation may cause a decrease in the CPP. If normovolemia is maintained, elevation to 30° has been shown to decrease ICP without compromising CPP or CBF in head-injured patients.

Care should be taken to avoid obstruction of cerebral venous return by cervical collars or endotracheal tube ties, and to keep the head maintained in the neutral position.

In patients with preserved cerebral autoregulation, elevation of MAP will lead to compensatory vasoconstriction with reduction of ICP.

**Table 5.1.** Treatment of elevated ICP

**Conventional measures**

1. Elevation of head and relief of potential venous obstruction
2. Elevation of MAP (if appropriate)
3. $P_aCO_2$ of 30–35 mmHg, or 25–30 mmHg if there are signs of brain herniation
4. Mannitol 0.5–1.0 g/kg q. 6 h prn and furosemide 20 mg prn. Keep serum osmolality <320.
5. Maintain hypovolemia; monitor CVP, if possible.
6. Ventriculostomy for drainage of CSF, if applicable.
7. Sedation with opiates, benzodiazepines and/or propofol
8. Fine-tune the level of PEEP, if applicable.
9. Maintain normovolemia.

**Aggressive measures (in patients refractory to conventional measures)**

1. Induction of hypothermia to 33–34 °C
2. Maximal EEG suppression with induction of propofol or barbiturate coma
3. Hyperventilation to $P_aCO_2$ of 20–25 mmHg (monitor $S_{jv}O_2$ or $P_{br}O_2$)
4. Hypertonic saline (3% or 7.5% 25–50 ml/h); monitor serum sodium

**Extreme measures**

1. Decompressive craniectomy
2. Excision of infarcted tissues ± lobectomy

This can be accomplished with maintenance of normovolemia and infusion of phenylephrine at 1–10 μg/kg/min, or norepinephrine at 0.05–0.2 μg/kg/min.

## Hyperventilation

Because of the exquisite sensitivity of CBF to $P_aCO_2$, hyperventilation will reduce CBF, and concomitantly cerebral blood volume (CBV), resulting in an acute decrease in ICP. Although the acute reduction in ICP and improvement in CPP is theoretically desirable, and hyperventilation has been traditionally used as an effective treatment modality, in recent years the concern for the risk of cerebral ischemia has curtailed its use. CBF studies have demonstrated that even moderate hyperventilation may increase brain regions with CBF below the ischemic threshold [3]. Reduction of jugular venous oxygen concentration ($S_{jv}O_2$) and brain tissue $PO_2$ ($P_{br}O_2$) have also been repeatedly demonstrated in studies in head-injured patients. Moreover, in the only randomized controlled trial conducted on this therapeutic modality, prophylactic hyperventilation has been shown to be associated with adverse outcome. Thus the Brain Trauma Foundation Guidelines suggest that hyperventilation should not be used for the

management of patients with head injury, unless the ability to monitor independently for evidence of cerebral ischemia is available (CBF, $S_{jv}O_2$ or $P_{br}O_2$). In addition, because of normalization of pH in cerebrospinal fluid, the efficacy of hyperventilation on CBF, CBV and ICP declines after 24 hours. However, despite these studies, the issue of hyperventilation remains controversial. Whereas it is clear that a low $P_aCO_2$ would lead to a reduction in CBF, resulting in regions with CBF approaching or below the ischemic threshold, the definitive evidence of "ischemia" is lacking. Using positron emission tomography, Diringer et al. were unable to demonstrate any decrease in cerebral metabolic rate or change in the pyruvate–lactate ratio with acute hyperventilation, suggesting that the low basal metabolic rate of brain-injured patients paradoxically "protects" these patients from the low CBF [4]. As we await more definitive evidence on hyperventilation, $PaCO_2$ is best maintained at 35-40 mmHg. In acute situations where there is impending or ongoing brain herniation, hyperventilation to $P_aCO_2$ of 20–30 mmHg is warranted. However, this should be viewed as a temporizing measure while waiting for definitive therapy. For maintenance, $P_aCO_2$ should be kept at 30–35 mmHg. Xenon CT and SPECT (single-photon emission computed tomography) may be useful in gauging regional CBF response to hyperventilation.

## Elevation of Blood Pressure

In patients with intact cerebral autoregulation and decreased intracranial compliance, decrease in systemic blood pressure will lead to compensatory vasodilation and an increase in CBV [5]. This will lead to a further decrease in CPP, with a spiraling downhill effect and progressive decrease in net cerebral perfusion. On the other hand, patients with impaired cerebral autoregulation may exhibit an increase in ICP with increase in blood pressure. Since it is not possible to predict the presence or absence of autoregulation, it is important to maintain an adequate or even elevated systemic blood pressure to delineate the ICP response.

## Reduction of Brain Mass

Because of the presence of the blood–brain barrier, which is relatively impermeable to sodium and chloride ions, the movement of water into and out of the brain cells is primarily determined by the osmotic gradient. An effective osmotic diuretic that is frequently used to treat elevated ICP is 20% mannitol. Given as a bolus at 0.5–1.0 g/kg, the action is immediate in onset, but peaks at 30 minutes, lasting for about 90 minutes. The loop diuretic, furosemide, potentiates the actions of mannitol, may also have direct ICP lowering effects, and is often given as an adjunct. The effects of mannitol on systemic hemodynamics are complex, with initial reduction of systemic vascular resistance, followed by intravascular volume expansion, which may be accompanied by systemic hypertension. Patients with poor cardiac function may develop acute pulmonary edema with infusion of mannitol. With the onset of diuresis, contraction of intravascular volume occurs, and this would result in hypotension if fluid replacement is inadequate. The complications from mannitol therapy include fluid overload, dehydration and renal failure.

During mannitol therapy, electrolytes and serum osmolality should be monitored frequently, and serum osmolality should not exceed 320 mOsm. Although the primary mechanism of mannitol is based on the osmotic gradient, it may also cause reflex vasoconstriction

and reduce CSF production. Patients who become refractory to mannitol often would respond to hypertonic saline infusion (3% or 7.5%). Despite numerous clinical reports attesting to its efficacy, there have been no randomized clinical trials on the use of hypertonic saline, and rebound intracranial hypertension is a potential complication.

In patients with vasogenic edema associated with tumor, steroids are effective, and dexamethasone 10 mg is generally given every 6 hours. Steroids in general are considered to be contraindicated in patients with traumatic brain injury and ineffective in patients with subarachnoid hemorrhage or ischemic stroke. In patients with spinal cord injury, high-dose methylprednisolone has been shown to improve functions when given within 8 hours. In most centers, when seen within 3 hours, these patients are given methypredisolone 30 mg/kg bolus, followed by 5.4 mg/kg/h for 24 hours, and for 48 hours if seen between 3–8 hours (NACIS III). The improvement is, however, marginal, and many query if the benefits outweigh the risks of pneumonia and infection. Nevertheless, in view of the efficacy of steroid in spinal cord injury, the use of high-dose methylprednisolone in head injury is being re-examined, and a randomized trial aiming to enroll 20,000 patients is currently under way [6].

## Reduction of CSF volume

Twenty-five percent of patients with subarachnoid hemorrhage from a ruptured aneurysm will develop acute hydrocephalus with elevation of ICP. Insertion of ventriculostomy with controlled drainage of CSF is an effective treatment of ICP. Some of these patients will eventually require a ventriculo-peritoneal shunt. Placement of a lumbar subarachnoid drain can also reduce CSF volume, but at the increased risk of brain herniation. This is less useful in patients with head injury, as the ventricles are frequently compressed, making them inaccessible and drainage less effective.

## Sedation and Paralysis

Adequate sedation is essential in all patients with elevated ICP in order to minimize agitation and movement, and to improve tolerance of the endotracheal tube. Coughing or gagging on the tracheal tube or during tracheobronchial suction can cause rapid, extreme elevations in ICP. Neuromuscular paralysis effectively prevents this but at the expense of eliminating neurological examination as a monitor of the patient's condition. In addition, prolonged pharmacological blockade may result in the development of myopathy and persistent paralysis. Moreover, neuromuscular blocking agents (NMBs) should only be used in patients who are adequately sedated in order to avoid paralysis in an awake patient. Intermittent dosing and periodic discontinuation, coupled with careful monitoring of the degree of neuromuscular blockade, should allow regular neurological assessment.

## Propofol

Sedative drugs that decrease ICP via an effect on cerebral metabolism and CBF include most of the intravenous anesthetic agents except ketamine. All have a depressant effect on the central nervous system, resulting in a dose-related decrease in level of consciousness and metabolic rate. Propofol has a similar metabolic and vascular profile to barbiturates, causing a dose-related decrease in cerebral metabolic rate and coupled decrease in CBF, resulting in a reduction in ICP in patients with cerebral metabolic activity. However, in some studies the decrease in CBF exceeded the concomitant decrease in metabolic rate. Its pharmacokinetic profile, with a short half-life, makes it a particularly suitable sedative agent in neurosurgical patients, allowing prompt neurological assessment within 2–3 hours of discontinuation of the infusion in usual doses (50–150 μg/kg/min). In a multicenter trial, propofol was efficacious in reducing ICP although the study failed to show an improvement in neurological outcome. In high doses (>300 μg/kg/min), it can be used to induce pharmacological coma with burst-suppression on electroencephalogram to achieve maximal metabolic suppression for control of ICP. In children, when used as a continuous infusion for a prolonged period, propofol has been reported to be associated with the development of a metabolic syndrome that is characterized by acidosis, rhabdomyolysis, cardiac failure and a high mortality rate [7]. More recently, a similar syndrome has also been reported to occur in head-injured adults treated with propofol >5 mg/kg/h [8]. In both children and adults, the actual incidence of this syndrome is unknown and the pathophysiology remains unclear. However, given the high mortality reported in children, and apparently conclusive data in a clinical trial (as yet unpublished), the use of propofol infusion in children is currently not advised. In adults, where indicated, the benefits of propofol outweigh this potential risk and should not be withheld from patients in the neurointensive care unit. However, prolonged infusion for more than 1 week, at doses greater than 5 mg/kg/h, is not advised, and the infusion should immediately be discontinued should any acidosis or cardiac dysfunction develop. In addition, propofol in high doses will result in systemic hypotension, often necessitating the use of vasopressors for blood pressure support.

## Etomidate

Although etomidate had been used in the past as a sedative agent, it should not be given by infusion as it inhibits corticosteroid synthesis by the adrenal glands. It causes less cardiovascular depression than propofol or barbiturates and has been used in intermittent dosage in less stable patients. It reduces ICP by its effects on CBF and CVR.

## Dexmedetomidine

Dexmedetomidine is a selective alpha-2-receptor agonist, and has recently been approved for use as a sedative agent for cardiac patients in the intensive care unit. Although not well investigated in neurosurgical patients, its pharmacological profile suggests that it may be a useful sedative in this group of patients. When given as an infusion at 0.6 mg/kg/h, most patients are well sedated but arousable, with minimal respiratory depression. It causes cerebrovasoconstriction and should reduce ICP, although the reduction in CBF is not matched by reduction in cerebral metabolism. Our own studies show that autoregulation and $CO_2$ reactivity are not affected by sedative doses of dexmedetomidine (unpublished data). In experimental ischemia it has been shown to reduce the number of damaged neurons in transient global ischemia in gerbils, and following focal cerebral ischemia in rats. The mechanism of action is thought to be via a reduction in norepinephrine release. Additionally, it appears to enhance the disposal of glutamine by oxidative metabolism in astrocytes, thus reducing the availability of glutamine as a precursor of neurotoxic glutamates. As yet, there have been no clinical trials on its use as a sedative agent in the neurointensive care unit, but the lack of significant respiratory depression makes it a very appropriate sedative in spontaneously breathing patients with poor intracranial compliance.

## Barbiturates

Barbiturates reduce ICP by suppressing cerebral metabolism and, correspondingly, CBF. They do this both directly and by reducing seizure activity. Both pentobarbital and thiopental have been used to induce barbiturate coma. Their use is usually reserved for those patients whose intracranial hypertension has been refractory to other treatments. Similar to other sedatives, thiopental use is associated with systemic hypotension and should only be used in normovolemic patients. Two randomized controlled trials have assessed the efficacy of thiopentone for the treatment of raised ICP in patients with head injury. One trial showed a reduction in ICP that was significantly greater in the group treated with barbiturates, but with no improvement in long-term outcome. The second trial found that the ICP was controlled in approximately one-third of the treatment group, and that in those patients who responded, long-term outcome was also improved. A proportion of patients treated with barbiturates show no decrease in ICP. This may be due to uncoupling of cerebral metabolic rate of oxygen consumption from CBF, and is an indicator of poor prognosis.

## Hypothermia

Hypothermia reduces cerebral metabolism and CBF, with resultant reduction in CBV and ICP. It may also be neuroprotective by decreasing the release of excitotoxic amino acids. Despite initial enthusiasm reported with the therapeutic use of moderate hypothermia in a single-center trial, a multicenter, randomized controlled trial could not demonstrate any beneficial effects, although a subset of patients aged less than 45 years, who were admitted hypothermic and randomized to hypothermia, had better results than patients who were rendered normothermic [9]. A new trial focusing on younger patients

commenced in 2003. Despite the lack of proof of definitive benefits, most studies demonstrate a favorable ICP response to hypothermia. Moreover, the beneficial effects of therapeutic hypothermia on neurological outcome were recently demonstrated in patients who suffered cardiac arrest from sudden ventricular fibrillation. For now, therapeutic hypothermia should be used as an effective and useful adjunct for the control of ICP.

## Decompressive Craniectomy

Decompressive craniectomy is indicated in patients with persistent elevated ICP refractory to medical treatments. In patients with unilateral swelling following hematoma evacuation or tumor resection, hemicraniectomy or removal of a large cranial flap with dural patching has been successful in reducing ICP. In patients with cerebral edema of both hemispheres, bilateral craniectomy may be necessary. Rarely, removal of damaged tissue or lobectomy may be performed as a last-ditch effort to decrease the intracranial contents in the most severe cases of intracranial hypertension. This procedure appears to be effective both for traumatic brain injury as well as for swelling secondary to stroke or subarachnoid hemorrhage. A multicenter trial to assess its efficacy as an early treatment for traumatic brain injury will determine its future role as a definitive treatment for intracranial hypertension [10].

## Use of Positive End-expiratory Pressure in Patients with Elevated ICP

Positive end-expiratory pressure (PEEP) is frequently used to improve oxygenation in patients with respiratory distress syndrome or loss of lung volume due to a variety of pulmonary diseases. Theoretically, this can increase intrathoracic pressure, which in turn impedes venous inflow from the head, causing increase in ICP. However, this appears to be only clinically relevant if the patient has good intrathoracic compliance and poor intracranial compliance. Its safety was recently demonstrated in patients with acute stroke [11]. In practical terms, when properly indicated, PEEP up to 10 mmHg seldom causes significant elevation of ICP. However, it remains prudent to monitor the ICP response to PEEP in patients, particularly when PEEP >10 mmHg is used.

# Management of Blood Pressure/Cerebral Perfusion Pressure

## Head Injury

Optimal CPP–ICP management in the head-injured patient should be predicated on: (1) prevention of secondary injury and (2) promotion of recovery and repair of damaged neurons. Although maintenance of adequate CPP is the obvious and intended goal, there is controversy about the precise level of blood pressure required to achieve this goal. Because of the lack of randomized clinical trials, at least in the context of head injury, several approaches have been suggested, with all reporting improved results in their series. There are currently five approaches to the treatment of severe head injury that have been advocated: (1) guidelines issued by the Brain Trauma Foundation, (2) ICP management (Marshall approach), (3) CPP management (Rosner protocol), (4) "Lund therapy", which maintains low systemic pressures (MAP >50 mmHg) and normal colloid osmotic pressure to avoid vasogenic cerebral edema (prostacyclin to improve microcirculation) [12], and (5) the "cerebral ischemia model" (Robertson option), which relies upon the use of jugular venous oxygen saturation ($S_{jv}O_2$) monitoring to avoid global cerebral ischemia. These different options are summarized in Table 5.2. Although there is not a unified approach, with the exception of the Lund therapy, the consensus appears to be CPP at >60 mmHg [13] and MAP at >80 mmHg. Phenylephrine and norepinephrine are the most common agents used to support blood pressure in these patients. Both agents have negligible direct effects on the cerebral vasculature. Commonly used vasoactive agents are listed in Table 5.3.

**Table 5.3.** Vasoactive agents

| **Vasopressors/inotropes** |
| --- |
| Phenylephrine: 1–10 μg/kg/min |
| Norepinephrine: 0.05–0.2 μg/kg/min |
| Dopamine: 1–20 μg/kg/min |
| Dobutamine: 1–20 μg/kg/min |
| Vasopressin: 0.01–0.04 units/min |
| **Vasodilators/hypotensive agents** |
| Labetalol: 5-10 mg bolus q. 10 min, infusion at 50–100 mg/h, titrated to BP and HR |
| Esmolol: 500 μg/kg bolus, 3–15 mg/kg/h |
| Clonidine: 0.1 mg q. 4 h |
| Enlapril: 0.625–2.5 mg q. 6 h |
| Hydralazine: 10–20 mg q. 2 h prn |
| Sodium nitroprusside: 0.1–10 μg/kg/min |

**Table 5.2.** Comparison of four different approaches and the Brain Trauma Foundation guidelines for the management of acute head injuries

| | Approach: ICP | CPP | Threshold for MAP/SBP | Therapy for ↓CPP | Ischemia monitors |
| --- | --- | --- | --- | --- | --- |
| BTF guidelines | <20–25 | >70 | SBP >90 | Colloid, dopamine, phenylephrine | $S_{jv}O_2$, CBF, AVDO$_2$ if using hyperventilation |
| ICP (Marshall approach) | <20 | >60 | SBP >80 | N/A | Not routine |
| CPP (Rosner protocol) | | >70–80 | MAP >90 | Phenylephrine, norepi, colloid | Not routine |
| Lund therapy | <20–25 | >40–60 | N/A | N/A | Not routine |
| Cerebral ischemia (Robertson option) | <20 | >70 | MAP >90 | Colloid, dopamine, phenylephrine | $S_{jv}O_2$, CBF, AVDO$_2$ |

ICP, intracranial pressure; CPP, cerebral perfusion pressure; BTF, Brain Trauma Foundation; MAP, mean arterial pressure; SBP, systolic blood pressure; CSF, cerebrospinal fluid; STP, sodium thiopental; norepi, norepinephrine; $S_{jv}O_2$ jugular venous oxygen saturation, CBF cerebral blood flow; AVDO$_2$, arteriovenous oxygen difference.

## Subarachnoid Hemorrhage

In patients with ruptured and unsecured aneurysms and in good grade, blood pressure should be controlled and maintained at normal or slightly reduced values to reduce the risk of re-bleeding. Labetalol and beta-blockers have no effect on CBF and are the hypotensive agents of choice. In patients refractory to this treatment, the addition of clonidine or enlapril generally would control the blood pressure. In difficult cases, intravenous sodium nitroprusside may be necessary. Agents such as nitroprusside, hydralazine and nicardipine are cerebral vasodilators, and thus must be used with caution in patients with poor intracranial compliance or increased ICP. Continuous monitoring of ICP will enhance safety in these patients. In patients with elevated ICP and in poor grades, ongoing cerebral ischemia is an important consideration and blood pressure may have to be maintained at normal levels appropriate for the patient, albeit at the expense of increased risk of bleeding. Prompt surgical treatment will minimize this complication.

Patients in vasospasm will require hypertensive therapy to improve cerebral perfusion. The optimal blood pressure should be guided by the patient's clinical conditions and the magnitude of vasospasm. In general, systolic blood pressure of 140–160 mmHg is maintained for patients with mild vasospasm, and 160–180 mmHg for patients with evidence of moderate-to-severe vasospasm. Occasionally, even higher blood pressure may be required. A therapeutic dilemma occurs when vasospasm occurs in patients with unsecured aneurysms. However, therapeutic hypertensive therapy should not be withheld in these patients as the risk of hemorrhage appears to be very small.

## Hemorrhagic and Ischemic Stroke

In patients with hemorrhagic stroke, control of blood pressure is important to prevent further hemorrhage. However, it is important to rule out the occurrence of hypertension secondary to increase in ICP (Cushing's response), in which event the mean arterial pressure should be reduced gradually, and not below 130 mmHg in known hypertensive patients, and lower (100 mmHg) in previously normotensive patients. On the other hand, mild-to-moderate hypertension (160–180 systolic and 90–100 diastolic blood pressure) should be left untreated in patients with ischemic stroke. Vasopressors to support blood pressure may be necessary.

## Arteriovenous Malformation

Unlike cerebral aneurysms, increase in systemic blood pressure has not been identified as an etiological factor in hemorrhage in patients with arteriovenous malformations (AVMs). Control of blood pressure while the patient is awaiting surgery following hemorrhage is therefore relatively unimportant. However, because of the chronic adaptation of the adjacent blood vessels to a low pressure system, following resection of AVM, patients may develop hyperperfusion syndrome at normal blood pressure. Control of blood pressure at a normal or slightly reduced level is therefore crucial in the post-operative management.

# Monitoring in the Intensive Care Unit

## Basic Monitoring

### Neurological Examination

Physical examination of the neurological system, although a non-parametric and subjective tool, is rapid and easy to perform and is useful in the detection of changes in the patient's neurological status. Its importance should not be overlooked and it should be a basic skill of all staff involved in the care of the neurological patient. Inter-observer variation is common but may be minimized by the use of quantitative examination methods. Mental status, motor/sensory assessment and coordination testing may all be rapidly evaluated in the conscious patient. Both conscious and unconscious patients should be assessed for pupillary size and light response, deep tendon reflexes and response to peripheral noxious stimuli. Pupillary deviation and flexor or extensor posturing may also be present.

The desire for quantification of neurological status has led to the development and wide-

**Table 5.4.** Glasgow Coma Scale

| Eye opening | | Verbal response | | Motor response | |
|---|---|---|---|---|---|
| Spontaneous | 4 | Oriented | 5 | Obeys commands | 6 |
| To verbal | 3 | Inappropriate | 4 | Localizes pain | 5 |
| To pain | 2 | Incomprehensible | 3 | Flexion/withdrawal | 4 |
| None | 1 | Makes sounds | 2 | Flexion/abnormal (decorticate) | 3 |
| | | None | 1 | Extension (decerebrate) | 2 |
| | | | | None | 1 |

spread use of scoring scales, such as the Glasgow Coma Scale (Table 5.4), originally developed for use in the head-injured patient. In addition to establishing a baseline, these scales are most useful when performed regularly in order to give a more objective impression of deterioration or improvement over a period of time.

Sedatives and analgesics given in the intensive care unit should ideally have a short duration of action, and should be allowed to dissipate once a day to facilitate assessment of the neurological status.

## Monitoring of Intracranial Pressure

Although there are no data from randomized trials, it is generally accepted that monitoring and aggressive treatment of elevated ICP can minimize secondary ischemia and improve outcome. Thus the use of intracranial devices for the continuous measurement of ICP has become standard practice in the care of neurological patients in whom an elevated ICP is an issue. These devices include intraventricular catheters, subarachnoid bolts, epidural systems and fiberoptic intraparenchymal devices. Ventriculostomy catheters and fiberoptic intraparenchymal devices appear to give comparably accurate measurement of ICP (Fig. 5.2). Ventriculostomy catheters are generally considered to be the gold standard for ICP monitoring. This type of catheter has the additional advantage of allowing drainage of CSF to lower ICP.

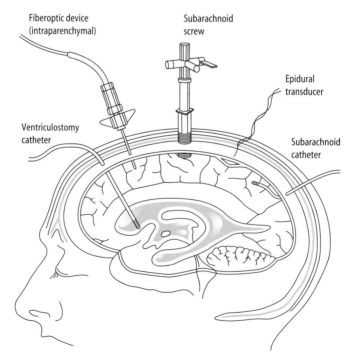

**Fig. 5.2.** Methods of monitoring intracranial pressure.

However, it is associated with a higher risk of infection compared with the fiberoptic intra-parenchymal catheters. Subarachnoid monitors should be placed on the same side as the lesion in order to avoid inaccuracy due to pressure differential between the two hemispheres. Computerized recording and display of the transduced ICP pressure wave is now standard with most multimodal bedside patient monitors: the 'real-time' pressure wave and analysis of any trend in pressure may be viewed and compared with other monitored signs such as systemic blood pressure or central venous pressure (CVP).

## Indications for ICP Monitoring

An ICP monitor may be useful in the management of any neurosurgical patient in whom a raised ICP is suspected, although it is in the management of severe head injury that its utility is most established. In those patients with moderate head injury in whom non-neurosurgical surgery is essential, an ICP monitor may also provide the only indication of deterioration of the patient whilst anaesthetized. Maintenance of an adequate CPP is only possible with knowledge of the ICP and systemic blood pressure in order to avoid secondary ischemic insults. ICP measurement also facilitates the ability to gauge response to therapeutic measures and gives early warning of the expansion of mass lesions. In general, ICP monitoring is indicated in all patients who are comatose with brain injury, and in patients with deteriorating neurological status with an abnormal CT scan. As mentioned above, many consider ICP monitoring desirable in patients with moderate head injury requiring prolonged surgical procedure under general anesthesia. In addition, routine post-operative ICP monitoring following major neurosurgical procedures is performed in some centers. The only absolute contraindication for ICP monitoring is the presence of uncorrected coagulopathy.

## ICP Tracings

The nature and characteristics of ICP waves were extensively described in 1960 by Lundberg from his observation of ICP monitoring in neurosurgical patients. He described three wave-types: A-waves or plateau waves, B-waves and C-waves.

A-waves, termed "plateau waves" for their characteristic shape, are associated with both an increase in CBV as a result of vasodilation and a decrease in CBF. They manifest in an abrupt rise in the ICP to levels of 60–80 mmHg for a duration of 5–20 minutes and are an indicator of poor prognosis (Fig. 5.3).

Rosner and Becker showed that plateau waves in cats with mild brain trauma are preceded by a decrease in systemic blood pressure to approximately 70–80 mmHg and that CBV increases exponentially with this decrease. In association with poor intracranial compliance, this increase in CBV is accompanied by an exponential rise in ICP, seen as the plateau wave. Plateau waves may be abolished with an increase in CPP or with maneuvers to improve intracranial compliance.

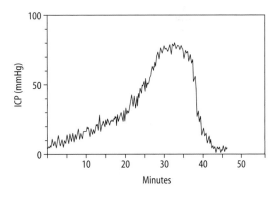

**Fig. 5.3.** Example of an A-wave.

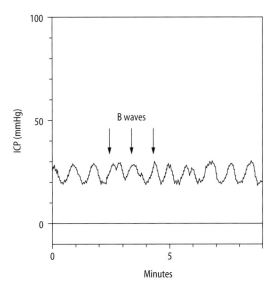

**Fig. 5.4** Example of a B-wave.

The B-waves described by Lundberg are repeating waves of usually 10–20 mmHg with a frequency of 0.5–2 waves/min, and reflect fluctuation in CBV owing to vasomotor waves of the regulating vessels. They usually indicate decreased intracranial compliance (Fig. 5.4).

C-waves were considered by Lundberg to reflect arterial Traube–Hering waves and to indicate decreased intracranial compliance.

## Advanced Monitoring

### Monitoring of Cerebral Oxygenation/ Metabolism

*Jugular Venous Oximetry, Tissue PO$_2$, and Near-infrared Spectroscopy*

As cerebral ischemia and secondary injury are the common factors leading to deterioration, monitoring of some indices of cerebral oxygenation would provide guide to appropriate therapy. By placing a fiberoptic oximetric catheter into the jugular bulb, cerebral venous oxygenation can be monitored continuously, providing an index of the balance between cerebral blood flow (supply) and cerebral metabolic consumption of oxygen (demand) ($CMRO_2$ = $CBF \times AVDO_2$, or $AVDO_2 = CMRO_2/CBF$). In essence, it is the arteriovenous oxygen content difference that represents the balance between supply and demand. However, if hemoglobin concentration stays relatively constant, and we ignore the contribution of dissolved oxygen, then the jugular venous saturation ($S_{jv}O_2$) effectively reflects the adequacy of CBF relative to oxygen consumption [$AVDO_2$ = Hgb × 1.39 × (1– $S_{jv}O_2$)]. Thus, a high $S_{jv}O_2$ implies luxury perfusion, and a low value reflects increased extraction, or inadequate delivery relative to the degree of consumption. It has been demonstrated that multiple episodes of desaturation below 50% are associated with poor prognosis in head-injured patients. Paradoxically, a high $S_{jv}O_2$ also indicates a poor prognosis as the brain is no longer extracting oxygen. However, it is a global measurement and does not and cannot reflect regional ischemia. Thus it is a highly specific but very insensitive monitor. Despite these limitations, when used properly it yields information that can help management, and has become a standard monitor in the care of the head-injured patient in many centers.

Combining this with lactate measurement enhances its value as a monitor. The potential complications of this technique include bleeding and thrombosis, none of which has proved to be clinically significant. The most predominant cause of jugular venous desaturation is probably excessive hyperventilation. Treatment of a low $S_{jv}O_2$ should include a careful examination of all systemic and cerebral factors (Fig. 5.5).

Tissue $PO_2$ electrodes are miniature Clark electrodes that can be inserted into brain parenchyma to measure tissue $PO_2$ ($PbrO_2$). The placement of these electrodes necessitates the drilling of burr holes, and is therefore more invasive than jugular oximetry. However, they provide regional measurement and can be inserted into brain tissues considered to be at risk. There are two types of electrodes that are commercially available: the Neurotrend and the Licox. The Neurotrend monitors $PCO_2$ and pH in addition to $PO_2$ (requiring a larger burr hole) whereas the Licox only measures $PO_2$. Both are combined with ICP and temperature monitors. The normal values of $P_{br}O_2$ are 25–30 mmHg. Values below 15 mmHg are associated with poor prognosis, and values less than 10 mmHg are usually incompatible with survival. It is debatable whether $P_{br}O_2$ truly reflects tissue oxygenation or a balance between the delivery and consumption of oxygen at the local level. Studies with $P_{br}O_2$ have repeatedly demonstrated that increase in $F_iO_2$ consistently causes an immediate rise in $P_{br}O_2$. Although this is considered beneficial by some, others consider it may be more related to $P_aO_2$ than to brain tissue oxygenation.

Near-infrared spectroscopy measures tissue oxygenation non-invasively using reflectance oximetry. Briefly, a light source is placed on the scalp, and light reflected from the scalp and brain is measured by optodes placed at a distance from the light source. Theoretically this can monitor not only oxygenation saturation, but also the amount of desaturated hemoglobin, regional CBV and the cytochrome redox state. Although attractive in theory, the many drawbacks, including variable optical path, contamination by scalp and bone, interference by ambient light, and the necessary placement on the forehead, have limited its usefulness as a clinical monitor. Extensive development and refinement are required before it can become a functional monitor.

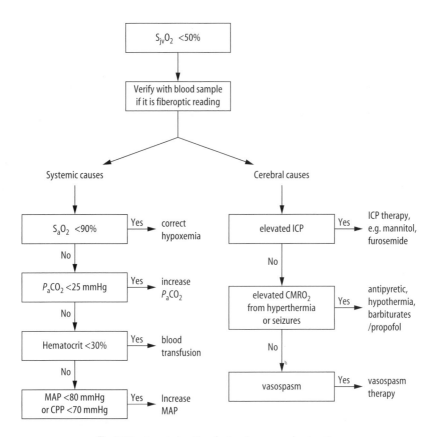

**Fig. 5.5** Treatment algorithm for jugular venous desaturation.

## Microdialysis

With placement of an intraparenchymal microdialysis catheter, it is now possible to do bedside measurement of local cerebral metabolite/neurotransmitter, including that of lactate, pyruvate, glucose and glutamate [14]. These microdialysis measurements complement other cerebral monitoring by confirming or refuting the presence of cerebral ischemia.

## Positron Emission Tomography (PET)

PET can measure CBF, CBV and oxygen consumption, as well as glucose consumption. It is, however, expensive and remains an investigative tool. Recent PET studies of head injuries show that some patients may develop regional hyperglycolysis during the early stages of head injury.

## Monitoring of Cerebral Blood Flow

Numerous methods have been employed to assess both global and regional CBF. This information has been used to evaluate autoregulation and $CO_2$ reactivity, to ensure adequate CBF, to assess the effect of treatments in modifying CBF, and to assess CBF as an outcome predictor. Although many methods are available, as yet there is no functional bedside method for the measurement of CBF that can be performed repetitively in a clinically useful manner. Several semi-quantitative methods are nevertheless clinically useful.

## Quantitative Global and Regional CBF

*Kety–Schmidt Technique* The gold standard for global CBF measurement is the Kety–Schmidt technique of nitrous oxide washin. Although first described in 1945, the technique remains valid today. It measures global hemispheric blood flow, necessitates cannulation of the jugular bulb, thus allowing derivation of cerebral metabolic rate for oxygen, and can be performed at bedside.

*Radioactive Xenon Washout* The Xenon133 washout method is derived from the Kety–Schmidt technique, and is probably the most commonly used bedside technique today. Xe133 can be administered by inhalation or intraarterial injection, but is most commonly given by intravenous injection. Multiple detectors placed next to the head allow measurements of regional CBF. Accuracy may be impaired in low-flow conditions, and areas with no flow cannot be detected (the "look-through phenomenon").

*Stable Xenon CT* Quantitative CBF can also be determined using stable xenon (30%) by inhalation and CT. Flows at multiple regions of interest can be measured. Transportation to the CT suite is necessary, and stable xenon is expensive and, at 30%, has significant cerebral vasodilatory effects. Repetitive measurements are possible and evaluation of therapeutic response to treatments aiming to modify CBF may be carried out with this method.

*CT Perfusion Scan* Quantitative CBF can also be obtained using contrast CT. The computer algorithm examines the transit time of contrast and derives the regional CBF. Compared with stable xenon, only limited slices can be obtained. This technique also allows repetitive measurements, making it possible to assess the patient's response to therapeutic maneuvers such as hyperventilation or augmentation of blood pressure.

*Positron Emission Tomography* As mentioned above, PET can measure regional CBF, metabolism and volume. This is, however, expensive and, with limited availability, remains primarily an investigative tool.

### Local CBF

*Laser Doppler* Continuous monitoring of CBF is possible using laser Doppler flow probes. This, however, involves implantation of a probe via a small burr hole directly into the brain parenchyma and can only measure local CBF in a volume of 1 mm$^3$.

### Semiquantitative/Qualitative Cerebral Blood Flow

*Single-Photon Emission Computed Tomography (SPECT)* Using Technetium$^{99}$ isotope administered intravenously, relative regional distribu-

tion of blood flow can be quantified. However, absolute CBF cannot be derived. This technique is relatively non-invasive, involves less radiation than a CT scan, and is useful in the assessment of cerebral ischemia secondary to vasospasm.

*Transcranial Doppler* The transcranial Doppler (TCD) was introduced by Rune Aaslid in 1982. Using a 2 MHz pulsed Doppler, flow velocities of the basal cerebral arteries can be measured in a non-invasive manner. Although actual CBF cannot be derived from the velocities, valuable information can nevertheless be obtained that can aid patient management. When the diameter of the insonated vessel stays constant, changes in flow velocity reflect corresponding change in flow. Under normal conditions, the basal cerebral arteries, being conductance vessels, vary little in diameter with physiological vasodilation or vasoconstriction, conditions that depend on change in resistance vessels. On the other hand, pathological constriction of the conductance vessel will lead to a dichotomy, with increase in flow velocity paradoxically reflecting a decrease in flow, as in the case of vasospasm following subarachnoid hemorrhage. TCD has been found to be useful in the management of vasospasm, allowing early diagnosis and assessment of therapy.

### Vasospasm vs Hyperemia

Increase in flow velocity as diagnosed by TCD can be secondary to development of vasospasm or hyperemia, with obvious different clinical implications. This is particularly relevant in patients with traumatic subarachnoid hemorrhage (SAH), since 20–40% may develop vasospasm. To distinguish vasospasm from hyperemia, the ratio of intracranial flow velocity to extracranial internal carotid flow velocity (Lindegard index) is frequently used. Hyperemia is considered to be present when the index is less than 3. Mild vasospasm occurs when the index is greater than 3, moderate vasospasm when the index is 5–7, and severe vasospasm when the index is greater than 7.

### Non-invasive Assessment of ICP

Significant elevation of ICP compromising cerebral perfusion results in a characteristic flow pattern on TCD with low diastolic flow velocities. Increasing ICP will result in correspondingly decreasing diastolic velocity, culminating in a "reverberating flow" pattern, with forward flow during systole, and backward flow during diastole, signifying the onset of intracranial circulatory arrest. Based on these considerations, many investigators have proposed using TCD as a non-invasive monitor of ICP, and preliminary results are promising.

### Autoregulation Testing

Patients who suffer traumatic brain injury or SAH frequently develop impaired cerebral autoregulation, increasing the risk of brain injury with sudden changes in systemic blood pressure. Elevation of blood pressure may increase the risk of vasogenic edema, whereas decrease in blood pressure may result in cerebral ischemia. Elucidation and quantification of the state of autoregulation would facilitate clinical management of these patients. Furthermore, it has been shown that delayed ischemic deficits are more likely to develop in patients with the combination of vasospasm and impaired cerebral autoregulation, as determined by TCD.

A number of different methods have been investigated. These include:

*Spontaneous relationship between blood pressure and flow velocity changes.* With intact cerebral autoregulation there is a negative correlation between changes in blood pressure and change in flow velocity, and a positive correlation when autoregulation is impaired. By monitoring both blood pressure and flow velocity simultaneously over multiple time epochs, the state of cerebral autoregulation can be qualitatively determined.

*Transient hyperemic response.* When autoregulation is intact, compression of the extracranial internal carotid artery for 7–10 seconds will result in a transient hyperemic response in the ipsilateral middle cerebral artery.

*Dynamic autoregulation.* When autoregulation is intact, a transient decrease in blood pressure effected by sudden deflation of inflated thigh cuffs will cause a very brief decrease in middle cerebral artery flow velocity, rapidly returning to baseline value.

*Static autoregulation.* Below the upper limit of autoregulation, elevation of systemic blood pressure using a vasopressor

(phenylephrine) will not affect cerebral artery flow velocity when autoregulation is intact.

### Imaging Modalities

Computed tomography of the brain is the most important diagnostic imaging modality in the care of the critically ill neurological patient. Patients with traumatic head injury may require daily CT during the initial course, and more often if the neurological status is fluctuating. It is important to obtain CT whenever there is sudden deterioration in the neurological status or sudden increase in ICP to rule out surgically correctable causes. Magnetic resonance (MR) imaging is more helpful in delineating infarcts and ischemic lesions, particularly with diffusion-weighted and perfusion-weighted imaging. However, it is time consuming and generally not as available as CT. Angiography is essential in the establishment of vasospasm and institution of interventional treatment.

## Monitoring Electrophysiological Functions

### EEG and Evoked Potentials

EEG and evoked potentials may be useful for diagnostic purposes. In patients suspected of having seizures, a diagnostic EEG may be helpful. In patients with status epilepticus treated with muscle relaxants, continuous EEG monitoring to guide pharmacological therapy is essential.

In patients with severe head injury, EEG is of relatively little value, whereas somatosensory evoked potentials (SSEPs) can provide important prognostic information. With unilateral or bilateral absence of cortical SSEP, the outcome is uniformly fatal. Preservation or early recovery of normal SSEP is compatible with high degree of recovery. Brainstem evoked potential, in combination with cortical SSEP, may allow assessment of the integrity of brainstem function and the site of injury to be located.

### Electrocardiographic and Cardiac Monitoring

Patients with isolated severe neurological injury can develop ECG changes. In patients with aneurysmal SAH, 40–60% of the patients may exhibit ECG abnormalities comprising of ST segment changes or arrhythmia. Acute left ventricular dysfunction can also occur, and in some patients acute pulmonary edema can develop. Frank myocardial necrosis secondary to SAH has been documented, although it is exceedingly rare. Patients with poor clinical grades are more likely to have ECG abnormalities as well as ventricular dysfunction, but there is poor correlation between these two abnormalities. Cardiac enzymes should be measured in patients with ECG changes to rule out myocardial infarction, and echocardiograms should be performed in patients with clinical ventricular dysfunction. Central venous pressure monitoring is indicated in these patients and, despite recent studies questioning the value of pulmonary artery catheter placement, measurement of filling pressures may facilitate the management of patients in vasospasm.

## Management of Vasospasm

Angiographic vasospasm occurs in up to 70% of patients after aneurysmal SAH, although only about 30–40% of patients become clinically symptomatic. Although nimodipine prophylaxis improves the neurological outcome of patients, it neither decreases the incidence nor alters the magnitude of vasospasm. Vasospasm typically occurs on day 3 after SAH, peaks on day 7, and generally subsides by the end of 14 days. Vasospasm is the main cause of delayed ischemic deficit, resulting in brain infarction or death. Early vasospasm results in elevated flow velocities, which can be detected by TCD, but the diagnosis must be confirmed with angiography in symptomatic patients. SPECT can detect regional differences in perfusion and facilitate management. Currently, the only medical treatment for symptomatic vasospasm is augmentation of cerebral perfusion by elevation of blood pressure, and cardiac output. Although its value has not been established with randomized clinical trials, triple-H therapy (hemodilution, hypervolemia, hypertension) is a standard management therapy for severe vasospasm in many neurointensive care units. This entails aggressive fluid therapy to maintain pulmonary wedge pressure at 14–16 mmHg, systolic blood pressure at 160–180 mmHg, and hematocrit at 30. Patients not responding to therapy may be candidates for angioplasty with or without papaverine infusion. Patients with vasospasm secondary to traumatic SAH generally respond to the same treatment regimen, although the risk of development of vasogenic edema may be higher.

## Fluid and Electrolytes

To maintain adequate cerebral perfusion, it is important to maintain normovolemia. The practice of keeping neurological patients dehydrated to minimize cerebral edema is outdated, and in head-injured patients is associated with poor outcome [15]. Fluid balance tallying total input and output should be monitored daily, and insensible loss of 500–800 ml per day should be allowed. Patients with head injury often suffer multiple injuries that may result in significant blood loss, contributing to hypovolemia and hypotension. On the other hand, patients who suffer SAH can develop acute decrease in circulating blood volume unrelated to blood loss. Patients with hemorrhagic or ischemic stroke may also be hypovolemic, and the volume status cannot be assessed by the presence or absence of systemic hypertension. A thorough history and clinical examination is crucial to the establishment of the correct diagnosis. To ensure normovolemia, isotonic fluids or normal saline should be given, although the latter, when given in large amounts, would inevitably lead to hyperchloremic metabolic acidosis.

In patients with partially disrupted blood–brain barrier (BBB), colloids have a theoretical advantage, and their benefits in reducing edema can be demonstrated in experimental focal cerebral ischemia. However, there is no clinical evidence of its efficacy. Moreover, meta-analysis of clinical trials suggests that the use of colloids for resuscitation of critically ill patients is associated with an increase in mortality. If colloids are to be used, albumin is preferred to hetastarch, as the latter can interfere with coagulation system and may cause bleeding in susceptible neurological patients, despite being given in small amounts. Monitoring of central venous pressure or pulmonary wedge pressure would help to guide fluid therapy, particularly in the management of patients in vasospasm. Anemia should be treated promptly to maintain adequate oxygen delivery. The optimal hemoglobin concentration for patients with brain injury has not been determined. In critically ill patients it has been demonstrated that, with the exception of patients with significant coronary artery disease, a conservative transfusion strategy is associated with better results than a liberal strategy, and transfusion to a hematocrit value of higher than 25–27 is not warranted. However, until data on patients with neurological disease are available, it remains prudent to maintain hemoglobin at about 10 g or hematocrit at 30.

In patients with severe head injury and stroke, as well as SAH, the presence of hyperglycemia is associated with a poor prognosis. Although stress is clearly a contributing factor, hyperglycemia itself can contribute to poor outcome. Thus hyperglycemia should be treated vigorously.

Neurological patients are prone to development of electrolyte disturbances; thus they should be measured daily, and appropriate replacements made. In particular, because of the relative impermeability of the BBB to ions, change in serum sodium and osmolality can have profound influence on movement of water across the BBB into neurons, and can exacerbate brain swelling/dehydration, causing coma and/or seizures.

## Hypo- and Hypernatremia

Both hyponatremia and hypernatremia can occur in the neurological patient. The two major causes of sodium disturbances are: (1) iatrogenic and (2) CNS pathology related. Iatrogenic causes include administration of hypotonic fluids and the use of thiazide diuretics. Although normal hemostatic mechanisms will regulate sodium and water balance to maintain serum sodium within the normal range, persistent administration of hypotonic fluids, particularly in patients with poor renal functions or low cardiac output syndrome, will result in hyponatremia. The tonicity and composition of usual intravenous fluids are listed in Table 5.5. Following SAH, hyponatremia is particularly common, although only hypernatremia has been noted to be associated with a poor outcome. Disease-related causes include the development of diabetes insipidus, the syndrome of inappropriate antidiuretic hormone (SIADH), and cerebral salt-wasting syndrome (CSWS). It is extremely important to distinguish between the last two entities as the treatment is vastly different. With SIADH, the patient retains fluid, and excretes urine with high serum sodium and osmolality. Thus the appropriate treatment for SIADH is fluid restriction with or without diuretics, whereas with CSWS the

**Table 5.5.** Electrolyte composition of crystalloid and colloid fluids

| Fluids | Osmolality (mOsm/kg) | Na (mEq/l) | Cl (mEq/l) | K (mEq/l) | Ca (mEq/l) | Mg (mEq/l) | HCO3-* (mEq/l) | Glucose (gm/l) | pH | Oncotic pressure (mmHg) |
|---|---|---|---|---|---|---|---|---|---|---|
| **Crystalloid** | | | | | | | | | | |
| Plasma-lyte | 294 | 140 | 98 | 5 | | 3 | | | 7.4 | |
| 0.9% NS | 308 | 154 | 154 | | | | | | 5.7 | 0 |
| 0.45% NS | 154 | 77 | 77 | | | | | | | 0 |
| 3% NS | 1024 | 513 | 513 | | | | | | | 0 |
| 7.5% NS | 2566 | 1283 | 1283 | | | | | | | 0 |
| Lactated Ringer's (LR) | 273 | 130 | 109 | 4 | 2.7 | | 28 | | 6.7 | 0 |
| D5LR | 525 | 130 | 109 | 4 | 2.7 | | 28 | 50 | | 0 |
| D5W | 252 | | | | | | | 50 | 4 | |
| D5NS | 560 | 154 | 154 | | | | | 50 | | |
| D5 0.45%NS | 406 | 77 | 77 | | | | | 50 | | 0 |
| Normosol | 295 | 140 | 98 | 5 | 0 | 3 | | | 7.4 | |
| Mannitol (20%) | 1098 | | | | | | | | | 0 |
| **Colloid** | | | | | | | | | | |
| Hetastarch (6%)in NS | 310 | 154 | 154 | | | | | | 5.5 | 30 |
| Albumin (5%) | 290 | | | | | | | | | 20 |

NS, normal saline
*Lactate in these fluids is converted to bicarbonate.

patient is usually hypovolemic as well as hyponatremic. Release of natriuretic peptides following SAH contributes to the development of CSWS, and the resultant hypovolemia and hyponatremia may exacerbate symptomatic vasospasm. Both atrial natriuretic peptide and B-type natriuretic peptide are acutely elevated after SAH, while the role of C-type natriuretic peptide remains unclear. The appropriate treatment for hyponatremia associated with hypovolemia in patients with SAH is volume replenishment with normal saline and increased salt intake. In symptomatic patients the use of hypertonic saline is warranted, although the rate of correction should not exceed 1–2 mEq/l/h to minimize the risk of development of central pontine myelinolysis. Fludrocortisone is a useful adjunct; it reduces natriuresis and expands intravascular volume.

The use of mannitol can also result in hyponatremia and hypokalemia. In addition, change in serum magnesium and phosphates frequently occur in critically ill patients, necessitating appropriate replacement therapy.

## Pneumonia, Antibiotics and Mechanical Ventilation

Pulmonary complications are common and are a major cause of morbidity and mortality for patients requiring neurointensive care. In one study on patients with SAH, half the deaths attributable to medical causes were pulmonary in origin. Risk of pneumonia appears to peak within the first 3 days (early-onset pneumonia or EOP) and has been found to be associated with trauma and, in non-trauma patients, with a Glasgow Coma Scale (GCS) of less than 9. In this cohort of patients, the organisms responsible for EOP were Staphylococcus aureus (33%), Haemophilus (23%), other gram-positive cocci (22%) and other gram-negative bacilli (19%). A second peak occurred on days 5 and 6; in this group, gram-negative bacilli other than Haemophilus spp. accounted for 45.4% of organisms isolated. EOP appears to be related to aspiration of gastric contents occurring at the time of, or soon after, injury or ictus. Late-onset pneumonia is more likely to be ventilator-associated pneumonia, and caused by organisms which have colonized the airways. Appropriate antibiotic therapy should be guided by systemic manifestations, cultures and sensitivity of organisms. Occasionally, empiric therapy with a broad-spectrum antibiotic is indicated. Daily chest X-ray is important in intubated patients, and broncho-alveolar lavage is indicated in patients not responding to antibiotic therapy or spiking a fever while on antibiotic therapy.

Patients with high cervical spinal cord injury frequently develop acute respiratory failure because of the sudden loss of intercostal muscles. Thus it is not surprising that tracheal intubation and mechanical ventilation are frequently indicated in these patients. Other indications include: depressed level of consciousness, inability to maintain or protect airway, respiratory failure, pneumonia, sepsis and pulmonary edema. Unconscious or obtunded patients are at risk of aspiration and development of pneumonia and adult respiratory distress syndrome (ARDS). In addition, many patients may require intubation and ventilation for imaging or angiography procedures. Pulmonary edema can develop from fluid overload and/or cardiac failure. Neurogenic pulmonary edema can develop in patients with acute traumatic brain injury, SAH or acute cervical spinal cord injury, presumably on the basis of severe sympathetic stress, leading to pulmonary vasoconstriction, with increase in pulmonary vascular permeability and disrupted capillary endothelium. Some patients also develop acute ventricular dysfunction. Although diuretics may be helpful, improvement is mainly dependent on dissipation of the sympathetic stress, and recovery of cardiac function, with or without inotropic support. Placement of a pulmonary artery catheter and echocardiographic examination of the heart is indicated in these patients. Weaning off ventilatory support in neurological patients should be no different from that in other patients. When weaning parameters are met using standard criteria (tidal volume, rapid shallow-breathing index, negative inspiratory pressure), the patient should be extubated. There is no standard method of weaning in these patients, and either intermittent mandatory ventilation or spontaneous continuous positive airway pressure can be used. Extubation should not be delayed because of depressed level of consciousness; the delay results in increased rate of nosocomial pneumonia and prolongs hospital stay.

In patients fulfilling the diagnostic criteria of ARDS, protective lung strategy with small tidal volume, high frequency and low airway pressure is indicated. This may lead to $CO_2$ retention, resulting in cerebral vasodilation and increase in ICP. Optimal management in these patients requires both careful consideration of both organs and a balancing of the relative risks and benefits of protective lung therapy vs high $CO_2$ to arrive at the appropriate strategy.

## Gastrointestinal Complications

Neurological patients are at increased risk of gastrointestinal bleeding or perforation. In one cohort of non-trauma neurosurgical ICU patients, 6.8% had endoscopically or surgically documented evidence of post-operative GI complications. The majority had bleeding, but two patients had both bleeding and perforation. Multivariate analysis suggested five risk factors of independent significance: (1) the presence of SIADH, (2) pre-operative coma, (3) the presence of post-operative complications, (4) age over 60 years, and (5) pyogenic infection of the CNS. Pre-operative coma was the only significant factor to predict the occurrence of life-threatening GI complications. Thus prophylaxis with a proton pump inhibitor or $H_2$ antagonists is routinely indicated in these patients.

Patients on broad-spectrum antibiotics may also develop pseudomembranous colitis, which usually subsides with discontinuation of antibiotic therapy.

## Anticoagulation Prophylaxis

Obtunded neurological patients are at risk of development of deep venous thrombosis (DVT). Unless contraindicated, all patients should be maintained on subcutaneous heparin or low-molecular-weight heparin in addition to compressor stockings. Contraindications include active intracerebral hemorrhage and impending surgery. Post-operatively, it is safe to restart subcutaneous heparin after 48 hours. Doppler ultrasound to rule out DVT in the lower extremities should be performed when indicated.

Pulmonary embolism occurs not infrequently in these patients, and any sudden deterioration in gas exchange or systemic hemodynamics should prompt investigations. Spiral pulmonary CT is a good diagnostic test and, when confirmed, systemic heparinization is indicated. Where this is contraindicated because of intracerebral hemorrhage, placement of a filter in the inferior vena cava is appropriate.

## Nutritional Support

Early nutritional support for critically ill patients is considered important. Specific guidelines have been issued for patients with traumatic brain injury (Brain Trauma Foundation, 2000). In general, enteral feeding via a nasogastric or nasoduodenal tube should commence within 24–48 hours of admission into the ICU. For patients who require long-term nutritional support, percutaneous endoscopic gastrostomy should be performed.

## Seizure Prophylaxis

The presence of intracranial lesions predispose patients to risk of seizures, although the role of seizure prophylaxis is not established for all conditions. Patients with traumatic head injury should be treated with dilantin for 1 week, as prophylaxis is effective for early but not for late post-traumatic seizure disorders. Patients undergoing aneurysm surgery should be maintained on dilantin during the perioperative period. For acute seizures, intravenous lorazepam 0.1 mg/kg or midazolam 0.1–0.15 mg/kg is generally effective. Propofol and thiopental are also effective agents, but their use would generally necessitate tracheal intubation. Phenobarbital or thiopental can be used to control status epilepticus, and dosage should be guided by electroencephalography monitoring as well as by serum levels.

## Temperature Control

Because of the risk of nosocomial infections, fever is very common in patients in the neurointensive care unit. Moreover, patients with neurological illness may have dysfunction of the temperature control mechanism and develop fever without infections. Although the role of hypothermia in neuroprotection remains to be defined, it is generally accepted that hyperthermia is detrimental to neuronal recovery. In addition, it is now recognized that a gradient may exist between body temperature and brain temperature; thus temperature of the brain may be underestimated, increasing the risk of neurological injury. Thus aggressive treatment of fever is warranted.

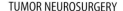
# References

1. Czosnyka M, Smielewski P, Piechnik S, Steiner LA, Pickard JD. Cerebral autoregulation following head injury. J Neurol 2001;95:756–63.
2. Thees C, Scholz M, Schaller MDC, Gass A, Pavlidis C, Weyland A et al. Relationship between intracranial pressure and critical closing pressure in patients with neurotrauma. Anesthesiology 2002;96: 595–9.
3. Coles JP, Minhas PS, Fryer TD, Smielewski P, Aigbirihio F, Donovan T et al. Effect of hyperventilation on cerebral blood flow in traumatic head injury: clinical relevance and monitoring correlates. Crit Care Med 2002;30:1950–9.
4. Diringer MN, Videen TO, Yundt K, Zazulia AR, Aiyagari V, Dacey RG Jr et al. Regional cerebrovascular and metabolic effects of hyperventilation after severe traumatic brain injury. J Neurosurg 2002;96:103–8.
5. Rosengarten B, Ruskes D, Mendes I, Stolz E. A sudden arterial blood pressure decrease is compensated by an increase in intracranial blood volume. J Neurol 2002;249:538–41.
6. Edwards P, Farrell B, Lomas G, Mashru R, Ritchie N, Roberts I et al. The MRC CRASH Trial: study design, baseline data, and outcome in 1000 randomised patients in the pilot phase. Emerg Med J 2002;19:510–14.
7. Bray RJ. Propofol infusion syndrome in children. Paediatr Anaesth 1998;8:491–9.
8. Cremer OL, Moons KG, Bouman EA, Krjijswijk JE, de Smet AM, Kalkman CJ. Long-term propofol infusion and cardiac failure in adult head-injured patients. Lancet 2001;357:117–18.
9. Clifton GL, Miller ER, Choi SC, Levin HS, McCauley S, Smith KR Jr et al. Lack of effect of induction of hypothermia after acute brain injury. N Engl J Med. 2001;344:556–63.
10. Coplin WM. Intracranial pressure and surgical decompression for traumatic brain injury: biological rationale and protocol for a randomized clinical trial. Neurol Res 2001;23:277–90.
11. Georgiadis D, Schwarz S, Baumgartner RW, Veltkamp R, Schwab S. Influence of positive end-expiratory pressure on intracranial pressure and cerebral perfusion pressure in patients with acute stroke. Stroke 2001;32:2088–92.
12. Naredi S, Olivecrona M, Lindgren C, Ostlund AL, Grande PO, Koskinen LO. An outcome study of severe traumatic head injury using the "Lund therapy" with low-dose prostacyclin. Acta Anaesthesiol Scand 2001;45:402–6.
13. Robertson CS. Management of cerebral perfusion pressure after traumatic brain injury. Anesthesiology 2001;95:1513–17.
14. Hutchinson PJ, Gupta AK, Fryer TF, Al-Rawi PG, Chatfield DA, Coles JP et al. Correlation between cerebral blood flow, substrate delivery, and metabolism in head injury: a combined microdialysis and triple oxygen positron emission tomography study. J Cereb Blood Flow Metab 2002;22:735–45.
15. Clifton GL, Miller ER, Choi SC, Levin HS. Fluid thresholds and outcome from severe brain injury. Crit Care Med 2002;30:739–45.

# III

# Techniques

# 6

# Neuroendoscopy

Jonathan Punt

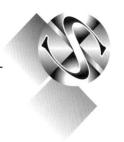

## Summary

Advances in optical technology and in neuroimaging, together with a rising interest in minimally invasive techniques, have resulted in the establishment of modern neuroendoscopy. As with most neurosurgical technologies, there is a regrettable dearth of Class I evidence and, although there are areas in which the benefits appear to be self-evident, this is unsatisfactory. Neuroendoscopic third ventriculostomy is currently the primary treatment of choice for selected cases of non-tumorous and tumorous hydrocephalus; the only demonstrable benefit on present evidence is freedom of complications from implanted devices. There are particular applications in the management of shunt complications, intraventricular and paraventricular tumors, and non-tumorous cysts. The future may bring more sophisticated applications in conjunction with image guidance. Proper training is essential and the technique should probably remain within the hands of a restricted number of specialists. Unstructured propagation is likely to be associated with avoidable morbidity. Prospective studies are required to evaluate the hazards as well as the benefits in comparison with older approaches. Regulatory authorities should monitor morbidity until the position is clear.

## Historical Landmarks

It is interesting to reflect that even 'high-tech' neurosurgery has its origins in the versatile skills and open minds of the earliest neurosurgeons in the first two decades of the last millennium, and that more recent technological advances have enabled latter day pioneers of voyages into the intracranial compartments to venture further and more effectively, creating a renaissance in this elegant therapeutic modality. The history of neuroendoscopy has been described elsewhere [1], and is seen to be a study in miniature of the ways in which techniques wax and wane in surgery, more often riding on the ebb and flow of fashion than on the hard facts of evidence-based science.

In 1910, Lespinasse reported to a Chicago medical society that he had employed rigid cystoscopes to perform choroid plexus ablation on two hydrocephalic infants; one child died post-operatively but the other survived for 5 years. Eighty-four years later, the phrase "minimally invasive endoscopic neurosurgery" was coined.

In 1920, at Massachusetts General Hospital, Mixter performed the first endoscopic third ventriculostomy on a 10-month-old baby, using a urethroscope and a sound. Although follow-up was for less than 1 year, he takes credit for obtaining manometric and dye injection proof of patency of the ventriculostomy. Amongst the few neurosurgeons who persisted with endoscopic neurosurgery, the most notable were Putnam, who persevered with endoscopic choroid plexectomy, and Scarff, who also employed endoscopic third ventriculostomy.

The 1950s saw the advent of the first implantable valved shunting systems for the treatment of hydrocephalus, and inevitably the interest in neuroendoscopy waned. However, even before widespread disenchantment with the fickle nature of hydrocephalus shunts had set in, this first era of neuroendoscopy was marked by important papers by Scarff [2], the results of which are summarized in Table 6.1. An interesting observation was that, whereas when 618 patients treated surgically by choroid plexectomy or third ventriculostomy, without an implanted device, were compared with 1,087 patients treated by a shunt, there were equivalent operative mortalities of about 15% and early success of about 65%, the late complication rates were 3–5% without a shunt but 35–100% with a shunt. This early experience still holds true as, although the early mortality of both types of surgery has fallen, it serves to emphasize that, in discussing the optimum treatment for any particular patient with hydrocephalus, one has to consider not only the acute efficacy and hazard, but also the late morbidity.

Major improvements in visibility came with the solid glass rod endoscope and the cohesive fiberoptic bundle. Vries in the USA, followed by Jones in Australia, Sainte-Rose in France, and the present author in the UK, saw the potential for a return to a neuroendoscopic approach to the treatment of hydrocephalus, while Griffith in the UK also perceived a wider application of neuroendoscopy both within and outside of the ventricular system, coining along the way the term "endoneurosurgery" [1].

# Instrumentation [3]

Modern neuroendoscopic techniques are enabled by, and are dependent upon, purpose-built neuroendoscopes utilizing high-quality optical systems and dedicated instrumentation. Although there are a number of neuroendoscopes available, there are three basic patterns: rigid, flexible and, more recently, the disposable Channel™ neuroendoscopes. The comparative features are detailed in Table 6.2. Individual surgeons will inevitably have their own preferences based upon the usual range of experiences, prejudices, purchasing opportunities and persuasiveness of sales people. However, it is important in selecting neuroendoscopes to consider the use to which they will be put. The most commonly performed intraventricular procedure will always be third ventriculostomy; for some surgeons that may be the only neuroendoscopic operation that they adopt. The superior visibility, ease of use, and simplicity of orientation make a rigid endoscope or the Channel™ neuroendoscope the most frequently employed devices. Although flexible neuroendoscopes are relatively unpopular, they come into their own when procedures are to be performed at two anatomically distinct sites, such as tumor biopsy coupled with third ventriculostomy. Similarly, if there are unusual anatomical conditions such as those encountered in patients with hydrocephalus associated with the dysraphic states or particularly narrow interventricular foramina, then a flexible neuroendoscope may be the only safe and practical choice. This is particularly the case in pediatric practice.

For tumor biopsy, the size of the specimen is important so as to give the neuropathologist the maximum material for diagnosis and to minimize the effects of crush artifact; the

**Table 6.1.** Comparison of surgical treatments for hydrocephalus [2]

|  | CP | NTV | Shunts |
|---|---|---|---|
| *n* | 95 | 529 | 1087 |
| Follow-up (years) | up to 27 | 7.5 (avg) | 2 (avg) |
| Operative mortality | 15% | 15% | 10% |
| Success | 60% | 70% | 60% |
| Adverse late effects | – | 3% | 57% |
| Alive at 5 years | – | 30% | 2% |

CP, choroid plexectomy; NTV, neuroendoscopic third ventriculostomy

**Table 6.2.** Features of neuroendoscopes: rigid vs flexible vs disposable

| Type of endoscope | Advantages | Disadvantages |
|---|---|---|
| Rigid | Excellent optics<br>Ease of use<br>Good instrumentation<br>Durable<br>Relatively inexpensive | Larger size<br>Restricted range of angulation |
| Flexible | Manoeuverable<br>Smaller size | Disorientation<br>More difficult to use<br>Poorer optics<br>Poorer instrumentation<br>Smaller biopsies<br>Fragile<br>Relatively expensive |
| Channel™ (disposable) | Very easy to set up<br>Good optics<br>Relatively small caliber<br>Excellent instrumentation<br>Inexpensive<br>Convenient, safe single use | Restricted range of angulation |

present author finds the generous caliber of biopsy forceps permitted by the Channel™ neuroendoscope to be superior.

The range and quality of adjunctive instrumentation continue to increase, and currently include monopolar and bipolar diathermy, biopsy and grasping forceps, scissors, dissecting hooks, aspirating needles, catheters and inflatable balloons. The laser has advocates, and the author has found the KTP laser (Laserscope UK) to be particularly appropriate to neuroendoscopy. More specialized viewing endoscopes have been developed for endoscope-assisted ventricular shunt insertion and for endoscope-assisted microneurosurgery. A fine malleable endoscope is the most useful adjunct in aneurysm surgery and in some skull-base procedures. For transnasal endoscopic pituitary surgery, the endoscopes and allied instruments used in endoscopic sinus surgery are the most appropriate. An absolute requirement is a competent irrigation system in order to maintain good visibility. There is no evidence that special 'physiological' irrigating fluids are advantageous. The author's practice is to employ normal saline, irrigated under simple pulsed pressure that is operated by a footswitch and passed through a blood warmer.

A camera, a monitor and a fiberoptic light source are required. Ever since the first endoscopic photographs of the living human cerebral ventricles were taken in Philadelphia in 1922, the value and attraction of a photographic record have been recognized. The ability to make good-quality videocassette recordings cannot be overstated. Not only are they useful for training and teaching purposes, but also they are of great value to the surgeon for self-education and improvement on the rather steep learning curve involved. Recordable DVDs are replacing videocassettes.

# Neuroimaging

Cranial ultrasonography can be usefully employed in babies with an open anterior fontanelle. It is extremely operator dependent, but with care, skill and experience it can provide much information on ventricular size and configuration and the relationships between fluid-filled intracranial spaces. Post-operatively, a 5 MHz and color Doppler ultrasonogram can demonstrate CSF flow [4].

Computed tomography (CT) remains the mainstay of much diagnostic imaging in neurosurgery. CT can be used as a satisfactory basis for planning many neuroendoscopic procedures, but there is no doubt that magnetic resonance (MR) is superior because of its multiplanar functionality, the better demonstration of blood vessels, the identification of membranes between fluid-filled spaces, and the ability to detect CSF flow.

A sequence of particular value, which is proprietary to Siemens MR scanners, is "constructive interference in the steady state" (CISS): this is of superior quality in demonstrating structures with one or more interfaces with CSF, such as the floor of the third ventricle, membranes within the ventricular system, and paraventricular cysts and subarachnoid structures [5]. Patients with hydrocephalus in association with the dysraphic states may have very complex ventricular anatomy, which will be best understood if examined by MR with CISS. The avoidance of ionizing radiation, especially in younger patients who may well require repeated imaging, is a further advantage. MR is therefore the modality of choice for pre-operative planning and for post-operative evaluation. Close collaboration and good communication between neurosurgeon, neuroradiologist and neuroradiographer will be rewarded by a more effective analysis of cases and an optimized, and safer, neuroendoscopic approach. Some practitioners have found the employment of intraoperative positive-contrast ventriculography of value in confirming patency of third ventriculostomies.

# Neuroendoscopic Procedures and Applications

The operative interventions in which neuroendoscopy can play a definitive or supportive role can be classified by site and disease into: those within the internal cerebrospinal fluid spaces – principally the cerebral ventricles, those within the brain parenchyma, and those outside the brain in the subarachnoid or subdural spaces or extracranial skull base (Table 6.3).

Although most neuroendoscopic operations are minimally invasive, they should not be regarded as "minor procedures". They should only be undertaken in fully staffed and equipped neurosurgical operating rooms by surgeons who are prepared to proceed to an open operation if necessary. Nursing and resident medical staff must be available for post-operative observation and supervision as for any other intracranial neurosurgical operation. The operations most commonly undertaken relate to the management of hydrocephalus.

**Table 6.3.** Neuroendoscopic indications and procedures

| Anatomical site | Condition | Treatment |
| --- | --- | --- |
| Intraventricular | Hydrocephalus | Primary treatment |
| | | NTV |
| | | Shunt insertion |
| | | Aqueductaplasty |
| | | Choroid plexectomy |
| | | Shunt complications |
| | | NTV |
| | | Shunt liberation |
| | | Marsupialization |
| | | Shunt removal |
| | Tumors | Biopsy |
| | | Removal |
| | Cysts | Marsupialization |
| | | Drainage |
| Parenchymal | Hematomas | Evacuation |
| | Abscesses | Drainage |
| Extracerebral | Subdural collections | Drainage |
| | Aneurysm | Assisted craniotomy & clipping |
| | Skull base tumors | Assisted craniotomy & excision |
| | | Microvascular decompression |
| | | Transnasal excision |

NTV, neuroendoscopic third ventriculostomy

## Neuroendoscopic Third Ventriculostomy (NTV)

NTV can be employed as the primary treatment of hydrocephalus (primary NTV) or as an alternative to shunt revision in the management of shunt complications (secondary NTV). NTV is the most frequently undertaken neuroendoscopic procedure. Ideally, pre-operative MR is acquired to give the necessary anatomical details and to assist in the evaluation for suitability and the operative approach.

Although techniques will differ in detail from one surgeon to another, the principles are fairly constant. The intention is to make an opening in the floor of the third ventricle and thereby create an internal fistula between the ventricular system and the basal subarachnoid spaces. Although the full procedure can best be understood by reference to video clips [3], there are a number of critical technical points that are worthy of attention. Under general orotracheal anaesthesia, the patient is placed supine with mild-to-moderate flexion of the head and neck. A burr hole is placed accurately on, or just anterior to, the coronal suture in the mid-pupillary line. The lateral ventricle is located with a brain cannula, which is then replaced with the neuroendoscope.

Most neuroendoscopes are inserted through a sheath. If a disposable plastic 'peel away' sheath is used, it is best not to peel it apart or fix it to the scalp as the additional mobility afforded by keeping the sheath free can be an advantage. The sheath can be used to direct a flexible neuroendoscope or can be advanced through the interventricular foramen so as to protect its margins. The foramen of Monro is navigated carefully, without damaging the choroid plexus, the thalamo-striate vein or the fornices. The configuration of the foramen of Monro is quite variable. Correct selection of the point at which to incise the floor of the third ventricle is crucial so as to avoid the tip of the basilar artery. Careful attention to this critical vascular relationship on the pre-operative MR is recommended, as there is more anatomical variation than is generally appreciated. The correct site is on the anterior part of the floor of the third ventricle, slightly posterior to the pink vascular area that marks the pituitary infundibulum. Practices and opinions differ as to how best to make the opening. Some surgeons simply perforate the floor with the tip of a rigid endoscope [6]; others use biopsy forceps, diathermy or laser, with or without enlargement of the opening by an inflatable balloon [7]. Beneath the floor of the third ventricle lies Liliequist's membrane; it is variable in extent, and its superior attachment may lie anterior or posterior to the mammillary bodies. In the former case of pre-mammillary attachment, failure to open it may result in ineffective CSF drainage [8].

An opening of at least 4 mm is desirable, and it is advisable to pass the endoscope through the third ventriculostomy into the basal cisterns to confirm that the opening is of adequate proportions and that there is indeed an unencumbered passage into the interpeduncular or prepontine cistern. On withdrawing the endoscope into the third ventricle, an encouraging sign that is likely to presage a successful outcome is a gentle undulation of the margins of the ventriculostomy that is clearly different from the cardiac or respiratory cycle [9]. There is frequently a small amount of bleeding that settles with irrigation. Often, one can observe a progressive spontaneous enlargement of the ventriculostomy over the course of a few minutes. In general it is best to resist the urge to go on a tour of the ventricular system after completing the ventriculostomy, and it is preferable to leave the ventricles fairly plump rather than to aspirate them, so as to encourage flow through the opening.

In patients with neural tube defects, a number of anatomical peculiarities may be encountered. The interventricular foramen is frequently a rather oblique narrow triangle. The massa intermedia may be unusually large, but more significantly there may be an extra commissure running in the sagittal plane above the anterior part of the floor of the third ventricle obscuring the site of the intended ventriculostomy; there may be buckling of the floor of the third ventricle, and there can be multiple basal cistern subarachnoid adhesions. Many of these hurdles can be identified pre-operatively on CISS MR.

In performing a secondary NTV, particular attention should be paid to a variety of anatomical considerations that may make the procedure difficult, more hazardous, or even impossible. The skull can be pathologically thick in those who were shunted primarily in infancy, and can restrict the range of direction of approach when using a rigid neuroendoscope. There may be thick, calcific subdural membranes from past subdural hematomas. The wall of the lateral ventricle may be tough and thick, especially in those patients shunted for perinatal post-hemorrhagic hydrocephalus, those with slit-ventricle syndrome, and those who have suffered ventriculitis. The internal anatomy of the lateral ventricle can be bizarre. There may be synechiae related and unrelated to the presence of a ventricular shunt catheter. The usual landmarks leading to the interventricular foramen may be absent, especially in patients who have suffered intraventricular hemorrhage, or ventriculitis associated with meningitis or serious ventricular shunt infections. On occasion, the lateral ventricles can be subdivided by complete or incomplete septae. The septum pellucidum may be spontaneously perforated or absent. The interventricular foramen may be completely obliterated by gliosis or may have assumed an abnormal configuration. Alternatively, patients with very large lateral ventricles due to chronic shunt malfunction can have very large interventricular foramina that are so huge that the third ventricle is almost assimilated into the lateral ventricle. The third ventricle can also be very abnormal, with gliotic septae obscuring or frankly obstructing the pathways. The cavity of the third ventricle may be narrow.

The usual landmarks on the third ventricle floor may be quite unclear. The anterior part of the floor may be thick and opaque; fortunately, the vascular area that marks the recess of the pituitary infundibulum is usually preserved. The interpeduncular cistern may be densely obliterated by subarachnoid adhesions that may in themselves conceal the basilar artery and its branches and cranial nerves III and VI. Liliequist's membrane may be abnormally thick. The circle of Willis may be in an unusual position. The two most frequent variants are an unusual application of the basilar artery to the dorsum sellae and upper clivus, usually due to subarachnoid scarring, and an abnormal tortuousness of the anterior communicating artery, which may bulge into the anterior part of the third ventricle. Patients with intracranial tumors may have anatomical distortions due to the presence of tumor tissue or the effects of previous surgery and radiation therapy.

Regression of clinical symptoms and avoidance of an implanted diversionary CSF shunt indicate a successful outcome. Routine postoperative imaging is not mandatory. In 60% of cases ventricular size is unchanged despite relief of symptoms; ventricular volume may drop despite ventricular size remaining constant. A flow void through the ventriculostomy on appropriate MR sequences is confirmation of functional patency of the ventriculostomy and correlates with radionuclide studies; flow voids in the interventricular foramina and interpeduncular cistern indicate active CSF flow, but signal in the prepontine cistern alone reflects basilar artery pulsation.

## Results of NTV

One of the longest running and largest series is that accumulated in Sydney, Australia, which extends back to 1978. In a mixed series of 103 children and adults, there was an overall success rate of 61%, with no difference between those undergoing primary, as opposed to secondary, NTV [10]. In a purely adult series from Nottingham, UK, followed for a mean of 3 years, 80% of 63 patients were successfully treated by NTV [11]. In both of these series there was no difference between those having primary NTV and those previously shunted patients undergoing secondary NTV. In an earlier, predominantly pediatric, series from Nottingham, with a median age of 16 months, there was a success rate of 62% [1]. Smaller series have reported much higher success rates, but in highly selected cases. For example, a French center reported 33 successes in 35 previously untreated cases [12]; around 60% would seem to be the overall success rate in unselected cases across all ages. Although there is a wider range of experience for secondary NTV, most reported series from experienced operators report success in 60–80% of cases (Table 6.4). This probably reflects a

**Table 6.4.** Success rate of secondary NTV

| Series | [ref] | n | Success (%) |
|---|---|---|---|
| Jones, 1992 | [6] | 27 | 74 |
| Teo, 1996 | [19] | 54 | 72 |
| Nottingham, 1997 | | 47 | 77 |
| Cinalli, 1998 | [20] | 23 | 78 |
| Hopf, 1999 | [29] | 25 | 84 |
| Nottingham, 2001 | | 88 | 61 |

range of happenstance selection bias. There are, of course, clinical circumstances in which the patient is so dogged by shunt complications that even a relatively low chance of success makes an attempt at secondary NTV justifiable. In general, given the recurrent tendency of shunt complications, it seems reasonable to at least consider secondary NTV in every case of shunt malfunction, as proposed by some practitioners [13]. Such a strategy, adopted by some, does have implications in terms of staff and equipment [1].

Some series have recorded a higher failure rate in the very young (Table 6.5), 16 out of 25 NTVs failing in babies aged under 6 months [10]. This has led some surgeons to regard failure as being age-related to the point that some are most reluctant to use NTV in the first year of life. Although overall success rates of 23% for those undergoing NTV in the first year of life [14], and 32% for those born prematurely [15], have been reported, more recent studies have shown that the outcome relates more to the pathology than to age [1]. For aqueductal stenosis there is no difference in outcome between those aged younger than 6 months and those that are older [16], and success rates of more than 80% for congenital aqueductal stenosis have been achieved [17]. A particularly unfavorable pathology for which primary NTV should probably not be attempted is post-meningitic hydrocephalus. However, the low success rate for this pathology, and also for the unfavorable post-hemorrhagic hydrocephalus, is less marked at a later age, and subsequent secondary NTV for shunt failure is always worth considering [16].

Other patients for whom both primary and secondary NTV is particularly successful are those with midline tumors [18] and those with myelomeningocele [19], with success rates of up to 100% and 80% respectively.

## Neuroendoscopy in the Management of Shunt Complications and Complex Hydrocephalus

Apart from secondary NTV, neuroendoscopy has other contributions to make in the management of shunt malfunction. Firstly, it should not be overlooked that secondary NTV can still be used to provide ventricular drainage following treatment of shunt infections. Most neurosurgeons manage shunt infections by the technique of shunt removal, interval external drainage with antibiotics, and then shunt insertion; the last stage can often be replaced by NTV [1, 20].

Loculation of the cerebral ventricles is a serious complication of intraventricular hemorrhage and infection, which can be the cause of much morbidity and mortality and frustrated neurosurgical endeavor. Although the surgery looks seductively easy on viewing the imaging, the reality is very different – neuroendoscopic deloculation can be one of the most challenging procedures. The absence of normal anatomy, the unexpected thickness and the vascularity of the septa, and the tendency for the operative field to become rapidly like a souvenir of the Eiffel tower in a snowstorm all make for great difficulties. Pre-operative planning should always include MR, preferably with CISS or equivalent sequences. Intraoperative guidance by ultrasound may assist if there is an appropriate sonographic window. Fenestrations should be as large as possible, and certainly greater than 1 cm in diameter. Cutting/coagulating diathermy is the tool of choice. Multiple procedures may be required.

The most dangerous variant is the loculated fourth ventricle. Unfortunately a neuroendoscopic approach is only rarely feasible as the cerebral aqueduct is usually densely occluded

**Table 6.5.** Success rate of NTV in infants

| Series | [ref] | n | Characteristics | Success (%) |
|---|---|---|---|---|
| Jones, 1994 | [10] | 25 | Age <2 years | 32 |
| Teo, 1996 | [19] | 11 | Myelomeningoceles | 9 |
| Buxton, 1998 | [14] | 27 | Age <1 year | 23 |
| Buxton, 1998 | [15] | 19 | Prematures | 32 |
| Hopf, 1999 | [29] | 4 | Age <1 year | 0 |
| Javadpour, 2001 | [17] | 21 | Age <1 year | 48 |

over most of its length. Occasionally there may be a simple membrane, division of which will restore communication between the third and the fourth ventricles. Again, MR with CISS is invaluable in defining the anatomy.

Neuroendoscopy can also be useful for liberating ventricular shunt catheters, either to make their removal safer, or as a definitive procedure if secondary NTV is not feasible [13]. It can be used to retrieve loose shunt components. This is also a situation in which cutting/coagulating diathermy is most useful to cut down on the ventricular catheter, just as would be done in dissecting out the extracranial portion of a shunt.

Slit-ventricle syndrome is another most unpleasant shunt complication in which neuroendoscopy may play a useful role. An initial subtemporal decompression may be effective in promoting sufficient ventricular enlargement to permit secondary NTV. Alternatively, patients may undergo shunt externalization, followed by a period of invasive intracranial pressure monitoring without CSF drainage, with those showing elevated or symptomatic intracranial hypertension then proceeding to NTV. The risk of acute deterioration mandates very careful observation.

The small ventricular size and relatively non-compliant ventricles do bring a risk of life-threatening cardiac dysrhythmias during NTV, so great care needs to be taken when irrigating.

## Neuroendoscopy in the Management of Non-tumorous Cysts

Neurodevelopmental arachnoid cysts in suprasellar, quadrigeminal, middle cranial fossa, interhemispheric septum pellucidum, and parenchymal locations have all been approached neuroendoscopically. The guiding principle is to marsupialize the cyst into an adjacent normal cerebrospinal fluid chamber or pathway. Pre-operative MR with CISS is again enormously helpful in planning an approach by displaying the fluid/cyst wall/fluid interfaces in three orthogonal planes. The next important principle is, wherever possible, to approach the lesion via a normal cerebrospinal fluid space or chamber. Even if this space is smaller than the cyst, the advantage of having some normal, and hopefully recognizable, anatomy greatly

exceeds the perceived difficulty in entering a space that may not be particularly dilated. Generous fenestrations of 1–2 cm are required, and are best made using cutting/coagulating diathermy. Suprasellar cysts are approached by the right frontal route to the lateral ventricle, and then via the interventricular foramen. The dome of the cyst is widely opened into the ventricular system (cysto-ventriculostomy) and the cyst then usually collapses, exposing the hitherto obstructed posterior third ventricle and aqueduct. There is debate as to whether the base of the cyst should then be opened into the interpeduncular cistern (cysto-cisternostomy) [12].

The author's approach is to perform both cysto-ventriculostomy and cysto-cisternostomy if the latter seems safe. However, if the area is very vascular, such that there is no very apparent safe route, then a generous cysto-ventriculostomy usually suffices. Quadrigeminal plate cysts can usually be opened into the third ventricle by an approach via the lateral ventricle and interventricular foramen, although on occasion there is an interface presenting into a lateral ventricle that can be accessed. Intraparenchymal cysts can often be marsupialized into a lateral ventricle. Other midline cysts may be made to communicate with the ventricular system or the subarachnoid space. Symptomatic cysts of the septum pellucidum may be approached via a lateral ventricle. If the cyst is punctured directly, the very different anatomy will warn the surgeon of the position and, with care regarding the midline vascular structures and the fornices, the cyst can be marsupialized into the third ventricle. Many of these cysts will require unique approaches and directions of attack that are not along straight lines; it is in this type of case that the flexible neuroendoscope really comes into its own and has considerable advantages over a rigid instrument. On occasion, small intraventricular third ventricle cysts of presumed ependymal origin, unsuspected from pre-operative imaging, have come to light in the course of performing a NTV; these can be readily opened up to relieve the hydrocephalus.

The place of neuroendoscopy in the management of colloid cysts of the third ventricle remains uncertain. Early reports concerned diagnostic rather than therapeutic interventions [1]. Subsequently it became clear that some colloid cysts could be dealt with endoscopically, and encouraging single-center reports continue to appear [21]. The debate tends to center on safety issues and the ability to achieve complete resection. Proponents of endoscopy, image-guided stereotactic drainage, and open micro-surgical resection continue to maintain their respective corners. These lesions are best tackled with a rigid or disposable Channel™ neuroendoscope because of the superior visualization and better instrumentation. As always, the direction and line of approach is all important; a pre-frontal entry point is required so as to be able to access the roof of the third ventricle and deal with the origin of the cyst. Dense solid cysts will continue to pose problems by any route other than an open transcallosal approach but, happily, are in the minority. The matter is clearly not going to be resolved without a randomized prospective study.

## Management of Intracranial Tumors

Certain intraventricular and paraventricular tumors can be approached endoscopically via dilated ventricles. One of the pioneering applications of the flexible neuroendoscope was in this field, and both pineal region and paraventricular tumors were biopsied through custom-made, flexible, fiberoptic neuroendoscopes. Interestingly, the authors of these papers did not consider the possibility of performing a concurrent NTV to relieve hydrocephalus.

The success rate for biopsy was low for those tumors that were not actually in the ventricular system, and this was attributed to the small size of the biopsies. Other problems are that many paraventricular tumors are still separated from the ventricular system by an intact layer of ependyma that must be breached if tumor tissue is to be obtained [3]. The relatively small size of the tissue samples is compounded by crush artifact. This is a particular problem with the flexible neuroendoscope and, wherever possible, a rigid or disposable Channel™ neuroendoscope is preferable because of the larger size of biopsy obtainable. One successful technique is to use a stereotactic biopsy needle passed though the endoscope (J. Firth, personal communication). In view of the age-related predilection for sites on and adjacent to the midline, neuroendoscopy has a considerable role in the management of pediatric brain tumors. The value of neuroendoscopy is not confined to children, and in a Nottingham series of 87 procedures in 77 patients, age ranged from 5 months to 70 years [18]. Relief of hydrocephalus by NTV remains a principal indication with a high level of success: 63 out of 66 cases (95%) in the short term, with durable shunt-free outcome in 55 out of 66 cases (83%). Neuroendoscopic tumor biopsies were successful in providing a tissue diagnosis in 17 out of 29 cases (61%) [18]. A very particular application is in pineal region tumors, in which there is the possibility of delivering "one-stop" neurosurgery that provides relief of hydrocephalus, tumor biopsy and cerebrospinal fluid sampling for tumor cytology and biochemical evaluation of germ-cell tumor markers.

Very high diagnostic accuracy has been documented [22]; under these circumstances there can be no justification in performing an open operation for pineal germ-cell tumors unless committed efforts have first been made to make the diagnosis by these alternative means. It has been stated that NTV is contraindicated in those patients who have undergone radiation therapy, both on the grounds of inefficacy and risk of complications [6]; this has not been the experience of the present author. NTV can be successfully used to relieve hydrocephalus due to posterior fossa tumors [18]. The ideal timing is yet to be defined; in patients with very chronic or massive hydrocephalus, there is a case for leaving an interval of a few days between NTV and definitive posterior fossa exploration. As a relatively small proportion of patients with hydrocephalus in association with a posterior fossa tumor will require a ventricular shunt following tumor resection, it is difficult to justify the routine performance of NTV in such cases, and it might be appropriate to reserve the procedure for those at greatest risk of persistent hydrocephalus, such as children under 5 years of age. The optimum strategy is yet to be established. However, when NTV is performed there is the added value of being able to inspect the ventricular system for possible metastases, to take samples of cerebrospinal fluid for tumor cytology, and, if a flexible neuroendoscope is used, to pass through the cerebral aqueduct and inspect the relationship of the tumor to the floor of the fourth ventricle.

Resection of intraventricular and parenchymal tumors remains a relatively infrequent practice owing to the limiting factors of hemorrhage, deteriorating visibility, length of operation and the limited range of available instruments.

A dual-portal approach has been piloted that uses one channel for illumination and visualization, and the other for the passage of instruments; complete resection was achieved in five out of six patients, one case being abandoned in favor of open operation due to hemorrhage [23]. Although there was no immediate reported morbidity, the potential hazards of multiple cortical punctures were a cause for concern. Extensive endoscopic resection of deep-seated parenchymal brain tumors has remained the practice of a very small number of committed neurosurgeons, often using highly sophisticated image-guided stereotaxy and laser ablation, or ultrasound guidance. Notwithstanding the high level of skill and elegance involved, the absence of any randomized trial data regarding disease-free remission or survival makes it difficult to evaluate and define the role of this technology in tumor management.

## Treatment of Non-tumorous Parenchymal Brain Lesions

The marriage of image-guided stereotactic localization with neuroendoscopy can be used to maximize evacuation of pus from intracerebral abscesses. However, a second procedure is often needed [24].

Endoscopic evacuation of intracerebral hematomas is also possible, and although one randomized study of drainage of subcortical hematomas in patients aged under 60 years with preserved consciousness suggested an advantage over best medical treatment, this is yet to be confirmed in larger trials [25].

## Endoscope-assisted Procedures

The development of small-caliber rigid endoscopes and malleable endoscopes has facilitated the marriage between neuroendoscopy and microneurosurgery. The overriding principles are to use the endoscope to bring light into the operative field, and to enable alternative lines of sight. Simultaneous images through the microscope and through the endoscope can be displayed on a single monitor. Particular applications are: the improved application of aneurysm clips, access to skull base tumors, microvascular decompression of the trigeminal and facial nerves through very minimal access approaches, and transsphenoidal pituitary surgery [26]. For those surgeons able to cope with the simultaneous integration of so much technology, and who can find space in the operating room for the additional equipment, the rewards do seem substantial in terms of enhanced visualization and accuracy.

## Complications

When the author introduced neuroendoscopy into the Nottingham neurosurgical department, he was concerned to register both outcomes and complications, not only for the purposes of scientific inquiry, but also to enable accurate data to be available to inform discussions with patients and colleagues when reaching decisions in management. The resultant purpose-built database "ENDOSPREAD" contained, in anticipation, a list of possible complications plus space for any unique or unexpected ones (Table 6.6)!

There was therefore some concern that, until relatively recently, there was an apparent dearth of reports regarding complications, despite word-of-mouth anecdotes of such momentous events as basilar artery injuries either requiring formal surgical repair or having fatal outcomes. Even stranger was that reports were not appearing of those that were successfully repaired. Following a number of verbal communications at international meetings, at which it became clear that very major complications of NTV – principally of a vascular nature – were not being reported, the ice finally broke [27]. These papers, from an extremely experienced leader in the field, served to acknowledge and define the position. The author's distinction between significant and insignificant complications was a helpful one, in that it provided a matrix and a benchmark for further analysis. In 173 procedures over a 2-year period, there was an incidence of 22 intraoperative events (13%); 7% of the patients suffered a significant complication. Insignificant complications are those such as

**Table 6.6.** Complications of neuroendoscopy (as coded & recorded in "ENDOSPREAD")

```
1 Intraoperative hemorrhage – operation abandoned
2 Intraoperative hemorrhage – operation continued
3 Hemorrhage – intraventricular
4 Hemorrhage – intracerebral
5 Hemorrhage – subdural
6 Hemorrhage – extradural
7 Infection – deep
8 Infection – superficial
9 Cranial nerve lesion – transient
10 Cranial nerve lesion – persistent
11 Neurological impairment – transient
12 Neurological impairment – persistent
13 CSF fistula – transient, requiring no more than suture
14 CSF fistula – persistent
15 Novel epilepsy <7 days from operation
16 Novel epilepsy >7 days from operation
17 Exacerbation of epilepsy <7 days from operation
18 Exacerbation of epilepsy >7 days from operation
19 Neuroendocrine – transient
20 Neuroendocrine – persistent
21 Cerebral infarct – asymptomatic
22 Cerebral infarct – symptomatic
23 ICU admission post-operatively
24 Death within 30 days of operation
25 EVD inserted – intraoperatively
26 EVD inserted – post-operatively
27 Intraoperative cardiac event
```

EVD, external ventricular drain

**Table 6.7.** The frequent or serious complications of neuroendoscopy

**Intraoperative complications**
Intraoperative hemorrhage causing procedure to be abandoned
Traumatic cerebral artery aneurysm
Intracerebral hematoma
Life-threatening cardiac dysrhythmias
Transient bradycardia
Transient hypertension

**Post-operative complications**
Death within 6 weeks
Cerebral infarction
New cranial nerve palsy
New neurological deficit
Subdural collections
CSF leak
Meningitis or ventriculitis
Superficial infection
Epilepsy
Hypothalamic damage

minor intraoperative bleeding that stops with irrigation and does not compromise the patient or the procedure. Significant ones are those that do, or might, have serious or lasting sequelae for the patient. It must be acknowledged that, whilst defining these categories is useful to the surgeon, in the mind of patients and families even a relatively small event such as a transient leakage of cerebrospinal fluid that resolves with a single suture is a cause for concern. Whereas the incidence of insignificant complications declined with experience, the occurrence of significant ones did not. The most frequent and the most serious complications are listed in Table 6.7.

Of some concern are reports of what appear to be sudden and unexpected deaths in patients who have undergone NTV. It is unclear whether these were truly without prodrome or whether the patients had been lulled into a sense of false security following successful NTV, and simply failed to seek medical attention when headaches or even visual symptoms recurred. They may therefore have been in no different a situation to the patient with a shunt who becomes a victim of failed follow-up.

# Strategies for Reducing Complications

The risk of damage to the basilar artery and its branches and to cranial nerves can be minimized by careful attention to: the local anatomy on pre-operative imaging; care in selecting a point on the floor of the third ventricle that is just posterior to the infundibular recess, rather than just anterior to the mammillary bodies; and a cautious technique for opening the floor of the third ventricle. It is worth reiterating that the only constant feature on the anterior third-ventricle floor is the pink, vascular area signaling the infundibular recess. The mammillary bodies in the first few months of life are surprisingly flat, and may only be identified by the very small whisker-like arteries running over them; the surface of the ventricular floor may be featureless or scarred as a result of previous infection or hemorrhage, or distorted by tumor invasion. Although a very fine ultrasound probe has been of value in identifying a 'safe', sonically silent area, the technology is very expensive and has not been generally adopted, even in specialist departments. There are strongly held views regarding the relative safety or otherwise of different instruments and methods for perforating the floor.

The argument against using laser or diathermy is the perceived risk of vascular damage, but no study has demonstrated an advantage in terms of either efficacy or safety for any particular method. The absence of any reporting system for adverse events, beyond individual personal or institutional systems, makes any such opinion difficult to confirm, but it is probably wise to keep any use of diathermy to a minimum, and to ensure that it is always used under direct vision. Similar strictures relate to the methods used for enlarging the opening. The most widely used is probably the balloon catheter, and as long as care is taken, it may well be safer than diathermy. Blunt hooks, as can be used through a disposable Channel™ neuroendoscope, appear to be safe and are most intuitive to the neurosurgeon, especially in the subarachnoid space. A sensible precaution would seem to be the practice of starting with a small, centrally placed opening and then looking through it into the space below the floor to check on position and the presence or absence of second membrane, adhesions, vessels or tumor. This will be easier to accomplish with a flexible neuroendoscope or a Channel™ neuroendoscope than with most rigid neuroendoscopes. The only safe rule is to abandon the procedure if the anatomy is not clear.

Throughout, the surgeon must be mindful regarding the irrigation, ensuring that there is easy egress of irrigate; with flexible and disposable Channel™ neuroendoscopes, the route of escape of the irrigate is between the endoscope and the inner wall of the plastic cannula. It is not difficult to allow the cannula to slip out of the ventricle, under which circumstance there will be no way for irrigate to escape.

At moments of high tension the surgeon may inadvertently pinch the plastic cannula, occluding it, allowing irrigate to accumulate in the ventricles with resultant rise in intracranial pressure. This will be particularly dangerous if the neuroendoscope is within the narrow confines of the third ventricle. Such circumstances can cause cardiac dysrhythmias, especially if the ventricular walls are stiff.

Whereas it is always tempting to take a wander through the ventricular system, especially with a flexible neuroendoscope, the surgeon should avoid the enticement of 'ventricular tourism' (with acknowledgement to Professor Christian Sainte-Rose) and withdraw from the operative scene. The cerebral ventricles should be left full so as to encourage flow through the NTV. Attention to the wound and its closure is worthwhile: in babies and infants with thinner, less well developed scalp tissues, the author now uses a small scalp flap of the size that would be used for insertion of a ventriculostomy reservoir, thus avoiding having a scalp incision directly over the dural incision. Formal closure of the dura is said to help eliminate cerebrospinal fluid leakage (G. Cinalli, personal communication), and the scalp is closed in layers.

The anesthetist must concentrate on the monitoring, and must be alert to the possibility of cardiovascular changes and the need to report them immediately to the surgeon.

A pilot study employing sophisticated statistical analysis failed to show any increased risk of epilepsy in children undergoing NTV [28].

# Training

Neuroendoscopy carries a steep learning curve and involves the acquisition of a variety of novel skills, including those relating to: the selection of patients; the imaging; the operating room set-up; the equipment; the practice of operating from a monitor with only two-dimensional images; working in close concert with an assistant; and being alive to a number of parameters that have to be monitored. There are also a number of hard-learned tips that are better assimilated in advance, rather than re-discovered anew.

Neuroendoscopy also lends itself to workshop training. In recognition of this, a number of 'hands-on' courses have been established, such as those in Mainz, Germany; St Louis, USA; and London, England. From the time that the author first established the Nottingham neuroendoscopy course, now held at the Royal College of Surgeons of England, London, it has been apparent from personal feedback that participants have benefited from attendance. It has been of particular significance when some senior neurosurgeons have decided that neuroendoscopy is not for them. Complementary to training workshops and in-service training with an established practitioner is the possibility of gaining experience by proxy from libraries of video clips on CD-ROM [3]. The development of computer 'virtual' surgery training will be of value, and is under development in Aalborg, Denmark (J. Haase, personal communication).

# Research and Future Directions

## Research Questions in Neuroendoscopy

The modern era of neuroendoscopy encapsulates some of the lessons to be learnt about the introduction of new technology, especially when it is suggested that it may replace existing methods. The natural enthusiasm of the surgeon to be amongst the first to offer the patient an alternative that may be 'better' runs hard on the commercial keenness of the salespeople to sell new and expensive kit. In some cultures and health systems, the ability to provide the latest facility may impact upon the income of the surgeon. In other societies, those who fund the purchase of new equipment may hide behind a pretend shield of "Where's the proof?" as a means of preventing progress. Meanwhile, those who are in a position to introduce the new technology do so, accumulate and present results, and begin to assume fixed positions regarding the value of the "new way". By this time it is probably too late in practical, though not in ethical, economic or scientific terms to run the studies that would be needed to seek the evidence in favor, or against. This is particularly so when existing methods are less than perfect, as is the case with hydrocephalus shunts.

So, is NTV "better" than a shunt? There are many who think so, including the present author, based simply upon the premise that shunts are vicarious, and that to be without the risk, or the actuality, of the misery of their complications is a better position in which to live one's life. Whether NTV is a better treatment per se for the hydrocephalic brain, complications of therapy aside, is not known.

One non-randomized, retrospective study comparing 30 children treated by NTV with 38 treated by ventriculo-peritoneal shunts found no difference between the two groups in neurological, endocrine, behavioral or social outcome [7]. As our aspirations for our patients become greater, it is appropriate that studies should be established to identify which method of treatment is better for the young brain in terms of neurodevelopment, and for the adult brain in terms of neuropsychological function.

For some categories of very young patient the success rate for NTV is low, but the complication rate of shunts is also high; a randomized study here would also be appropriate.

It is not known whether the apparently good results published from centers in which there are acknowledged experts in neuroendoscopy can extend to a whole population of neurosurgeons and their patients, yet this is a crucial point if advice is to be given on a national or international basis. A prospective study capturing all patients treated by NTV needs to look at this wider picture. With the concerns regarding complications, this could be matched with a central registry of adverse events. It is noteworthy, as an observation only, albeit not capable of analysis, that in Nottingham in an early study of 47 children and young people undergoing 51 secondary NTVs, there were only three significant complications (6%) [1]; yet in a series extending into a later epoch, of 63 adults undergoing 66 NTVs, there was a total complication rate of 17.5%, with an 11% serious complication rate [11].

Without any imputation, one operational change that occurred between the earlier study and the one including later patients was that the number of surgeons performing NTV rose from three consultants to six consultants plus a number of supervised trainees. This may mean nothing, but the question still needs to be asked as to whether this is a technique that can be pursued safely by all surgeons, or whether it should be subject to sub-specialization.

There are certain specific applications of NTV that could be addressed in prospective studies, e.g. the value of "routine" NTV in children with posterior fossa tumors, or the efficacy of NTV in treating syringomyelia when that condition is associated with ventriculomegaly.

With regards to other neuroendoscopic procedures, there is a clear place for a randomized study of endoscopic vs open resection of third-ventricle colloid cysts.

These study proposals will require multi-center collaborative studies. An encouraging start was made by Professor Bernhard Bauer (Hanover, Germany) and Professor Shizuo Oi (Tokyo, Japan) when they inaugurated the International Study Group on Neuroendoscopy (ISGNE) in Hyogo, Japan, in October 2001.

## Future Developments

The major requirements are in the fields of instrumentation and guidance. The present armamentarium could usefully be expanded to enable better methods of lifting and incising tissues. Methods of image enhancement should be brought to bear so as to increase the information available from images obtained, especially with fiberoptic neuroendoscopes.

Concerns regarding transmissible disease are likely to grow, such that there will be demands for completely disposable instrumentation; the neuroendoscope designers and manufacturers should anticipate this need. Although several surgeons have found a useful dialogue between neuronavigation and neuroendoscopy, the present position is far from ideal, and there is a need for real-time intraoperative neuronavigation that would enable more accurate localization when dealing with complex anatomy. All of these developments will require a closer working relationship between the surgeons and the companies involved.

## Acknowledgements

The author wishes to record the generosity of the following, whose fund-raising efforts enabled the establishment of neuroendoscopy at Nottingham University Hospital: the late Anthony Ozolins and his family, the family of the late Helen Ringrose, and the family of the late Emma Clayton.

## Copyright Warning

## Key Points

- *Advances in optical technology and in neuroimaging have resulted in the establishment of neuroendoscopy – a minimally invasive technique.*
- *There is a dearth of Class I evidence of the benefits and risks of this technique.*
- *Neuroendoscopic third ventriculostomy is currently the primary treatment of choice for selected cases of non-tumorous and tumorous hydrocephalus.*
- *The only demonstrable benefit on present evidence is freedom of complications from implanted devices.*
- *There are particular applications in the management of shunt complications, intraventricular and paraventricular tumors, and non-tumorous cysts.*
- *Proper training is essential and the technique should probably remain within the hands of a restricted number of specialists.*
- *Unstructured propagation is likely to be associated with avoidable morbidity.*
- *Regulatory authorities should monitor morbidity until the position is clear.*
- *Prospective studies are required to evaluate the hazards as well as the benefits in comparison with older approaches.*
- *The future may bring more sophisticated applications in conjunction with image guidance.*

## References

1. Punt J, Vloeberghs M. Endoscopy in neurosurgery. Minim Invasive Ther & Allied Technol 1998;7:159–70.
2. Scarff JE. Evaluation of treatment of hydrocephalus. Report of third ventriculostomy and endoscopic

cauterization of choroid plexuses compared with mechanical shunts. Arch Neurol 1966;14:382–91.

3. Punt J, Vloeberghs M, Terrett M. An introduction to neuroendoscopy. A computer based tutorial system on CD-ROM. Nottingham: HyperTech/2nd Messenger, 1996.

4. Wilcock DJ, Jaspan T, Punt J, Kwok BCT. CSF flow through third ventriculostomy demonstrated with colour Doppler ultrasonography. Clin Radiol 1996; 51:127–9.

5. Laitt RD, Mallucci CL, McConachie NS, Jaspan T, Vloeberghs M, Punt J. Constructive interference in steady state 3D Fourier Transform MRI in the management of hydrocephalus and third ventriculostomy. Neuroradiology 1999;41:324–7.

6. Jones RFC, Teo C, Stening WA et al. Neuroendoscopic third ventriculostomy. In: Manwaring KH, Crone KR, Dante MD, editors. Neuroendoscopy, 1st edn New York: Liebert; 1992; 63–77.

7. Sainte-Rose C. Third Ventriculostomy. In: Manwaring KH, Crone KR, Dante MD, editors. Neuroendoscopy. 1st edn. New York: Liebert; 1992; 47-62.

8. Buxton N, Vloeberghs M, Punt J. Liliequist's membrane in minimally invasive endoscopic neurosurgery. Clin Anat 1998;11(3):187–90.

9. Jones RFC, Kwok BC, Stening WA, Vonau M. The current status of endoscopic third ventriculostomy in the management of non-communicating hydrocephalus. Minim Invasive Neurosurg 1994;37(1):28–36.

10. Jones RFC, Kwok BCT, Stening WA, Vonau M. Neuroendoscopic third ventriculostomy. A practical alternative to extracranial shunts in non-communicating hydrocephalus. Acta Neurochir Suppl 1994; 61:79–83.

11. Buxton N, Ho KJ, Vloeberghs M, Macarthur D, Punt J, Robertson I. Neuroendoscopic third ventriculostomy for hydrocephalus in adults: report of a single unit's experience with 63 cases. Surg Neurol 2001;55:74–8.

12. Decq P, Yepes C, Anno Y, Djindjian M, Nguyen JP, Keravel Y. L'endoscopie neurochirurgicale. Indications diagnostiques et therapeutiques. Neurochirurgie 1994; 40(5):313–21.

13. Mallucci C, Vloeberghs M, Punt J. Neuroendoscopic third ventriculostomy: the first-line treatment for blocked ventriculo-peritoneal shunts? Child's Nerv Syst 1997;13:498.

14. Buxton N, Macarthur D, Mallucci C, Punt J, Vloeberghs M. Neuroendoscopic third ventriculostomy in patients less than one year old. Pediatr Neurosurg 1998;29:73–6.

15. Buxton N, Macarthur D, Mallucci C, Punt J, Vloeberghs M. Neuroendoscopy in the premature population. Child's Nerv Syst 1998;14:649–52.

16. Cinalli G, Saint-Rose C, Chumas P, Zerah M, Brunelle F, Lot G et al. Failure of third ventriculostomy in the treatment of aqueductal stenosis in children. J Neurosurg 1999;90:448–54.

17. Javadpour M, Mallucci C, Brodbelt A, Golash A, May P. The impact of endoscopic third ventriculostomy on the management of newly diagnosed hydrocephalus in infants. Pediatr Neurosurg 2001;35:131–5.

18. Macarthur DC, Buxton N, Punt J Vloeberghs M, Robertson IJA. The role of neuroendoscopy in the management of brain tumours. Br J Neurosurg 2002;16:465–70.

19. Teo C, Jones R. Management of hydrocephalus by endoscopic third ventriculostomy in patients with myelomeningocele. Pediatr Neurosurg 1996;25(2): 57–63.

20. Cinalli G, Salazar C, Mallucci C, Yada JZ, Zerah M, Sainte-Rose C. The role of endoscopic third ventriculostomy in the management of shunt malfunction. Neurosurgery 1998;43:1323–9.

21. Longatti P, Martinuzzi A, Moro M, Fiorindi A, Cartieri A. Endoscopic treatment of colloid cysts of the third ventricle: 9 consecutive cases. Minim Invasive Neurosurg 2000;43(3):118–23.

22. Pople IK, Athanasiou TC, Sandeman DR, Coakham HB. The role of endoscopic biopsy and third ventriculostomy in the management of pineal region tumours. Br J Neurosurg 2001;15:305–11.

23. Jallo GI, Morota N, Abbott R. Introduction of a second working portal for neuroendoscopy. A technical note. Pediatr Neurosurg 1996;24:56–60.

24. Hellwig D, Bauer BL, Dauch WA. Endoscopic stereotactic treatment of brain abscesses. Acta Neurochir Suppl 1994;61:102–5.

25. Auer LM, Deinsberger W, Niederkorn K, Gell G, Kleinert R, Schneider G et al. Endoscopic surgery versus medical treatment for spontaneous intracerebral hematoma: a randomized study. J Neurosurg 1989;70: 530–5.

26. Grotenhuis JA. Endoscope-assisted microneurosurgery – a concise guidebook. Nijmegen: Machaon, 1998.

27. Teo C, Rahman S, Boop FA. Complications of neuroendoscopic neurosurgery. Child's Nerv Syst 1996;12(5): 248–53.

28. Svendsen F, Bassi S, Punt J. Seizures after neuroendoscopic third ventriculostomies. Child's Nerv Syst 2002;18:259.

29. Hopf NJ, Grunert P, Fries G, Resch KDM, Perneczky A. Endoscopic third ventriculostomy: outcome analysis of 100 consecutive procedures. Neurosurgery 1999; 44(4):795–806.

# 7

# Principles and Practice of Image-guided Neurosurgery

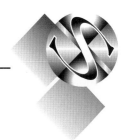

Kristian Aquilina, Philip Edwards and
Anthony Strong

## Summary

Image-guided neurosurgery depends on the registration of pre-operatively acquired images with the physical space of the patient on the operating table. With the aid of a computer workstation and a tracking device, the neurosurgeon is able to obtain a three-dimensional, visual, real-time image of a registered probe in relation to the patient's anatomy and pathology. Image guidance facilitates localization of target structures and their anatomical relations and allows the pre-operative planning of the ideal, minimal risk, trajectory. It has become a useful tool in the surgical management of intracranial tumors and has also been applied to arteriovenous malformations, pericallosal aneurysms, epilepsy surgery, intracranial endoscopy and spinal surgery. The principal problem is the system's dependence on pre-operatively acquired images; perioperative updating of these images by perioperative magnetic resonance imaging overcomes this difficulty.

## Introduction

No neurosurgeon needs to be reminded of the challenge posed by the need to identify and localize accurately structures on the brain surface and within the brain that are critical for neurological function, and which may be indistinguishable visually from adjacent, non-critical structures. Indeed, perhaps a frequent – but usually unspoken – question from a patient to their surgeon is: "How are you going to find your way around in there?". The practice of safe and effective neurosurgery rightly places increasing emphasis on the need to minimize risk. Reliable navigation in and around the brain, and the localization of surgical targets, are important contributions to the achievement of this goal.

A variety of technical approaches are available to the surgeon, and although much developmental work has taken place in several centers, involving collaborations between physicists, software engineers and surgeons, the commercial market has matured recently. Surgeons have some degree of choice of systems and technical solutions, and have a duty to understand both the nature of the procedures that contribute to neuronavigation, and the factors that determine reliability and accuracy. It is also important that evolution of the technology is driven not by technical advances but by specifications influenced primarily by surgeons.

In this chapter we shall set out the principles and methodological approaches that underlie the concept of image-guided neurosurgery, review and assess the state of development of applications to specific surgical procedures, and briefly consider potential future developments.

We believe that the term "stereotaxy" should be confined strictly to procedures in which a stereotactic frame is used, and that the term "image-guided neurosurgery" is a much more appropriate description of the subject; thus "frameless stereotaxy" is inappropriate, not least because it implies a degree of accuracy that is available only in frame-based systems.

# Methodological Approaches

In this section we will describe the standard methodology of alignment of images to the patient on the operating table, and consider the factors affecting accuracy and performance of image-guided surgery systems. Finally we provide a set of principles by which neuronavigation systems can be evaluated and compared.

## Statement of the Problem

In conventional surgery pre-operative images are largely used for diagnosis only and are present in theater only as a series of slices on a light-box. The positional relationship between these images and the patient's anatomy is established only in the mind of the surgeon. The three-dimensional nature of modern imaging techniques (e.g. MRI and CT) is under-utilized in such a scenario.

The aim of image-guided surgery is to align the 3D pre-operative images to the patient on the operating table and to present the accurately aligned image data to the surgeon in a manner that aids navigation. The technical problem can be stated as follows. We have accurate 3D information about patient anatomy and pathology from pre-operative scans. We wish to establish a correspondence between the image data and the physical space of the patient in order to present the surgeon with well-aligned anatomical information using a suitable visualization scheme.

## Method

In order to align pre-operative images to the patient on the operating table, it is first neces-

sary to define a physical coordinate system with respect to the patient. In frame-based methods, these coordinates are defined by the arc system on the frame itself, whereas in image-guided neurosurgery a coordinate measuring device is used. Various technologies have been proposed for this purpose, including mechanical arms, radiofrequency transmitter/receiver coils, ultrasound spark gaps and optical trackers. We will consider the relative merits of these devices in the next section.

Having defined a physical coordinate system in theater, the problem is now to align the pre-operative images to the patient in order to present the surgeon with image data that correspond to the patient's anatomy. This is achieved by identifying corresponding features in the pre-operative images and on the surface of the patient. These features will generally be landmarks, but may also include the skin surface or, as the operation proceeds, bone surface. The process of establishing correspondence between the image and the patient is termed "registration".

### Defining the Patient Coordinates

#### Stereotactic Frames

Frame-based stereotactic neurosurgery has been an established clinical routine since the 1950s. Here, the patient coordinate system is defined by an arc device that attaches to the frame. The frame carries high-contrast imaging markers and is rigidly bolted to the patient's skull prior to imaging. An entry and target point is defined in the images, and the arc angles are calculated to achieve this trajectory according to the manufacturer's instructions. The bulky and somewhat invasive nature of such frames has limited their application. Since only a target and trajectory can be defined, frames are generally used only for biopsies or placement of electrodes or cannulae. They are widely regarded as highly accurate, though some studies have suggested that the accuracy may be overstated [1].

#### Mechanical Arms

The first frameless neuronavigation device to be widely used was the "Faro Arm", a mechanical device that attaches to the side of the table. Encoders on each of the axes of the arm enable calculation of the tip position. Problems with such a device are that the range of movement is somewhat limited, that any movement of the head clamp requires re-registration, and that the inherent accuracy was found to be somewhat lower than that of other methods. Marketed as the "ISG wand", this mechanical localizer was a critical component in the first regular applications of image-guided surgery [2].

### Ultrasound Localization

The first example of frameless navigation was a system developed by Roberts et al. [3]. This system used a microscope both to register the images to the patient and to provide the guidance information. The localization system was based on ultrasonic spark-gap transducers. These emit a very short ultrasound pulse, which can be detected by three or more microphones in the operating room. The time delay for the sound pulse to reach each microphone gives a measure of distance and hence localizes the spark gap. Others have developed this technology for conventional pointer-based guidance [4]. Some problems have been encountered owing to variations of the speed of sound with temperature and air flow. This localization system was implemented in the Picker Viewpoint system, but was subsequently replaced by optical tracking.

### Optical Tracking

With either three linear cameras or two 2D cameras, if a point can be located in each view, the 3D location of the point relative to the cameras can be calculated. This is the basis of a number of tracking systems. The localized points are either active (bright infra-red-emitting diodes, IREDs) or passive (highly reflecting spheres). In smaller camera systems, such as the Polaris or IGT systems, each IRED can be localized with an accuracy of 0.2–0.4 mm. With the Optotrak – a larger and more expensive version – accuracy is 0.1–0.2 mm. The main difficulty with optical tracking is that line-of-sight between the cameras and tracked objects must be maintained. However, the high accuracy and stability of these systems have meant that optical tracking is now the technology of choice for most commercial image-guided surgery systems.

## Registration

Having defined a coordinate system for the patient, we now need to align the pre-operative images to this reference space. This is achieved by defining features in the pre-operative images that can also be identified by our localization device on the surface of the patient. Point-like landmarks are the most common type of feature and these are generally referred to as "fiducials". The fiducials may be purely anatomical points on the skin surface, skin-affixed markers or bone-implanted fiducials. The choice of fiducial depends on the accuracy required by the application.

For early pointer-based guidance we have used anatomical landmarks such as the nasion, the medial and lateral canthi, the external angular processes, the tip of the mastoid process and the occipital protuberance. Experience tells us that these can be located at best to within 3–5 mm, achieving a registration error of similar magnitude. Skin markers have been reported to provide a registration accuracy of 2–4 mm when used with great care. Inaccuracies can occur due to movement of the skin surface either with head repositioning, with application of protective eye covers, or with the force of the pointer used for registration. Care must be taken to protect the upper face after registration, and to mark the center of the marker whilst applying as little force as possible to the skin surface.

The only validated and approved method that provides sub-millimetric accuracy is to use bone-implanted markers [5]. Though this is clearly a rather invasive process, it does provide the most accurate registration for neuronavigation.

## Patient Immobilization and Tracking

Whatever the technology used, patient tracking is relative to some reference frame; the frame is an array of tracked targets that are locked in constant orientation with the patient's head. This can be the reference frame of the device itself, as is the case with mechanical localization. A more common approach is to attach an optical tracker to a Mayfield or similar clamp. To maintain accuracy it is advisable to keep this tracker as close as possible to the surgical field without hampering the procedure. It has also been proposed to attach a tracker either to the patient's palate or the upper teeth [6]. This allows freer movement of the patient's head for interventions where a head clamp is inappropriate. The use of a reference frame is essential, and permits movement of the head relative to the tracking cameras, or vice versa, without loss of registration.

## Accuracy Considerations

When performing point-based registration, there are a number accuracy metrics that can be described. It is very important when talking about the accuracy of a particular system that the measurements used are clear and that their meaning is understood. In a paper by Fitzpatrick et al., the three main error metrics associated with point-based registration are described and a derivation of the most important statistic is given [7]. We will describe their results and the implications thereof for image-directed neurosurgery in this section. It is vital that any surgeon using point landmarks as a means of registration for image guidance understands these results.

### Error Metrics

We will call the point landmarks "fiducials". The first statistical measure of error we will describe is the "fiducial localization error" (FLE). This is simply the accuracy with which one can generally locate a given fiducial. An estimate of FLE for a particular fiducial must take into account the accuracy with which the point can be found by the user in the images and on the patient, as well as the intrinsic accuracy of the localization device.

The second metric is the "fiducial registration error" (FRE). This is the root mean square (rms) residual error on the fiducials after transformation. For example, if we have a set of points in image coordinates and their corresponding physical locations, we can calculate a transformation from image to physical space. By transforming the image points, we have two sets of points that should coincide: the transformed image points and their measured physical positions. Because there are errors in our measurements, these points do not coincide exactly and the distances between them provide the FRE. It is common, because it is easy to calculate, for commercial systems to quote FRE either as an rms or as an error on each point. As we shall see, however, FRE is not a good measure of registration accuracy.

The third, and most clinically relevant, metric is the "target registration error" (TRE). This is the accuracy with which a point other than our fiducials can be located. If we are performing an electrode placement heading for a specific target, the TRE is a measure of the accuracy with which we can locate that target given the registration we have obtained from our fiducials. This is clearly the error in which we are most interested.

Fitzpatrick et al. [7] have found a formula relating TRE to FLE and the configuration of the landmarks, as follows:

$$\langle TRE^2(r) \rangle = \frac{\langle FLE^2 \rangle}{N} \left( 1 + \frac{1}{3}\sum_{k=1}^{3}\frac{d_k^2}{f_k^2} \right)$$

where there are n fiducial points, where fk is the rms distance of the fiducials to the principal axis, k, of the point distribution, and where dk is the distance from this same axis to the target point, r. In image-guided neurosurgery we are interested in reducing the TRE. From this equation we can see that there are two methods of achieving this. One is to increase the number of fiducials used; the other is to increase the spread of these fiducials.

For systems that quote FRE only, there may be a temptation to ignore landmarks that have a high FRE and reduce the set until the mean FRE falls below a given value. This is a very poor method of achieving registration. It will tend to mean that a poor configuration of landmarks will remain, perhaps all being close together or all close to lying along a line. Though a low FRE may result from this process, the associated TRE, especially at a distance from these landmarks, may be very poor indeed. Landmarks with high FRE should only be discarded if there is a good reason for thinking that they are outliers, e.g. if a skin marker has clearly moved.

Manufacturers of IGS systems should be encouraged to incorporate the above equation into accuracy assessments provided to the surgeon. Until this is the case, it is paramount that surgeons are aware of the issues affecting the true target accuracy of navigation.

# Clinical Applications

## Brain Biopsy

Accurate biopsy of brain lesions has been possible since the introduction of stereotactic frames. The frame, however, restricts access to the surgical field, interferes with instruments, and requires immediate pre-operative imaging. It gives no feedback to the surgeon and requires multiple calculations that are not always intuitive and simple. It is also inconvenient to the patient. Stereotactic biopsy in the lateral temporal lobe is contraindicated with some frames, where the needle track is liable to traverse the Sylvian fissure, placing the middle cerebral artery at risk. The development of frameless image-guided systems was an important step in increasing the user friendliness of localization systems. Light-emitting diodes (LEDs) attached to the biopsy needles allow their precise tracking by the camera within the operating space, and holding arms have been developed to maintain biopsy needles rigidly in the correct position. The ideal trajectory to approach and biopsy the lesion can be worked out pre-operatively and stored in the workstation. The development of trajectory and targeting software allows the needle to be advanced according to such a pre-planned pathway, with real-time 3D visualization of the position of the needle tip within the brain.

Brain biopsy procedures require a higher accuracy than is necessary for most other procedures performed under image guidance. The use of scalp-applied or even skull-implantable fiducial markers, as well as the holding of the patient's head in a rigid Mayfield head holder, is important. The accuracy now given by most systems is better than 2 mm, but the limitation imposed by the thickness of the image slices remains.

In a study by Barnett et al. [8], 218 biopsy procedures were performed using scalp-applied fiducial markers. The average minimum lesion diameter was 27.7 mm and the average depth from the scalp was 39.8 mm. Lesions included glial tumors, metastases, lymphomas, meningiomas and demyelination. The procedure yielded a diagnosis that supported the clinical and radiological findings in 96.3% of cases. This was comparable to the accuracy achieved by frame-based stereotactic systems. The most significant complication was intracerebral hemorrhage, which occurred in five cases, two of which required craniotomy. It was noted that the diagnostic accuracy for posterior fossa biopsy, at 70% (7 out of 10 patients), was much lower than that for supratentorial lesions; it was suggested that scanning the patient in the prone position and the application of skull-implantable fiducials would increase the accuracy.

## Surface Lesions

For access to lesions on the brain surface, guidance with registered images allows the performance of a small craniotomy, planned to give maximal exposure of the tumor and at the same time decreasing the extent of exposure. The disruption of normal tissue is minimized. Most importantly, an accurate craniotomy decreases the brain retraction required. This is of particular value in convexity meningiomas, where excessive brain retraction leads to post-operative swelling, which may be difficult to control and may lead to significant morbidity. A lower degree of brain manipulation decreases the risk of a post-operative intracerebral hematoma. In meningioma surgery, a smaller bone flap also decreases the intraoperative blood loss. The brain shift associated with surface lesions has been studied [9,10]. It is more predictable than for deeper lesions, and consists of bulging of the lesion and the surrounding brain on opening the dura; this is associated with an outward movement of the deep brain/tumor interface. The cortex at the resection site sinks back on completion of resection.

## Skull Base and Pituitary Surgery

Tumors of the skull base have a high propensity to invade osseous boundaries and distort anatomy, obscuring surgical landmarks in a region crowded with critical neurovascular structures. Image-guided surgery is becoming an important tool in the resection of complex skull base tumors, particularly in the petroclival and parasellar regions, as well as in the foramen magnum and the jugular foramen [11].

When compared with other lesions, such as vault meningiomas, cerebral gliomas and non-gliotic intra-axial lesions, skull base lesions are associated with substantially lower degrees of post-imaging, intraoperative brain shift. This implies that the accuracy of frameless image-guided methods is higher for such lesions [9].

Sure et al. [11] evaluated the role of neuronavigation in a series of 10 skull base tumors. The value of pre-operatively acquiring both CT and

MRI scans, with subsequent fusion of the two image sets on the navigation workstation, was described. The CT scan allowed accurate patient-to-image registration on the basis of bony landmarks. The MRI scan allowed detailed evaluation of soft tissue and bony distortion by the tumor. A registration error of less than 2 mm was obtained in each of the 10 cases.

The workstation facilitates selection of the optimal skull base approach for maximal resection of the lesion. Sure et al. [11] found it particularly useful in deciding whether a pterional or an orbitozygomatic approach would give the better access to a given parasellar lesion. In posterior fossa surgery, it allows precise definition of keyhole craniotomies in relationship to the underlying dural venous sinuses. Neuronavigation also allows a clear pre-operative indication of how much tumor can be excised safely, depending on the proximity of the tumor to important structures.

Intraoperatively, early identification of important anatomical landmarks, such as the clinoid processes in anterior fossa surgery, and the petrous apex, the arch of the atlas, the vertebral artery, the occipital condyle and the bone cells in the posterior fossa, is useful. Major vessels and critical neural structures can be identified early during intratumoral decompression, facilitating their preservation when displaced by, or encased within, the tumor mass. It allows the neurosurgeon to calculate the position of the instrument within a large tumor cavity devoid of landmarks. A better understanding of the topography of complex anatomical structures is afforded; this is relevant, for example, when the petrous portion of the carotid artery is being protected during drilling of invaded or eroded petrous temporal bone. Bony infiltration by skull base meningiomas is sometimes not grossly identifiable, even under the microscope, and image guidance then allows a more complete tumor resection.

In one of the few studies that also takes account of the overall cost effectiveness of image guidance, Elias et al. [12] described the role of CT-based neuronavigation in transsphenoidal surgery for pituitary tumors. The maintenance of an appropriate midline trajectory is vital in transsphenoidal surgery. Intracranial entries into the anterior fossa floor and through the clivus have been reported. Whereas intraoperative fluoroscopy only provides sagittal guidance, the neuronavigation system gives constant 3D information and allows adjustments in both the sagittal and the coronal planes during the approach to the sella. Attachment of reflective markers to ring curettes and their calibration within the navigation system allow the neurosurgeon to identify the sellar boundaries and to delineate the cavernous sinus and the carotid artery on each side. The system, however, cannot reliably demonstrate soft and potentially mobile tissues within the sella once excision of the adenoma has begun. Use of the image-guidance system to dynamically assist in, or confirm, the complete removal of the adenoma necessitates the incorporation of some form of intraoperative image updating.

The usefulness of such a system in defining and confirming the midline trajectory is particularly evident in re-operations. Disruption of important midline landmarks, such as the vomer, the anterior nasal spine and the rostrum of the sphenoid, renders such operations hazardous. Image guidance allows the neurosurgeon to approach the sella with increased confidence and goes a long way to increase the safety of the procedure.

In an effort to decrease the additional cost ($318 per procedure) and the time requirement in the setting up and registration of the system (mean of an extra 12 minutes per procedure), the same neurosurgical unit has evaluated frameless fluoroscopy-guided transsphenoidal surgery using the FluoroNav Virtual Fluoroscopy System (Medtronic Sofamor Danek Inc., Memphis, TN) [13]. A dynamic reference arc was attached to the headholder fixed to the patient's cranium. A calibration device containing multiple light-emitting diodes was attached to a standard C-arm fluoroscope. This device supplies information regarding the relationship of the C-arm and the reference arc to the computer. Frontal and lateral videofluoroscopic images were then obtained, calibrated and stored in the computer. With a referenced probe, the surgeon was then able to refer to the stored images and visualize its position in real time. The principal advantages of this system are: (1) radiation exposure to the patient is reduced (fluoroscopy is only used once at the beginning of the procedure, and there is no preoperative CT scan); (2) the fluoroscope can be removed from the theater before draping the patient, cutting down on radiology costs;

and (3) as in CT-guided neuronavigation, this system allows more confident maintenance of the midline in re-operations. The cost of each procedure was calculated to be $750 less than for the CT-guided system, primarily because no pre-operative navigation protocol imaging is required; the mean increase in set-up time was only 7.2 minutes.

## Intrinsic Brain Tumors and Functional Mapping

Image-guided surgery has become an integral component in the surgical management of brain tumors. The clear advantages include: the possibility of performing a smaller craniotomy centered directly over the pathology; localization of tumors deep within the cortical surface with minimal disturbance of the surrounding brain tissue; definition of the relationships of the tumour to eloquent cortex and other important structures; and definition of the tumor–brain plane, especially when this is poorly visible at surgery, such as in low-grade astrocytomas. The completeness of resection may also be enhanced, although this is controversial unless some form of intraoperative image updating is also used. The opportunity to plan the optimal approach to the tumor pre-operatively is also valuable.

The integration of functional data into the anatomical image data set was the next logical step in the development of image-guided surgery systems. If the function of relevant eloquent brain in the vicinity of a lesion can be mapped onto the MR image on the workstation, maximal resection with minimal neurological morbidity is facilitated. The potential to increase the safety of the procedure is evident. It is not always possible to accurately identify eloquent brain regions perioperatively with reference to standard anatomical landmarks, as tumors may cause significant gyral displacement and distortion of surface cortical anatomy.

Intraoperative, invasive, functional mapping using cortical stimulation techniques is time consuming and requires modification of the anesthetic regimen. Patients need to be awake for assessment of language function, but light anesthesia without muscle relaxation is adequate for motor mapping. Unlike pre-operative non-invasive mapping, this technique does not allow pre-operative planning and risk evaluation.

Magnetoencephalography (MEG) and functional MRI (fMRI) have been successfully used to obtain functional information that was subsequently integrated with the pre-operatively acquired image data set. In the former [14], cortical neuromagnetic signals are generated by repetitive sensory and motor stimulation; in practice, this involves mechanical stimulation of the index finger or repetitive finger-tapping movements. These signals are picked up and localized by a biomagnetometer, consisting of two 37-channel sensors placed over the scalp. Electrical sources can be localized with high spatial and temporal accuracy. The locations of the sensory and motor cortex are therefore identified, and, using a contour-fit algorithm, the MEG results can be overlaid onto the MR images. Lesions close to the motor cortex were successfully removed in 50 patients [14], with procedure-related neurological impairment in only one patient. Perioperative somatosensory evoked potentials agreed with the co-registered MEG localizations to a high level of concordance.

Functional MRI is non-invasive and uses widely available equipment [15]. Unlike MEG, it does not detect neural activation directly, but identifies a region within the cortex that is metabolically activated during the repetitive performance of an activity such as finger tapping. Performance of the task causes a substantial increase in cerebral blood flow in the corresponding brain region, sufficient in fact to lead to a decrease in the level of deoxyhemoglobin in the veins draining that region. This is detected as an increase in the T2-weighted MR signal. The signal-to-noise ratio is low, and many repetitions are required to generate each image slice. The fMRI image is then fused with the anatomical data set. In a study in which 12 patients underwent excision of lesions near the motor cortex, the prediction error ranged from 0 mm to 10 mm. This was considered to be satisfactory, as the target was the precentral gyrus rather than a single point on it. Intraoperative confirmation using somatosensory evoked potentials and phase reversal to identify the sensory and motor cortices respectively showed that fMRI identified the region correctly in each case. All of the tumors were excised without causing new neurological deficits [15]. Interestingly, patients with severe peri-lesional edema consistently showed a higher prediction error. This may be related to impairment of vascular autoregulation with decreased activation-dependent changes in cerebral blood flow in regions of high edema. It was also noted that distortion of the fMRI images could be a problem when the region of interest is closely related to bone, as may occur with the inferior temporal lobe.

Identification and mapping of white matter tracts is now also possible [16]. Image-fusion software then allows the accurate fusion of these maps with the anatomical image data set. The presence of the axonal membrane and the neurofilamentary cytoskeleton restricts the diffusion of water to the long axis of the fiber tracts – anisotropy. Diffusion-anisotropy MRI identifies the restricted diffusion as a hyperintense area, delineating in three dimensions the position and direction of the tract. In four patients presenting with tumors displacing the pyramidal tract, this technique was helpful in the perioperative identification of the tract. As in fMRI, peri-lesional edema poses a problem, as there is no restriction of diffusion direction in edematous foci; tract identification is then difficult. It has been suggested that this method can also be used to map the optic radiation and the commissural fibers if these structures are relevant to the procedure.

## Movement of the Brain During Surgery

A critical limitation of image-guided surgery, particularly relevant to tumor resection, is the reliance on a pre-operatively acquired image data set. Progressive movement or distortion of the brain during the procedure means that the pre-operative image becomes progressively outdated as the surgery proceeds [10]. Reliance on the image-guided system would lead to errors in the intraoperative delineation of tumor location and borders, as well as in the relationship of the tumor to adjacent eloquent cortex. Brain distortion, relative to the pre-operative image, is due to the release of cerebrospinal fluid (CSF), pressure changes on skull opening, unopposed gravity, ventricular compression, brain retraction and tumor resection. Patient positioning, the physiological effects of diuretics and mechanical ventilation are also relevant.

Dorward et al. [9] studied the magnitude and direction of post-imaging brain distortion in 48 cases; maximal brain shifts were found to be greater than 1 cm in magnitude. The degree of shift depended on the size of the tumor, the degree of midline shift, and the presence of peritumoral edema; significant differences were identified between meningiomas, gliomas, non-glial intra-axial lesions and skull base lesions.

Nabavi et al. [10] studied post-imaging brain deformation in 25 patients using a 0.5T vertically open bore MR imager. Baseline imaging was performed after positioning; further images were taken after dural opening and initial CSF drainage, after tumor resection, and after dural closure. Software allowed image overlapping on the same coordinates to facilitate comparison between the images. In this study, brain shift was shown to have a high degree of inter-individual variability and was a continuous and dynamic process, evolving separately and differently in distinct brain regions. It was noted that the direction of deformation might even reverse within relatively short time-frames. The occipital and parietal lobes were seen to be less mobile than the frontal and temporal lobes. It is clear that brain biomechanics are still far from understood, and although software may be designed to predict unidirectional surface shifts secondary to gravity and CSF loss associated with small surface lesions, predictions of multidirectional subsurface movements associated with larger lesions are unlikely to be accurate.

The effects of brain shift can be minimized by paying attention to some operative details, such as allowing as little CSF as possible to escape, by delaying aspiration of cystic tumor components, and by removing tumor adjacent to eloquent cortex first. The use of dehydrating agents such as mannitol should be avoided and the positioning of the patient should be such that the craniotomy site lies at the highest point.

## Intraoperative MRI

One solution to the problem of intraoperative brain movement is to combine guidance from registered pre-operative images with intraoperative MRI. This allows the acquisition of image updates intraoperatively; these updates are then fused with the pre-operatively acquired image data set. Several centers have reported their experience with such systems [17,18,19]. The difficulties and cost of modifying the usual operating theater set-up to suit the requirements of MR scanning are clear. Several options have been used in various centers:

The use of a vertical open-bore MRI scanner, allowing two surgeons to operate within the scanner. This avoids the need for patient movement but requires the use of non-ferromagnetic instruments as well as magnetic shielding of the operating room [19].

The use of a twin operating theater; surgery is performed in a conventional theater and the patient is transported to an adjacent MRI suite for imaging. The scanner can be rendered more cost effective by allowing its use for diagnostic scans unrelated to theater sessions [17].

The use of a single-shielded operating theater, with the surgery being performed in the fringe field of the magnet. Normal ferromagnetic instruments and microscopes are then allowed [18].

There is a steadily growing volume of literature on intraoperative MRI and it is not possible to discuss this topic in detail here. Its value was demonstrated in a recent study [17] in which 40 patients underwent image-guided resection of gliomas (WHO grades II–IV) using an image-guidance system. An intraoperative MRI scan was obtained after the surgeon felt that the planned extent of tumor resection was achieved. Of these patients, 53% were found on MRI to have had a less than optimal resection. It was noted from this study that patients with a tumor volume higher than 20cm$^3$ are more likely to have incomplete resections, probably because the degree of brain shift is much higher for larger lesions.

The intraoperative MRI system described by Hadani et al. [18] is characterized by a vertical-bore 0.12T open magnet that can be stored below the operating table when not in use. The patient's head occupies a fixed position relative to the magnet. With the magnet in the scanning position, real-time navigation can be employed using an MRI wand. This is independent of the optical tracking system and the magnet is the only reference point. Alternatively, the magnet can be lowered under the operating table once an image update has been obtained; optical tracking using the standard guidance set-up then allows navigation on the updated image data set. Image updating is independent of fiducials and skin markers, because the same relationship between the magnet and the patient is maintained throughout the procedure. Ferromagnetic instruments are used when the magnet is not in the scanning position.

There are several issues relating to intraoperative MRI that are still unclear. The presence of residual tumor on intraoperative images is ascertained on the basis of contrast enhancement around or within the resection cavity [17]. Increased permeability of the blood–brain barrier also occurs as a direct result of surgical manipulation, and indeed, surgically induced nodular as well as diffuse enhancement has been reported. This is probably more likely after contrast agents have been injected several times during the same procedure. The use of contrast agents that bind the tumor for a longer period of time and that are cleared from the circulation before the operation is begun has been investigated; iron oxide microparticles are phagocytosed by glioblastoma cells. It would then be possible to avoid administration of contrast agents just before or during the procedure. Bohinski et al. found that biopsy of residual enhancing tissue after partial glioma resection yielded tumor in 81% of cases [17]. Comparison with pre-operative contrasted scans is useful to differentiate tumor-induced enhancement from surgery-induced enhancement.

The edema associated with retraction is easily identifiable on T2-weighted imaging. As enhancement in the dependent part of the resection cavity might also be due to blood clot, it is essential that adequate hemostasis be secured prior to imaging. Blood is also identifiable on T2-weighted images. Oxidized cellulose in the cavity is another factor that interferes with the identification of tumor remnants. The debris of a metal drill produces significant artifact on MRI and it is preferable to use only diamond drills [19]. Even when all of these precautions are taken, however, definition of the borders of low-grade astrocytomas is still a challenge.

Other unanswered questions relate to the frequency of intraoperative scanning. Ideally one should obtain enough information to ensure that the image data set used for navigation is not outdated, and also to control resection of the target, without prolonging the operation or moving the patient unnecessarily. Should scanning be tied to critical events, such as the completion of tumor resection or the preservation of a functional region?

## Intraoperative Ultrasonography

The use of intraoperative ultrasonography to update the pre-operative image has been considered. Ultrasonography is inexpensive; also, it allows fast multiplanar examination and can reliably detect tumor remnants. Tracking of the ultrasound probe allows 3D reconstruction. However, the overall quality of soft-tissue visualization is not as good as that of MRI, and the fusion of the ultrasonic image with the MR image is still difficult to obtain.

## Outcome of Image-guided Surgery for Intrinsic Tumors

A more important question is whether a more complete resection of a high-grade glioma, as is possible with image-guided surgery, leads to a better prognosis. Recurrence of gliomas generally occurs at the site of residual tumor, and therefore gross total resection might increase the progression-free survival and improve the quality of life when compared with subtotal resection or biopsy. There is also evidence to suggest that the immediate complication rate after gross total resection is lower than that after biopsy or subtotal resection [20]. A systematic analysis of survival times, with and without target resection control for matched patients and tumors, is required.

## Epilepsy Surgery

Image guidance has been used in several aspects of epilepsy surgery, including the removal of deep lesions, selective amygdalo-hippocampectomy, callosotomy, temporal resection, cortical resection and the placement of depth electrodes [21]. The hippocampus and the corpus callosum are relatively fixed structures, and there is only minimal brain shift along the anteroposterior axis. Once hippocampal resection has begun, however, CSF drainage and the mesial displacement of the brain due to gravity lead to error in the mesio-lateral plane. According to Olivier et al. [21], this did not lead to interference with localization and gross total resection of the mesial structures.

In transylvian selective amygdalo-hippocampectomy, surgical orientation is achieved primarily through the exposure of anatomical landmarks, namely the uncus and the sulcus circularis insulae. This requires a wide opening of the Sylvian fissure with the associated risks of vessel injury and vasospasm. Image guidance allows orientation without the necessity to expose and identify such landmarks. Trajectories to the hippocampus and resection borders can be defined pre-operatively. Image guidance directs trans-sulcal dissection and also ensures complete resection of the relevant hippocampal structures; the outcome of epilepsy surgery has been shown to be closely related to complete hippocampal resection.

The location of focal cortical dysplasia is often difficult to identify macroscopically. Image guidance allows accurate anatomical correlation in cortical resections, and this becomes more accurate if the system is used concurrently with electrocorticography and motor mapping. It also facilitates the confirmation of the length of a callosal section, and in temporal lobectomy it aids a decision on the volumes of lateral temporal cortex and hippocampus that can safely be resected.

## Arteriovenous Malformations

Although the importance of neuro-endovascular therapy and radiosurgery in the management of arteriovenous malformations (AVMs) has been increasing steadily over the past 5 years, microsurgical excision still retains a primary role, particularly as it is the only treatment option that immediately eliminates the risk of bleeding. The frequent intimate relationship of AVMs to eloquent brain tissue has rendered neuronavigation techniques useful in surgical management, in an effort to reduce post-operative neurological morbidity.

Image-guided surgery based on a pre-operatively acquired MR scan allows pre-operative planning and identification of the ideal location and size of the skin incision and bone flap. For lesions with minimal gyral representation, it allows precise localization of the AVM through a small, optimally placed craniotomy. More importantly, it allows planning of the optimal surgical trajectory to the AVM, maximally avoiding eloquent brain tissue, particularly for AVMs located close to, or within, motor, sensory, speech or visual areas.

A recent study [22] described image-guided AVM surgery based on CT angiography rather than on MRI. Segmentation and 3D reconstruction of the AVM allowed exact definition of the nidus, as well as the draining veins and feeding arteries, in relation to the underlying brain tissue. Manipulation of the reconstruction through rotation and subtraction allowed multi-angle viewing of the relationships of the AVM vessels. Preliminary image-guided temporary clipping of the sulcal feeding arteries led to decompression of the AVM nidus in most cases, rendering easier the subsequent step of dissection along the previously localized draining veins. However, temporary clipping prior to complete feeder dissection is associated with a low risk of clipping en-passant vessels. Another limitation of this study was that only vessels larger than 3 mm in size could be identified – a direct result of the resolution limit of the segmentation process.

By demonstrating the configuration and margins of the nidus, image guidance decreases the risk of inadvertent surgical entry into the AVM. The plane between the AVM and the surrounding brain tissue can be readily identified, minimizing tissue manipulation and decreasing intraoperative bleeding.

It is still unclear, however, whether image-guided surgery for AVMs does in fact result in a lower morbidity when compared with standard, free-hand techniques.

## Surgery for Intracranial Aneurysm

Few surgeons see any indication for image guidance in the approach to the majority of intracranial aneurysms, usually located in the region of the supraclinoid segment of the internal carotid artery. However, aneurysms located more distally, in particular pericallosal aneurysms, can present a significant problem, and localization is facilitated by the use of image guidance.

## Endoscopic Surgery

Guidance from registered images has been used extensively in conjunction with endoscopic neurosurgery. Unlike frame-based stereotaxy, it allows free-hand movement of the endoscope

with real-time feedback of its tip position. The versatility of the software is such that a 'tool file' is available for each of the various instruments introduced through the sheath. A change of instrument only necessitates a change in the active tool file on the computer workstation. The pre-calibrated parameters and length of the instrument then allow representation of that instrument in the multiplanar views on the screen.

In a study by Schroeder et al. [23], the principal usefulness of guidance from registered images was in the selection of an ideal entry point and trajectory to the lesion with minimal injury to the fornices and eloquent brain. Most procedures were then performed under direct endoscopic visual control. The pre-operative trajectory planning was very useful when the ventricular system was small and when the posterior third ventricle had to be approached through a small foramen of Monro. In the management of arachnoid cysts, a trajectory penetrating as many of the septae as possible, as well as ensuring an optimal fenestration point, would be planned. In such situations, as well as in multi-loculated hydrocephalus, there are few, if any, anatomical landmarks, and there is a real risk of disorientation, particularly if the membranes are thick [23]. The value of image guidance in the maintenance of orientation was clear. In the endoscopic resection of colloid cysts, guidance from registered images facilitated the maintenance of a trajectory leading to the most lateral and anterior aspect of the foramen of Monro, without injury to the fornices or the caudate nucleus; this would, in turn, allow visualization of the roof of the third ventricle, rendering complete dissection of the cyst from its base easier.

The authors did not find pre-operative image guidance useful for endoscopic third ventriculostomy [23]. In this procedure the ventricles tend to be large, and a high degree of endoscope maneuverability is possible. Clear intraventricular landmarks, such as the thalamo-striate vein, the foramen of Monro and the choroid plexus, determine the orientation. The basilar artery can often be seen through the thinned-out floor of the third ventricle, and its position can be scrutinized from the mid-sagittal pre-operative MRI. The optimal position of the stoma is determined via visual information through the endoscope.

The problem of CSF drainage and brain shift remains, however. The authors advise positioning the patient with the cyst at the highest point. Other studies [18,19] have pointed to the value of intraoperative MRI-based updating of the pre-operative image data sets in such situations. The decompression of cystic lesions and multi-loculated hydrocephalus under continuous (every 3 seconds) MRI scanning has also been described [24]; the changes of the relationships on drainage and fenestration of the cysts can then be observed in real time. This, of course, requires an intraoperative MRI set-up.

## Spinal Surgery

The development of increasingly complex spinal surgical techniques and instrumentation has meant that 2D lateral intraoperative fluoroscopy is now considered to be insufficient for safe and effective insertion of implants. The application of the principles of intracranial neuronavigation to the spine is not straightforward, for several reasons. Registration of the spine cannot reliably depend on skin markers or fiducials, in view of the high mobility of the spinal column and the overlying skin. Indeed, registration needs to be performed intraoperatively on the exposed spinal anatomy of the segment requiring surgery, using points that are easily and accurately identifiable on the exposed spine and on the pre-operatively acquired images. These may include the superior and inferior portions of the spinous processes and the medial and lateral limits of the facet joint in the cervical spine, and the posterolateral aspect of the transverse process tips on each side in the thoracic spine. Problems may arise when the posterior elements of the relevant segment are disrupted by trauma or previous surgery. A minimum of three points is required for the vertebra in question. Because each level in the spine represents a separate and distinct anatomical structure, each vertebra should ideally be registered and tracked individually during surgery. The spine is mobile within the body and therefore the reference arc or LED array must be attached to the spine itself. In practice, this is clamped to a spinous process of the same, or an adjacent, vertebra for posterior approaches, and to a Caspar retractor for anterior approaches [25]. This is essential because the spatial relationships of adjacent spinal segments during pre-operative image acquisition (in the supine position) may be different from those during surgery, often in the prone position, particularly in situations of spinal instability such as high-grade spondylolisthesis and spinal fractures. Frequent perioperative confirmation of registration accuracy is advised; this is readily done by placing the activated probe on an easily identifiable bony point within the operative field and by ensuring that the cursor on the computer points to the corresponding point on the pre-operative image. A significant decrease in accuracy, usually recorded at around 2 mm, should prompt re-registration. The absence of clear bony landmarks and the flat 2D nature of the anterior vertebral bodies imply that accurate registration of the spine for anterior or anterolateral approaches remains difficult.

Virtual fluoroscopy technology (FluoroNav, Medtronic Sofamor Danek Inc., Memphis) does not require a pre-operative image. The C-arm is equipped with an LED attachment and a fiducial display that acts as a calibration target. The bony anatomy is first exposed; a reference arc is then attached to the spine. A lateral or anteroposterior image is taken. The fiducial display is used by the computer to register the anatomy instantaneously. Data from the optical camera allow the computer to identify the spatial relationships between the C-arm and the reference arc attached to the spine. This registered image then forms the basis on which navigation, using LED-marked instruments that appear on the image in real time, can proceed.

Probably the most important spinal application of image-guided surgery is the insertion of pedicle screws [26,27]. Pedicle screws confer high rigidity to a spinal construct, allowing the insertion of a shorter and more reliable construct, with maximal preservation of movement at the adjacent segments. In the lumbosacral spine, using perioperative radiography only, the rate of penetration of the pedicular cortex has been shown to be between 21% and 31%. Poor pedicle screw insertion is associated not only with neural injury, but also with fixation failure, particularly if the pedicle is fractured. Image guidance allows evaluation of the pedicular anatomy, the selection of the appropriate screw entry point, the identification of the optimal trajectory in the axial and sagittal planes, and also the ideal depth of insertion, allowing the longest bone purchase in the best-quality bone.

The surgeon is able to select the ideal screw diameter and length in the pre-operative planning phase; the computer provides a 3D view of the selected screw in the pre-operatively acquired image. It also provides a "target" window to facilitate screw insertion along the predetermined trajectory. In one of the earlier clinical studies in the use of image guidance for the insertion of lumbosacral pedicle screws [26], 137 out of a total of 150 screws were optimally placed. Only one screw was found to be in a significantly unsatisfactory position. No nerve root injuries were reported.

Image guidance is even more valuable in pedicle screw insertion into the thoracic spine [27]. Compared with its lumbar counterpart, the thoracic pedicle is smaller, has a more complex 3D morphology and has a variable cross-section in the coronal plane. There is a high degree of variability in the diameter, shape and angle of the thoracic pedicle. Moreover, its proximity to the pleura, nerve roots and the relatively fixed spinal cord means that inappropriate insertion is less forgiving. From clinical and cadaveric studies, up to 25% of thoracic pedicle screws were found to violate the pedicular cortex when perioperative fluoroscopy alone was used. In a recent study using post-operative CT evaluation, only 5 out of 266 screws inserted at all levels of the thoracic spine in 65 patients showed a structurally significant (defined as more than 2 mm) inadvertent violation of the pedicular cortex. These tended to cluster in the mid-thoracic spine. The majority of these misplacements occurred in severe traumatic fracture subluxations, implying that the increased inter-segmental mobility in these situations interferes with the accuracy of registration of the image-guidance system. The authors also advocate an alternative screw trajectory through the rib head into the vertebral body if the pedicle is smaller than 4 mm in its widest coronal diameter, or scaphoid in shape, or laterally directed. This information can only be gleaned through pre-operative pedicle evaluation on the image-guidance system.

Image guidance is also useful when there is a concurrent anterior construct, such as a Kaneda system, for example. Pedicle screw insertion then allows a rigid parallelogram of fixation [25].

Applications to the cervical spine have included anterior cervical diskectomy and vertebrectomy, transoral odontoid resection, and the insertion of C1–C2 transarticular screws and lateral mass plates [25]. In anterior cervical surgery, image guidance allows the identification of the lateral resection margins of osteophytes and their relationships to the transverse foramen, the vertebral artery and the nerve root foramen. The risks of vascular and neurological injury (to the nerve roots and spinal cord) for these procedures have been quoted as up to 5% and 1% respectively. Image guidance also reduces the risk of incomplete osteophyte excision.

Surgical difficulties in the C1–C2 region include the complexity of the anatomy, which may be distorted by inflammatory pannus or tumor, and a limited operative field. Image guidance allows the determination of the position of unexposed structures, minimizing the need for extensive exposures. Insertion of atlanto-axial transarticular screws can then be performed with a higher margin of safety and with increased confidence.

# Current Developments

There are a number of issues that remain to be tackled to improve the accuracy and delivery of neurosurgical guidance. An increasing amount of information is available to the surgeon in the operating theater, particularly from intra-operative imaging devices. This may be used to improve registration and provide information about structures beneath the available tissue surface. This becomes particularly important in the presence of tissue deformation, sometimes referred to as "brain shift".

There are several imaging devices that are routinely available to a neurosurgeon. They provide real-time information about the current position and shape of the patient. If these devices are calibrated to relate the image space to physical space, they can then be incorporated into a neuronavigation system. The simplest way that this can be achieved is to show the position of a pointer or tool in the intraoperative image.

X-ray guidance is an important part of the transsphenoidal approach. The use of X-ray images to register pre-operative CT data to the patient has been proposed for use in surgery of the head and spine. X-ray angiography may also provide useful information on current patient position.

Ultrasound is not generally used to guide neurosurgical procedures because of the poor quality of the images and the difficulty in identifying anatomical features. The real-time nature of the technique could prove useful in aligning pre-operative images to the patient, however. Ultrasound has been proposed for use in compensating for brain shift and also in improving rigid registration by finding the bone surface in spinal surgery.

Attention is also being paid to the ergonomics of surgical guidance. The systems have sometimes been seen as a cumbersome addition to an already crowded operating theater, and the interface between the system and the surgeon is often too complicated. Simplicity and ease of use are vital if image-guided neurosurgery is to become standard practice. Visualization of pre-operative images is an important factor in this regard, especially for microscopic procedures. The surgeon often finds that looking away from the operative view is distracting and inconvenient. Visualization of the target lesion and surrounding critical structures directly on the optical view of the patient, sometimes referred to as "augmented reality", is one way of avoiding this problem. In the MAGI (microscope-assisted guided intervention) system [28], this is achieved accurately and in stereo, offering the possibility of 3D perception of structures beneath the viewed surface (Fig. 7.1).

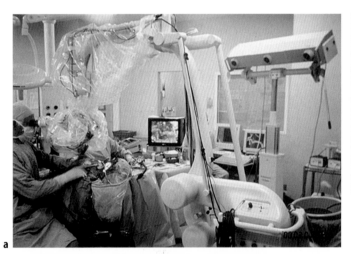

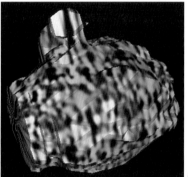

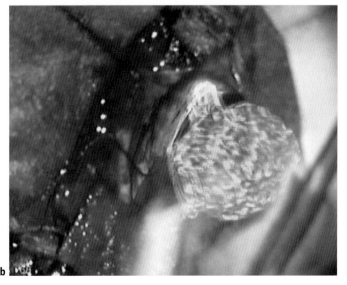

**Fig. 7.1.** The MAGI (microscope-assisted guided intervention) system in the operating theater. (**a**) An example overlay on the operative scene. (**b**) A rendering of the lesion from a similar viewpoint. (**c**) The views in (**b**) and (**c**) are seen by the surgeon in true stereo. The lesion is a vestibular schwannoma seen extending into the internal auditory meatus (IAM).

# The Future

In speculating about the future for image-guided neurosurgical interventions, it is interesting to consider whether registration of pre-operative images to the patient will still be important. The advent of interventional MRI has led some to suggest that the quality of intraoperative imaging will provide all the necessary information to carry out a surgical procedure. Visualization and interaction with this data is an important issue, however.

Incorporation of a navigational device into an interventional scanner is important. The surgeon wants to see the location of a pointer or surgical tool in the images without needing to re-scan with the tool in place. This flexibility will enable scans to be performed only when there is significant movement or tissue deformation.

Also, as the scope of intraoperative imaging widens, so does that of pre-operative imaging. There will be more accurate and more functional data available from pre-operative scans that may not be practical to obtain during a procedure. Ideally, the segmentation of relevant features will be done automatically in real time. This process may be more practically achieved by alignment with previously segmented images.

The challenge for future navigation systems will be to incorporate pre-operative and intraoperative data seamlessly into the neurosurgical process, with real time update of the pre-operative model to compensate for both rigid and non-rigid movement of the patient. The relevant features will be visualised by the surgeon without complicated interaction and ideally directly on the operative view of the patient. Advances in imaging, tracking, computational power, algorithms, perception and display devices will be required. Significant research effort is being directed towards all these areas and will hopefully make this a reality.

# Key Points

- *Image-guided neurosurgery involves the alignment of the patient in the operating space to a set of pre-operatively acquired images. Although accuracy issues need to be considered, it generally provides the ability to localize a target to within 2 mm.*

- *Image guidance facilitates the accurate localization of the target pathology or structures; the neurosurgeon can plan a smaller and more precise craniotomy and follow the ideal trajectory, minimizing the extent of brain exposure and retraction.*

- *The technique is particularly useful in the management of intracranial tumors, but is also being applied to vascular disease, particularly arteriovenous malformations and some aneurysms, epilepsy surgery, intracranial endoscopy and craniocervical and spinal surgery.*

- *Image guidance is very valuable in the insertion of spinal instrumentation, usually for fusion purposes. It facilitates the appreciation of pedicular anatomy and allows the choice of the ideal screw length and diameter prior to insertion.*

- *Current developments include the fusion of anatomical with functional images using functional MRI technology, and perioperative MRI, which allows the pre-operative images to be updated during surgery.*

# Acknowledgement

P. Edwards was supported by EPSRC under the MedLINK program (project M108) in collaboration with Leica, Heerbrugg and BrainLab, Munich.

# References

1. Maciunas RJ, Galloway RL, Latimer JW. The application accuracy of stereotactic frames. Neurosurgery 1994; 35(4):682–94.
2. Sandeman DR, Patel N, Chandler C, Nelson RJ, Coakham HB, Griffith HB. Advances in image-directed neurosurgery – preliminary experience with the ISG viewing wand compared with the Leksell-G frame. Br J Neurosurg 1994;8:529–44.
3. Roberts DW, Strohbehn JW, Hatch JF, Murray W, Kettenberger H. A frameless stereotaxic integration of computerised tomographic imaging and the operating microscope. J Neurosurg 1986;65:545–9.
4. Reinhardt HF, Horstmann GA, Gratzl O. Sonic stereometry in microsurgical procedures for deep-seated brain tumors and vascular malformations. Neurosurgery 1993;32(1):51–7.
5. Maurer C, Fitzpatrick MJ, Wang MY, Galloway RL, Maciunas RJ, Allen GS. Registration of head volume images using implantable fiducial markers. IEEE Trans Med Imaging 1997;6(4):447–61.

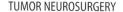

6. Hauser R, Westermann B, Probst R. Non-invasive tracking of patients' head movements during computer-assisted intranasal microscopic surgery. Laryngoscope 1997;211:491–9.

7. Fitzpatrick MJ, West JB, Maurer C. Predicting error in rigid-body point-based registration. IEEE Trans Med Imaging 1998;17(5):694–702.

8. Barnett GH, Miller DW, Weisenberger J. Frameless stereotaxy with scalp-applied fiducial markers for brain biopsy procedures: experience in 218 cases. J Neurosurg 1999;91:569–76.

9. Dorward NL, Alberti O, Velani B, Gerritsen FA, Harkness WFJ, Kitchen ND et al. Post-imaging brain distortion: magnitude, correlates and impact on neuronavigation. J Neurosurg 1998;88:656–62.

10. Nabavi A, McL Black P, Gering DT, Westin CF, Mehta V, Pergolizzi RS et al. Serial intraoperative magnetic resonance imaging of brain shift. Neurosurgery 2001;48:787–98.

11. Sure U, Alberti O, Petermeyer M, Becker R, Bertalanffy H. Advanced image-guided skull base surgery. Surg Neurol 2000;53:563–72.

12. Elias WJ, Chaddick JB, Alden TD, Laws ER. Frameless stereotaxy for transsphenoidal surgery. Neurosurgery 1999;45:271–7.

13. Jane JA, Thapar K, Alden TD, Laws ER. Fluoroscopic frameless stereotaxy for transsphenoidal surgery. Neurosurgery 2001;48:1302–8.

14. Ganslandt O, Fahlbusch R, Nimsky C, Kober H, Moller M, Steinmeier R et al. Functional neuronavigation with magnetoencephalography:outcome in 50 patients with lesions around the motor cortex. J Neurosurg 1999;91:73–9.

15. Schulder M, Maldjian JA, Liu WC, Holodny AI, Kalnin AT, Mun IK et al. Functional image-guided surgery of intracranial tumours located in or near the sensorimotor cortex. J Neurosurg 1998;89:412–18.

16. Coenen VA, Krings T, Mayfrank L, Polin RS, Reinges MHT, Thron A et al. Three-dimensional visualisation of the pyramidal tract in a neuronavigation system during brain tumour surgery: first experiences and technical note. Neurosurgery 2001;49:86–93.

17. Bohinski RJ, Kokkino AK, Warnick RE, Gaskill-Shipley MF, Kormos DW, Lukin RR et al. Glioma resection in a shared-resource magnetic resonance operating room after optimal image-guided frameless stereotactic resection. Neurosurgery 2001;48:731–44.

18. Hadani M, Spiegelman R, Feldman Z, Berkenstadt H, Ram Z. Novel, compact, intraoperative magnetic resonance image-guided system for conventional neurosurgical operating rooms. Neurosurgery 2001;48:799–809.

19. Black P McL, Moriarty T, Alexander E III, Steig P, Woodard EJ, Gleason PL et al. The development and implementation of intraoperative magnetic resonance imaging and its neurosurgical applications. Neurosurgery 1997;41:831–45.

20. Fadul C, Wood J, Thaler H, Galicich J, Patterson RHJ, Posner JB. Morbidity and mortality of craniotomy for excision of supratentorial gliomas. Neurology 1988;38:1374–9.

21. Olivier A, Germano IM, Cukiert A, Peters T. Frameless stereotaxy for surgery of the epilepsies: preliminary experience. J Neurosurg 1994;81:629–33.

22. Maucevic A, Steiger HJ. Computer-assisted resection of cerebral arteriovenous malformations. Neurosurgery 1999;45:1164–71.

23. Schroeder HWS, Wagner W, Tschiltschke W, Gaab MR. Frameless neuronavigation in intracranial endoscopic neurosurgery. J Neurosurg 2001;94:72–9.

24. Kollias SS, Bernays RL. Interactive magnetic resonance imaging-guided management of intracranial cystic lesions by using an open magnetic resonance imaging system. J Neurosurg 2001;95:15–23.

25. Bolger C, Wigfield C. Image-guided surgery: applications to the cervical and thoracic spine and a review of the first 120 procedures. J Neurosurg (Spine) 2000;92:175–80.

26. Kalfas IH, Kormos DW, Murphy MA, McKenzie RL, Barnett GH, Bell GR et al. Application of frameless stereotaxy to pedicle screw fixation of the spine. J Neurosurg 1995;83:641–7.

27. Youkilis AS, Quint DJ, McGillicuddy JE, Papadopoulos SM. Stereotactic navigation for placement of pedicle screws in the thoracic spine. Neurosurgery 2001;48(4):771–9.

28. Edwards PJ, King AP, Maurer CR, de Cunha DA, Hawkes DJ, Hill DLG et al. Design and evaluation of a system for microscope-assisted guided interventions (MAGI). IEEE Trans Med Imaging 2000;19(11):1082–93.

# 8

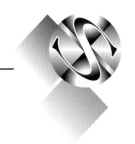

# Stereotactic Radiosurgery

Andras A. Kemeny, Matthias W.R. Radatz
and Jeremy Rowe

## Summary

Stereotactic radiosurgery is a novel method of treating well-defined targets in the brain, causing cell destruction, vascular occlusion or just functional changes within it. It is one of the fastest growing fields within neurosurgery. The range of appropriate indications has not yet crystallized but it is increasingly popular with patients, particularly those with a "high-risk" surgical lesion.

## Introduction

Stereotactic radiosurgery is a neurosurgical technique that utilizes focused radiation as a tool. It was introduced for functional neurosurgery but its applications have widened to encompass cerebral arteriovenous malformations and a wide range of well-defined benign and malignant intracranial neoplasms.

Although it may be considered by some to belong to the realm of radiotherapy rather than neurosurgery, neurosurgical trainees must become familiar with the basics of this technique and particularly with its indications and limitations.

The minimally invasive nature and the perceived, and in most cases truly, low risk of this treatment make it popular with patients and ensure that an increasing proportion of conditions traditionally requiring open surgery are treated by this technique.

## Historic Notes

The expression "stereotactic radiosurgery" (SRS) was coined by Lars Leksell, the Swedish neurosurgeon who first introduced this technique into neurosurgical practice. The term stands for a single fraction, stereotactically guided, high-dose radiation treatment on a small and well-defined volume of the brain. In this phrase (as in the method) he combined a number of important individual elements. The first, stereotaxy, the coordinate-based guidance technique in the brain, has developed from the initial endeavors of Victor Horsley and Robert Clark in 1908 and the first clinically used apparatus, devised by Spiegel and Wycis in 1947. Using this guidance system Leksell directed ionizing radiation to achieve the desired clinical effect. He included the term "surgery" to try and ensure that, as in open surgery, the selection of patients and targets would be done by neurosurgeons who were trained in neuroanatomy, neurophysiology and neuropathology and who were also familiar with the value and indications of the open surgical alternatives.

As the reader will know, Leksell greatly contributed to stereotaxy by designing his own simple and clinically easy-to-use frame. In order to reduce the invasiveness of even a precision-guided surgical procedure, he introduced ionizing radiation to substitute for the knife or needle. He began with photons from a 300 kV X-ray tube mounted on his stereotactic apparatus. In Berkeley, California, in 1950, Tobias had begun cross-firing the sella turcica with charged particles to suppress pituitary function, and work with proton beams was taken up at the Gustaf Werner Institute, Uppsala, in 1954, tested clinically from 1958 onwards, and subsequently in 1961 by Kjellberg, in Boston. In the late 1950s and 1960s, Leksell and Larsson explored the practicability of protons from the Uppsala synchrocyclotron, as well as the theoretical advantages of other particles, before deciding that gamma rays, from a heavily shielded static array of Co60 sources directed towards a central point by narrow collimators, provided the simplest and most practical system for daily clinical use. The first Leksell "gamma knife" was completed in 1967 and became operational in Stockholm in 1968. It was designed for treating functional targets, and thus intractable pain and movement disorders were the first indications. The introduction of stereotactic radiosurgery was initially received with skepticism. However, since that time, the gamma knife (as the later model became known owing to its ease of use and precision) found its way into the neurosurgical armamentarium in many centers around the world. Indeed, some purists are of the view that the phrase "gamma knife surgery" should be applied in order to emphasize the differences from other delivery methods of radiosurgery on one hand, and the crucial role of neurosurgeons in this intervention on the other. After the initial experience became better known, further "gamma units" were installed in 1984 and 1985 in Buenos Aires, Argentina and Sheffield, England, respectively. The next unit, installed in 1987 in Pittsburgh heralded an increasingly broad acceptance worldwide. According to data held at the manufacturer, by September 2001 more than 170,000 patients had been treated with a gamma knife worldwide.

Colombo and others modified the radiotherapy linear accelerator to provide a similar treatment technique. By virtue of the different technical properties, linear accelerator (Linac) radiosurgery has developed in many ways very differently from gamma knife surgery. In particular, at least in part due to the lesser degree of precision achievable with a Linac, a fractionated delivery of radiation was favored, and thus "stereotactic radiotherapy" (SRT) was born. This technique is a multi-fraction, stereotactically guided radiation therapy. Although it is possible to deliver SRT with the gamma knife, it is usually performed using a Linac.

In parallel with the developments in the radiation delivery technique, the imaging localization of the target has also undergone dramatic developments over the last five decades. The initial treatments were based on plain X-rays and pneumo-encephalography. With the introduction of computed tomography in the 1970s and magnetic resonance imaging in the 1980s, it became possible to properly delineate the pathological substrate of the treatment. Moreover, the precise identification of adjacent normal structures further dramatically improved the safety and efficacy of the technique.

# Principles of Radiosurgery

Stereotactic radiosurgery in all its forms consists of the following steps: stereotactic imaging, dose planning and dose delivery.

## Stereotactic Imaging

This requires the application of a set of standard reference points, or a "fiducial system", around the head followed by the acquisition of radiological images. The images obtained provide information about the precise spatial position of anatomical and pathological structures in relation to the fiducial system. The highest precision is achieved using a stereotactic frame fixed to the skull before imaging. It is usually carried out under local anesthetic for all adults unless claustrophobia prevents this. Children aged over 12 years are also treated with local rather than general anesthetic. Where the lesion is large, it is acceptable to use a less precise fiducial system, based on a dental imprint and straps to fix to the skull.

With the stereotactic frame in situ, images are taken to demonstrate the pathological lesion. In most patients this consists of a magnetic resonance imaging (MRI) scan. In the case of arteriovenous malformations (AVMs), a high-quality arterial angiogram is used. The recent trend is to combine these modalities in order to enhance the precision of outlining the margins of the lesion. Three-dimensional information is essential for precise delineation of the contours. Unfortunately, MR images, when used alone, contain potential spatial inaccuracies. These arise from non-linearities inherent in MR physics. Some can be improved by careful quality control and choice of sequences. Certain factors, for example metallic foreign bodies, in the patient, which will distort the local magnetic field and create image artifacts, cannot be overcome. In contrast, the physics of CT is linear and allows greater spatial accuracy. Therefore, in the case of smaller targets, a combination (fusion) of MRI scan and CT scan is used. Such image fusion combines the advantages of the superior soft-tissue definition of MRI scanning and the precision of CT scanning. Co-registration of MRI and angiography helps in determining the three-dimensional distribution of an AVM nidus. The added combination of functional imaging with functional MRI (fMRI) and positron emission tomography (PET), etc., is being explored on an experimental basis. Having defined the coordinate system and, within this, the contours of the target, the treatment can be planned.

## Dose Planning

The aim of this step is to match the radiation treatment as precisely as possible to the contour of the lesion. Inclusion of adjacent normal tissue would lead to side-effects and complications, whereas omission of part of the lesion reduces efficacy. The precision of this step is measured not only by the precision of hitting the target point but also by the degree of matching to the contour. The most refined indices of radiation conformity take into account both the amount of target, e.g. tumor, not receiving sufficient radiation dose and the proportion of normal tissue outside the target that would be needlessly irradiated [1]. These indices show a superiority of gamma knife planning to the alternative with a Linac [2].

In addition to matching the shape, particular care is taken to avoid passing the radiation beams through eloquent structures adjacent to the lesion or even at a distance (e.g. the lens in the eye). This is achieved by plugging some of the radiation sources in the gamma knife and

choosing the entry of the beams in linear accelerator techniques.

## Dose Delivery

### The Gamma Knife

The gamma knife uses an array of 201 Co60 sources, which are evenly distributed around a hemispherical source core. Each source (together with its associated collimator housing) produces a narrow beam of gamma radiation, and these are all directed towards a common focal spot at the center of the hemisphere ("isocenter"). The cross-firing of 201 radiation beams results in a sharp focus in which the central radiation intensity is high, and the intensity of dose falls rapidly with distance in any direction.

The size of the focal radiation field is controlled by the addition of secondary collimators, which are housed in a "helmet" situated at the head of the patient couch. Four collimator sizes are available, producing fields with nominal sizes of 4 mm, 8 mm, 14 mm and 18 mm.

A simple, single-field treatment requires the target tissue (e.g. entry zone of the trigeminal nerve for trigeminal neuralgia) to be accurately positioned at the center of the helmet collimator system where the fine radiation beams converge. This can be achieved with 0.1mm precision. The couch, helmet system and patient are then moved into the central body of the gamma knife. The treatment begins when the secondary collimators align with the sources.

Typically, the treatment of an intracranial lesion will require the overlapping of a number of foci or fields of radiation. After each field of radiation, the patient couch withdraws from the treatment position, and the position of the patient is adjusted to target an adjacent portion of the tumor. The latest C-model gamma knife offers an automatic positioning system for the head, both reducing human error and increasing precision. The ease with which this latest model affords treatment to many target points in succession encourages the planner to use a larger number of isocenters. This allows more complex plans using more isocenters to be formulated, the increased number of isocenters allowing greater conformity in matching the treatment volume to the tumor whilst sparing the surrounding tissues.

## Linear Accelerators

Linear accelerators, used for years in radio-therapy, have been modified by the addition of a secondary collimator system to perform radiosurgery. Single-focus multiple non-coplanar arc and conformal block techniques are the most widely used. These phrases need explanation to the neurosurgery reader. The former technique means that the radiation source is moved along a large arc, while point-ing to the same center (the so-called "isocen-ter"), then a similar arc is drawn tilted a few degrees away from the first one. A series of arcs are being used to maximize the dose to the center (the target) and minimize the exposure of the surrounding tissues. The second tech-nique involves manufacturing an irregularly shaped portal for the radiation, attempting to match the shape of the targeted lesion as if viewed from the direction of that beam. Similar blocks are made for each entry beam (usually five or six). A series of static, shaped beams are then used to irradiate the lesion from a number of angles. In order to improve conformality, in some centers multiple overlapping foci are used (in a similar fashion to that described for the gamma knife). However, the calculations and set-up of numerous fields are much more diffi-cult with the moving source of a linear acceler-ator than when using a gamma knife, and this deters most centers from using this technique.

More flexibility is incorporated into the system if the linear accelerator is adapted with a micro-multileaf collimator. The device con-sists of a series of individually motorized tung-sten leaves that can be positioned automatically to create any desired beam shape. This is effec-tively the same principle as the conformal block technique but avoids the need to make up spe-cific blocks for each use. The relatively short collimation length and radiation transmission between the collimator leaves are factors that may degrade the sharpness of the final radiation dose gradient and could result in higher doses to normal adjacent brain tissues. The high cost and complexity of these additions resulted in a slow initial acceptance of this method. In the intensity-modulated radiotherapy (IMRT) tech-nique, the dose is delivered in different intensi-ties across the lesion. The collimator leaves dynamically open and close under computer control to selectively expose or shield portions of the tumor according to predetermined limits. Treatment planning for IMRT is complex. All components of the treatment and planning thus require computer control. This promising tech-nique is in its early stages of development and is still under clinical evaluation.

## Suitable Targets

The physical properties of lesions best suited for SRS are:

> small size
> sharply defined margins, and
> favorable shape.

On size, it is customary to quote 3–3.5 cm maximum diameter as the upper limit. In spite of the high precision of targeting ("hitting" the target point: 0.1 mm for gamma knife and 1–2 mm for Linac) and conformal planning, the outer margin of the radiation field is not absolutely sharp. The radiation dose drops very rapidly at the margins but there is a definable penumbra, which receives potentially harmful radiation. The steepness of the margin becomes less with larger lesions. Also, the surface of the lesion increases in proportion to the square of the radius, and thus the volume of adjacent normal brain receiving potentially harmful radiation would become unacceptable for a large target. In these cases single-dose radiation has to be given in lower doses and thus efficacy suffers. This is true whichever equipment one uses.

The margins of the lesion have to be well defined. An infiltrative glioma or a diffuse AVM does not lend itself to precise dose planning. If these lesions are nevertheless treated, the treat-ment must be considered to be palliative, whereby the aim is to achieve an effect only in the limited volume covered by the treatment plan.

A very flat shape may also pose a dose-plan-ning problem. Examples of these lesions would include "en-plaque" extensions of meningiomas or dural AVMs.

There are many lesions that are adjacent to highly eloquent structures, e.g. the optic chiasm. Good dose planning can minimize the risk to those structures. The precise details of the tech-niques achieving this are beyond the scope of this review, particularly as they are equipment dependent. However, there is no particular advantage in this respect of any one delivery method. Even the most advanced dose planning would fail to achieve protection of the structure at risk in the situation where the eloquent tissue is in the middle of the tumor and thus in the center of the radiation field, for example an optic nerve meningioma wrapped around the still-functioning optic nerve or an AVM doing the same in Wyburn-Mason's syndrome. These lesions remain a challenge for management.

# Single Fraction and Fractionation

Fractionation is a well-established principle of radiotherapy, and describes fractionating or dividing the dose of radiation into many smaller increments. This reduces the effect of the radiation on the surrounding normal tissues. It is most effective when there is a high $\alpha/\beta$ ratio, i.e. when there is a marked difference between the radiosensitivity of the pathological target tissue and that of the surrounding structures. In conventional radiotherapy this is important, because the lack of localization means that the radiation field includes a large volume of normal tissue. Philosophically, gamma knife radiosurgery uses exactly the opposite approach: it relies on imaging, matching the radiation fields to conform precisely to the target tissue, and spares neighboring structures in this way, the actual radiation dose being given as a single unfractionated treatment. Intuitively, the stereotactic approach may be advantageous when the $\alpha/\beta$ ratio is not that high, typically the case with benign tumors, and hence the role of SRS in treating acoustic neuromas, meningiomas and AVMs. Conversely, fractionation (either with or without stereotaxy) may be more useful treating flat "en-plaque" tumors, large lesions, and pathology adjacent to radiosensitive structures such as the optic chiasm, where, even with image guidance, there is concern about the radiation delivered to the surrounding area.

Fractionation carries with it the disadvantage of necessitating multiple treatments. When it is used with stereotaxy, relocatable frames are necessary. These are inherently less accurate

than the single fixed frame used in SRS. The impact of these concerns in clinical practice, and the relative role of SRS and SRT, are yet to be ascertained.

# Pathologies

The gradual broadening of indications for radiosurgery was not driven by scientific considerations. Neurosurgeons, usually in charge of the gamma knife in their respective institutions, were all too aware of the complications encountered in open surgical management of their patients, and so the more "high surgical risk" conditions were referred for the alternative. This was the main explanation for the emergence and rise of AVM radiosurgery. The initial few, tentative, referrals were followed by increasing numbers when the general advantages of radiosurgery and the good results became apparent. The second driving force was the evolution that took place in the hearts and minds of patients who obtain information from the Internet and other sources. This is most apparent in patients with benign conditions, e.g. vestibular schwannomas. These patients have the time to research their condition and to enquire about side-effects and complications and compare those with different interventions. They encounter their brethren through patient organizations. Such personal observations may be biased but often prove decisive. Patients tend to make up their minds based on perception and emotional reasons and not leave to their surgeon or to chance the decision as to whether to have major brain surgery or undergo a day-case procedure. Patient pressure is a very powerful force.

Scientific evidence in the form of prospective randomized controlled trials is lacking for both surgery and radiosurgery for most pathologies. Given the problems in recruiting sufficient numbers for the trials, and problems with patients dropping out and crossing over, such data are unlikely to become available. On the other hand, case series provide useful data. The strength of radiosurgery publications is the easy reproducibility of the results in similar units; quite the opposite would apply to microsurgical results published only from centers of excellence, with average and poorer results never becoming available.

# Arteriovenous Malformations

The primary aim in the management of AVMs is to remove the risk of hemorrhage. This risk is 2–4% per annum, with approximately 25–30% mortality rate per bleed. In view of this risk, immediate removal of the lesion is the ideal treatment for those AVMs that can be operated upon with minimal morbidity, and indeed this is the practice in the UK and elsewhere for these lesions. The AVM is characterized by the size, position and venous drainage of the nidus. This allows a classification (Spetzler-Martin grade), which correlates with surgical mortality and morbidity. An AVM in a non-eloquent brain area, less than 3 cm in diameter in size and with superficial venous drainage (Spetzler-Martin grade 1) would be an "operable" lesion.

In emergency situations where a large hematoma requires urgent removal, the AVM is often removed during the same procedure. On the other hand, in these situations it may not be possible to obtain satisfactory angiographic images to plan surgery, and thus many end up with remnants demonstrated on post-operative imaging – requiring further treatment.

In operable, cold cases the risk of neurological complications in the hands of neurosurgeons specializing in this field may be low, and the risks of intracranial surgery (infection, seizures, pneumonia, deep venous thrombosis) and the unavoidable inconvenience (protracted hospital stay, discomfort of a craniotomy, a temporary ban on driving, etc.) may appear worth taking. Thus, surgery is accepted by many patients. However, one has to observe in an increasing proportion of patients the trend to seek less invasive alternatives.

The use of radiosurgery for "operable" AVMs remains controversial; indeed, this group of patients is the only one in which a "surgery vs radiosurgery" debate is still ongoing. Schramm & Schramm [3] performed a meta-analysis of published radiosurgery results for low surgical risk AVMs. His own excellent personal operative results appeared to be better than those for radiosurgery, if the analysis of the latter included the statistical risk of hemorrhage during the latent period, i.e. before radiosurgery would have had its effect. However, the rate of immediate new post-operative neurological deficits or worsening of pre-operative deficits was 27.4% – a figure many times that of gamma-knife-treated patients.

Unfortunately, not all AVMs are ideal or indeed suitable for elective surgery. The resulting problems are incomplete resection and surgical complications. Those with higher Spetzler-Martin grade have a higher neurosurgical risk and surgery has to be more cautious. This leads to not infrequent post-surgical remnants, particularly with AVMs located in the thalamus, basal ganglia and brainstem [4]. Despite the negative reporting bias, the evidence is clear that surgery for these deeply placed AVMs carries a high surgical risk [5].

Endovascular techniques are increasingly used for cerebral AVMs. Analysis of the technique and role of interventional radiology is beyond the scope of this chapter. Suffice it to say that a close cooperation with one's neuroradiologist is an essential factor in the successful management of AVMs.

Since the early reports by Steiner et al. [6], describing successful obliteration of AVMs by radiosurgery, many hundreds of abstracts of proceedings, papers and book chapters have appeared to prove the same [7, 8, 9]. Concerning the mechanism, the main effect of radiation is upon the endothelial cells within the nidus, with an additional effect of myofibroblast development in the connective tissue stroma [10].

It is broadly accepted that about 80–90% of AVMs undergo thrombo-obliteration after single-dose radiation (Fig. 8.1). The efficacy depends on the radiation dose given to the periphery of the lesion. In small ($<1cm^3$) lesions, this dose is usually 25 Gy, which can achieve close to 100% obliteration rate [11]. In cases of larger AVMs, the dose is kept lower in order to keep complications to around 5%. Series with a significant component of large malformations and utilizing lower doses have lower response rate, but even in those the success rate is around 65–75% [12]. It has to be emphasized that these series largely consist of patients referred for radiosurgery because the surgeon in charge of the patient considered open surgery to be of too high risk, usually owing to the eloquent position of the nidus ("inoperable").

The response shows a latency of 1–3 years, with only minor changes occurring in the third year. The risk of hemorrhage appears to decline

STEREOTACTIC RADIOSURGERY

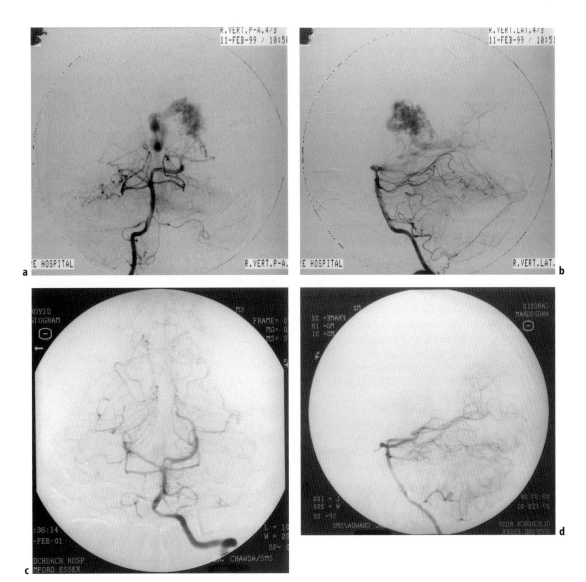

**Fig. 8.1. a–d.** Obliteration of cerebral AVM 2 years after gamma knife radiosurgery: 25 Gy peripheral dose used. **a** PA view. **b** Lateral view. **c** PA view after radiosurgery. **d** Lateral view after radiosurgery.

slowly after radiation but it is not eliminated fully until obliteration is complete. No doubt, the slow response during the latent period contributes to the safety of the method, avoiding pressure-breakthrough hemorrhage by altering the hemodynamics slowly. A speedier reaction could be achieved by higher radiation doses, but the incidence of permanent untoward neurological sequelae may then rise above 5%. The current dose regimens achieve this while achieving overall obliteration rates of 75%, or considerably better in more favorable cases.

It is not possible to give a strict system of criteria for suitability, as the decision as to which technique to use, or which one to use first, is multifactorial. The site, shape and size of the nidus, the angio-architecture, the patient's age, general health, etc., are all factors in this decision. Each case should be considered in a multidisciplinary fashion by a team that has all facilities (surgery, embolization and radio-surgery) available. Those centers where one or the other is unavailable should obtain an outside opinion before any treatment is carried out, even if this involves transmitting or posting images in order to utilize distant expertise.

The likelihood of complete AVM obliteration must be balanced against the need to avoid an unacceptable rate of radiation-related compli-cations after radiosurgery. Flickinger et al. [13] found that 30% of AVM patients had MRI changes adjacent to or within the irradiated volume at a median of 8 months after radio-surgery. However, though some mistakenly describe this as "radionecrosis", these radiolog-ical changes resolve within 2–3 years in the majority of patients. The explanation is proba-bly that the signal change is due to altered per-ilesional blood flow as the nidus gradually obliterates rather than to tissue damage [14]. It is more important to consider the neurological symptoms and signs rather than the radiologi-cal appearance. In a multicenter study of AVM patients, 8% of patients developed neurological sequelae (cranial nerve deficits, seizures, cyst formation) after radiosurgery [15]. Symptoms resolved completely in 54% of these at 3 years post onset. Good prognostic factors were no prior history of hemorrhage and symptoms of minimal severity. According to the prospec-tively maintained database of over 3,000 cases treated in Sheffield, the permanent clinical com-plication rate is 3.8% (data on file). These low-complication figures were obtained with gamma knife treatment. Linear-accelerator (LINAC) technology results in somewhat worse statistics [16].

Earlier reports on AVM radiosurgery sug-gested that the annual hemorrhage rate after radiosurgery prior to obliteration was greater than that occurring in the natural history of untreated AVMs. More recent reports, analyz-ing radiosurgical hemorrhage rates, found that radiosurgery did not change the annual bleed-ing rates during the latency interval [17, 18]. Karlsson et al. [19] reported 1,604 patients with a total of 2,340 patient-years at risk of a hemor-rhage. They detected a decrease in hemorrhage rates within 6 months after radiosurgery and patients who received higher radiation doses were conferred the greatest protection from bleeding. When considered together, these three reports with 2,000 patients and more than 3,000 patient-years at risk of hemorrhage document quite convincingly that radiosurgery does not increase the annual bleeding rate for AVM patients prior to obliteration. In fact, the data suggest that even patients with incomplete obliteration may have some protection against the risk of future bleeding. Nevertheless, the continued risk of hemorrhage during the delay in obliteration is a drawback of radiosurgery.

Some papers [20] highlighted the late radio-logical changes seen on MRI, noted many years after the malformations had been shown by angiography to be obliterated. In most cases this is merely an imaging finding, but in a selected small proportion of cases clinical symptoms may arise. Surgery for these cysts (including one case operated upon in our department) found no neoplastic change. The long-term signifi-cance of these fluid-filled cavities is uncertain but it is likely that most will be innocuous and similar to the porencephalic cyst seen after surgical removal of any large mass lesion.

## Other Vascular Malformations

Angiographically occult vascular malforma-tions (AOVMs) are often referred for radio-surgery. Treatment of cavernous venous malformations is, to some extent, controversial. Planning the treatment may be difficult because the true margins of the vascular anomaly are not obvious, even on MRI. The ring of hemosiderin may lead to an overestimate of the volume and thus increase the risk of complications. Indeed, the treatments planned on CT in the early years were associated with side-effects. The natural history of these lesions is still not clear and many, particularly the incidentally detected ones, are only observed. Those that are in a surgically easily accessible position are usually removed by microsurgery, particularly if they had bled or caused epilepsy. Those in an elo-quent site (brainstem, basal ganglia, etc.) may be good radiosurgical targets. There is increas-ing statistical evidence that the risk of hemor-rhage is reduced by radiosurgery. The difficulty in interpretation of the results lies in the fact that obliteration cannot be demonstrated radiologically. Epilepsy may also improve after treatment.

Radiosurgery is ineffective at best and may be harmful if pursued.

Pure vein of Galen malformations are best treated by endovascular methods. However, these should be distinguished from true AVMs with demonstrable nidus; the latter are treatable with radiosurgery.

# Vestibular Schwannomas (Acoustic Neurinoma)

The indications for the radiosurgical option evolved over the years. First we considered only the elderly and medically infirm who would not tolerate a long surgical procedure. The next group of patients – those with tumors in their only hearing ear or with bilateral tumors – were referred later as a result of the recognition of a perceived superior hearing preservation with radiosurgery. Similarly, facial nerve preservation may be difficult with surgery for recurrent tumors, so these were considered for radiosurgery. Finally, it became a primary choice for those who refused microsurgery in order to avoid the inconvenience and interruption of their daily life by open surgery. The latter group is undoubtedly influenced by the plethora of information available on the Internet both from other patients and from institutions.

Those patients with brainstem compression symptoms usually benefit from at least partial removal of the mass. Therefore, they should undergo open surgery rather than hoping for a slow decompression by eventual shrinkage of the tumor. The arbitrary upper limit of 3.5 cm maximum diameter is born out of the observation that a larger tumor cannot be irradiated with a therapeutically effective single dose without unacceptable cranial nerve neuropathies. There are, of course, anecdotal successes even amongst these large tumors.

The aim of radiosurgery is different from that of open surgery. It does not aim to remove the lesion, merely to control its growth. This control may be defined as "no growth compared with the pre-treatment size", or the looser definition advocated by some, where the criterion is "the absence of need for further intervention"; the latter is open to biased interpretation. The control rate is reported to be about 97–98%, with an actual reduction in size in 23–55% [21].

Involution of the tumor occurs slowly, through several years (Fig. 8.2). Considering the rates of residual and recurrent tumors seen even in the best published surgical series, not to mention the case material submitted for radiosurgery, tumor control with radiosurgery is at least as good.

Complications of radiosurgery can be immediate and late. In the first 24 hours, nausea and headache were seen, particularly in the early days of radiosurgery when larger radiation doses and less precise dose planning were used. The combination of conformal planning, delivering no more than 12–15 Gy peripheral dose, and perioperative steroid cover eliminated these side-effects. Late cranial neuropathies are dependent on peripheral dose and the size of the tumor. The latter is an important factor, as with larger tumor size a longer section of the nerves receives toxic dose. On the other hand, intracanalicular tumors may also pose a challenge. They are more difficult to delineate precisely, and the relative imprecision of MRI imaging may lead to complications. In these cases fusion with CT scan is particularly helpful.

Hearing preservation is reported in 30–75%, and as the fading of hearing is gradual, the result is dependent on length of follow-up. In our own material (in Sheffield) concerning unilateral vestibular schwannomas (VS), using the Gammaplan planning software, no higher than 15 Gy peripheral dose and at least 5 years' follow-up, hearing preservation was achieved in 75% of patients (submitted for publication). Over-enthusiastic reduction in the delivered dose may be counterproductive: losing tumor control would lead to morbidity through increased tension on the cranial nerves. One must not forget that, after all, most VS are originally diagnosed as a result of progressive hearing loss.

In considering tumor control and the management of patients after radiosurgery, it is important to understand the changes that occur with time after the treatment. Early on, around 1 year, the tumor is frequently larger. It is important not to rush into surgery as subsequently the tumor may well involute and shrink. At that time the cranial nerves may be at their most fragile, rendering the operation higher risk. Failure of tumor control should not be declared until 4–5 years after radiosurgery owing to the slow effect of the treatment.

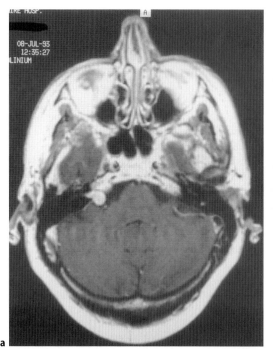

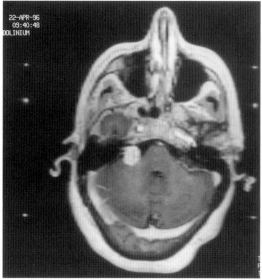

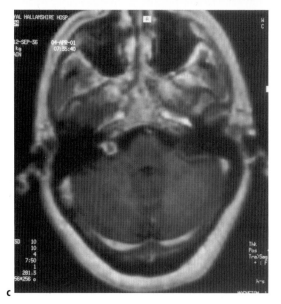

**Fig. 8.2. a–c.** Involution of vestibular schwannoma (VS) after gamma knife treatment with 13 Gy peripheral dose. **a** MRI scan of right VS at presentation. **b** Enlarged tumor at the time of radiosurgery. **c** Typical appearance 5 years after treatment.

There has been concern expressed about the late consequences of radiosurgery. Excision after radiosurgery may be more difficult due to scarring, even in later years, though the evidence for this is very weak and anecdotal. There is a possibility of malignant change in the irradiated schwannomas [22]. So far the statistics suggest that such a change is only a remote possibility, but long-term follow-up of these patients continues.

In summary, radiosurgery is an attractive alternative for patients with small and medium-sized VS, particularly if hearing and/or facial nerve preservation on the affected side is paramount. It is increasingly considered (at least by the patients) to be the primary procedure of choice for those with small tumors. It is often chosen to treat recurrent tumors. There are indications that recurrence after microsurgery may be the result of less radical removal in an attempt to achieve hearing preservation. In our material of over 500 acoustic neuromas referred for radiosurgery, 36% had one or more previous operations on their tumor. This is a particularly important group as, owing to the almost uniformly present post-operative hearing loss, they may not have new symptoms until the tumor is large and causes ataxia. One of the common criticisms of radiosurgery relates to the need for follow-up imaging – true, but the high proportion of post-surgical cases in our material suggests that vigilance is necessary even after excision; the notion that microsurgery is a "definitive treatment", without the risk of recurrence, is a myth. Long-term supervision is warranted after all treatments of these tumors, whether surgery or radiosurgery is applied.

# Malignancy

In principle, infiltrative tumors should not be considered to be suitable for a focal treatment. This statement is particularly true for high-grade gliomas that infiltrate far from the main mass. We rarely use this technique in such cases. However, in the case of metastases, local infiltration into the normal tissue is fairly limited and thus both surgery and radiosurgery confer a benefit by local cytoreduction. Furthermore, radiosurgery treatment has a penumbral effect, as opposed to the truly sharp boundary with surgical excision, and this may even result in superior local control compared with surgery alone. A multicenter randomized trial is in progress in Europe, which compares gamma knife radiosurgery alone to surgery with whole-brain radiotherapy.

This pathology is especially important for healthcare planners. During the course of their disease, 20–40% of cancer patients will develop brain metastases, and this predicts almost half a million patients with brain metastases per year in the USA alone. Given the number of cases,

the following question arises: "How many of these cases are appropriate for radiosurgery?" Appropriate is defined as "the patient stands a reasonable chance of obtaining a benefit in terms of control of brain disease and retention/improvement in quality of life with treatment". In order to identify a group of patients who might benefit from more aggressive treatment, such as radiosurgery, one can use the experience of the RTOG (Radiation Therapy Oncology Group) protocol 79-16, a radiation therapy protocol on brain metastases. The four factors predictive of improved survival were:

Karnofsky performance status ≥70%

Absent or controlled primary disease

Age <60 years

Evidence of metastasis to brain only

In our unit we use these criteria to include patients in the radiosurgery program, but also consider the number of metastases visible on MRI. We are reluctant to treat in cases where there are more than three lesions as the benefits of focal treatment are lost when there is an obvious generalized disease. Technically speaking, most metastases are close to ideal for radiosurgery. They are easily visible on imaging, they are rarely beyond the suitable size-range, and they are usually spherical with sharp outlines, therefore the matching of the shape of the lesion is easy. There is published evidence from a multicenter study [23] showing that there was a 2.84 times higher risk of local recurrence after LINAC treatment than after gamma knife treatment. The reason for this finding is controversial but it may question in the future the acceptability of LINAC use, as opposed to gamma knife use, for this indication.

It is particularly important in this patient group to state that the aim of radiosurgery is only to achieve local tumor control. This may be achievable in up to 90% of cases. Prospective randomized trials are needed to properly define the role of radiosurgery for cerebral metastases.

# Functional Indications

As mentioned in the introduction, radiosurgery was originally devised to be used for lesion making in functional indications. A wide range of interventions were carried out, including anterior capsulotomy for obsessive–compulsive disorder, thalamotomies for pain and movement disorders, and irradiation of the trigeminal ganglion for neuralgia. Subsequently, the technique became increasingly used for vascular and neoplastic lesions, as discussed above.

However, over the last few years the fastest growing indication for radiosurgery, particularly in the USA, has been trigeminal neuralgia. This revival was made possible by the development of imaging enabling the identification of, and thus targeting the entry zone of, the trigeminal nerve, or indeed the nerve itself. The reader will be familiar with the wide range of treatments and procedures in use for this condition. The reason to add another was the perceived surgical risk of microvascular decompression on one hand, and the recurrence rate with the alternative operations on the other. In practical terms the procedure is particularly straightforward as there is very little shape matching necessary when planning this treatment. Most gamma knife centers use a single 4 mm collimator field, prescribing 70 or 80 Gy to the isocenter. It was observed that irradiation of a longer section of the nerve using two adjacent fields may increase the risk of post-operative facial sensory impairment. In terms of efficacy, gamma knife surgery does live up to the expectations: in primary cases 85–90% pain-free state is achieved. The only drawback is the 3–12 weeks lag period before the cessation of pain. Salvage procedures after previous destructive operations are less effective but may result in good and excellent outcome (pain free with or without continued medication) in 65–70%. The permanency of the results appears to mirror microvascular decompressions rather than the percutaneous rhizotomies. Whether in the long run the recurrence rate remains as low as it appears at present is not yet clear. The risk of facial dysesthesia or numbness is low, and the other risks of surgery (e.g. cerebrospinal fluid rhinorrhea, meningitis, hearing loss, etc.) are avoided. The attraction of a day-case procedure under local anesthetic for an elderly or infirm patient is obvious.

After treating AVMs associated with focal-onset epilepsy, many observed an improvement or cessation of epileptic activity. This prompted treatment of small indolent lesions and good seizure-control results were observed. Since 1995, Regis presented several patients with

mesial temporal sclerosis who had been treated using focused radiation with the gamma knife. His results were very convincing, achieving seizure control in a high proportion of cases. Other centers, including the authors of this review, followed suit, treating small series of patients. Our experience showed that seizure control at 3 years following irradiation is very similar to that achieved with temporal lobe resections, and thus this method could be advocated for those who are unable or unwilling to undergo resective surgery. However, our observation was that there was a long, 12–36-month time lag to achieve the seizure-free state. Furthermore, some patients found it difficult to cope with the slow alteration of their seizure pattern and the appearance of frequent auras for some months. In our small series we have not observed permanent neurological deficit, but about 50% of patients required several weeks of dexamethasone treatment owing to focal cerebral swelling after about a year. The method certainly deserves to be exposed to wider scale trials, but its role is not yet established.

Sporadic reports are available concerning the revival of radiosurgery for traditional functional indications. Thalamotomies, anterior corpus callosotomies and even cingulotomies have all been described using radiosurgery. Admittedly, it would be attractive to make the lesions currently made using radiofrequency techniques without the need for a burr hole and physical penetration of the brain. The limitation of radiosurgery for these indications is the lack of feedback obtained by stimulation and recording. Although the need to adjust the target coordinates during open procedures is infrequent, the reassurance before making the lesion is required by most neurosurgeons. An additional problem is the relative variability of the size of the brain lesion made even with a standard radiation dose. These indications should be considered as experimental.

## Future Trends

The history of radiosurgery shows that, over the years, the greatest development has occurred in imaging. It is likely that this trend will continue at least for the foreseeable future. MRI techniques are likely to improve within years to allow the AVM nidus to be identified without arterial angiography. New protocols are already being developed (e.g. one in our unit, termed "MR-DSA") to be used for post-radiosurgery assessment of the nidus, although at present an apparent cure would still have to be confirmed by high-quality digital subtraction angiography.

The currently used planning software for the gamma knife technique and for some of the Linac techniques allows protection of adjacent eloquent structures. Automated planning will make these procedures even safer and easier in the future. It will be helpful to include functional information in the planning of treatment near important cortical structures, and a combination of structural MRI with functional MRI will no doubt be increasingly utilized. The role of PET is likely to grow, both in pre-operative work-up and post-radiosurgery assessment of tumors, in the same manner as it is currently used to differentiate between radionecrosis and recurrence after radiotherapy.

Delivery of focused radiation is also likely to change. The precision and reliability of the gamma knife is far superior to LINAC-based systems, but it is hoped that the latter techniques will add flexibility to treat larger lesions and those in extracranial positions. The role of fractionated delivery will be clarified. The potential for malignant changes and other late complications will also be explored in years to come.

# Key Points

- *Stereotactic radiosurgery delivers a high dose of radiation to well-defined targets in the brain. In most situations lesions of less than 3.5 cm maximum diameter are considered to be suitable.*

- *Thrombo-obliteration of AVMs is achieved in 60–95%, depending on size, and with 4–9% risk of neurological complications, depending on eloquence of the area.*

- *Vestibular schwannomas can be controlled in over 90% of cases, with 1% risk of permanent facial nerve deficit and 25% risk of hearing loss.*

- *Functional indications are still under evaluation.*

# Self-assessment

☐ What are the main indications for stereotactic radiosurgery?

☐ What are the two principal technologies used in delivery of the radiation?

☐ What are the main factors taken into account in the decisions regarding suitability?

# References

1. Paddick I. A simple scoring ratio to index the conformity of radiosurgical treatment plans. J Neurosurg 2000;93(suppl 3):219–22.

2. Borden JA, Mahajan A, Tsi JS. A quality factor to compare the dosimetry of gamma knife radiosurgery and intensity-modulated radiation therapy quantitatively as a function of target volume and shape. J Neurosurg 2000;93(suppl 3):228–32.

3. Schaller C, Schramm J. Microsurgical results for small arteriovenous malformations accessible for radiosurgical or embolization treatment. Neurosurgery 1997;40:664–72.

4. Lawton MT, Hamilton MG, Spetzler RE. Multimodality treatment of deep arteriovenous malformations: thalamus, basal ganglia, and brain stem. Neurosurgery 1995;37:29–36.

5. Morgan MK, Drummond KJ, Grinnel IV, Sorby W. Surgery for cerebral arteriovenous malformation: risks related to lenticulostriate arterial supply. J Neurosurg 1997;86:801–5.

6. Steiner L, Leksell L, Forster DMC, Greitz T, Backlund E. Stereotactic radiosurgery in intracranial arteriovenous malformations. Acta Neurochir (Suppl) 1974; 21:195–209.

7. Lunsford LD, Kondziolka D, Flickinger JC, Bissonette DJ, Jungreis CA, Vincent D et al. Stereotactic radiosurgery for arteriovenous malformations of the brain. J Neurosurg 1991;75:512–24.

8. Steiner L, Lindquist C, Adler JR, Torner JC, Alves W, Steiner M. Clinical outcome of radiosurgery for cerebral arteriovenous malformations. J Neurosurg 1992;77:1–8.

9. Colombo F, Pozza F, Chicrego G, Casentini L, De Luea G, Francescon P. Linear accelerator radiosurgery of cerebral arteriovenous malformations: an update. Neurosurgery 1994;34:14–21.

10. Szeifert G, Kemeny AA, Timperley WR, Forster DMC. The potential role of myofibroblasts in arteriovenous malformation obliteration after radiosurgery. Neurosurgery 1997;39:67–70.

11. Lunsford LD, editor. Stereotactic radiosurgery clinics of North America, vol 3, no. 1. Philadelphia: WB Saunders, 1992.

12. Yamamoto Y et al. Interim report on the radiosurgical treatment of cerebral arteriovenous malformations. The influence of size, dose, time, and technical factors on obliteration rate. J Neurosurg 1995;83:832–7.

13. Flickinger JC, Kondziolka D, Pollock BE, Maitz A, Lunsford LD. Complications from arteriovenous

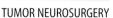

malformation radiosurgery: multivariate analysis and risk modeling. Int J Radiat Oncol Biol Phys 1997;38: 485–90.

14. Pollock BE. Patient outcomes after arteriovenous malformation radiosurgery. In: Lunsford LD, Kondziolka D, Flickinger JC, editors. Gamma knife brain surgery (Progress in neurological surgery, vol 14). Basel: Karger, 1998; 51–9.

15. Flickinger JC. Kondziolka D. Lunsford LD et al. A multi-institutional analysis of complication outcomes after arteriovenous malformation radiosurgery. Int J Radiat Oncol Biol Phys 1999;44:67–74.

16. Miyawaki L, Dowd C, Wara W et al. Five year results of LINAC radiosurgery for arteriovenous malformations: outcome for large AVMs. Int J Radiat Oncol Biol Phys 1999;44:1089–106.

17. Pollock BE, Flickinger JC, Lunsford LD, Bissonette DJ, Kondziolka D. Hemorrhage risk after stereotactic radiosurgery of cerebral arteriovenous malformations. Neurosurgery 1996;38:652–61.

18. Friedman WA, Blatt DL, Bova FJ, Buatti JM, Mendenhall WM, Kublis PS. The risk of hemorrhage after radio-surgery for arteriovenous malformations. J Neurosurg 1996;84:912–19.

19. Karlsson Lidquist C, Steiner L. The effect of gamma knife surgery on the risk of rupture prior to AVM obliteration. Minim Invasive Neurosurg 1996;39:21–7.

20. Yamamoto M, Jimbo M, Kobayashi M, Toyoda C, Ide M, Tanaka N et al. Long-term results of radiosurgery for arteriovenous malformation: neurodiagnostic imaging and histological studies of angiographically confirmed nidus obliteration. Surg Neurol 1992;37:219–30.

21. Flickinger JC, Lunsford LD, Coffey RJ et al. Radio-surgery for acoustic neurinomas. Cancer 1991;67: 345–53.

22. Hanabusa K, Morikawa A, Murata T, Taki W. Acoustic neuroma with malignant transformation (case report). J Neurosurg 2001;95:518–21.

23. Shaw E, Scott C, Souhami L, Dinapoli R, Kline R, Loeffler J et al. Single dose radiosurgical treatment of previously irradiated primary brain tumours and brain metastases: final report of RTOG protocol 90-05. Int J Radiol Oncol Biol Phys 2000;47:291–8.

# IV
# Tumors

# 9

## Low-grade Gliomas in Adults

Henry Marsh

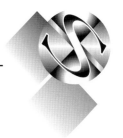

## Summary

The treatment of low-grade gliomas remains one of the most uncertain and controversial areas of modern neurosurgery. It is an increasingly important area because the widespread availability of MRI scanning has meant that more and more cases are being diagnosed. A small number of patients can be cured by complete surgical resection, and modern neurosurgical techniques, combined with awake craniotomy and intra-operative histology, have probably increased this number. Nevertheless, the majority of patients cannot be cured and the decision as to how best to treat them can be very difficult, especially since low-grade gliomas are very variable in their size, location, histology and biological behavior. Treatment decisions need to be made jointly by neurosurgeons and neuro-oncologists. Careful follow-up and explanation to the patient are often just as important as any treatment undertaken.

## Introduction

The term "low-grade gliomas" is used by neurologists and neurosurgeons to describe a group of intrinsic cerebral tumors arising primarily from astrocytes, oligodendrocytes or ependymal cells that are characterized by their relatively slow rate of growth and certain radiological appearances when compared with the commoner malignant or "high-grade" gliomas. The use of the term is often confusing since it is not a precise pathological definition. It is sometimes used to refer only to low-grade astrocytomas, but oligodendrogliomas, ependymomas, gangliogliomas and pleomorphic xanthoastrocytomas will sometimes be included as well. To add to the confusion, the pathology of these various tumors often overlaps, and "mixed oligoastrocytomas" or "ependymal differentiation in an oligodendroglioma", for instance, are quite often reported by pathologists on microscopic examination of biopsy specimens. Furthermore, there is no precise border between "low grade" and "high grade", and many tumors will be found, on histological examination, to contain cells of differing degrees of malignancy. Although "low-grade" tumors typically grow quite slowly, it is euphemistic to describe them as "benign" since the great majority of adults with these "low-grade" tumors will die from the disease within 10 years of the initial diagnosis, irrespective of any treatment that they might have received [1]. Death most frequently occurs as a result of the tumor eventually transforming into a more malignant form (in up to 80% of tumors, according to Russell and Rubinstein [2]) or occasionally as a result of slow but steady expansion of the tumor without obvious malignant change. Patients with these tumors, therefore, are best seen as suffering from a chronic, usually incurable, illness where treatment is only palliative in the great majority of cases.

Low-grade gliomas of all varieties account for about 15–20% of primary cerebral neoplasms in adults and most commonly present in young adults with epilepsy and without any neurological deficit. In the modern era of widely available and increasingly sensitive CT and MRI scanning, they are diagnosed more frequently, at an earlier stage, when the tumor is smaller, than in the past. Nevertheless, it is remarkable how large some of these tumors can become before they produce any symptoms. Only a small number of patients will have symptoms of raised intracranial pressure or a focal neurological deficit at the time of presentation. Their comparative rarity and long natural history have made it difficult to establish how best to treat them and there have been no controlled trials comparing different methods of treatment. The published literature is largely anecdotal and retrospective (see, for instance, the review by Marantz [3]). If low-grade gliomas as a whole are considered, evidence-based conclusions cannot be drawn as to whether treatment has any significant impact on life expectancy or not.

It must never be forgotten that the diagnosis of a brain tumor is quite devastating for the patient and the patient's family. They will hope for confident and certain advice from the neurosurgeon to whom they are referred. The neurosurgeon's difficulty in knowing what to advise, given the lack of evidence from any controlled trials, is made even more difficult by the fact that treatment is never entirely safe and is often very unpleasant. Most of the patients will be entirely well at the time of presentation, often having only suffered a single epileptic fit. Not surprisingly, therefore, opinions vary as to how best to treat these tumors, ranging from the so-called "conservative treatment" of doing nothing at all (other than treating the epilepsy with anticonvulsants), to minimal biopsy, to radical resection, with or without chemotherapy or radiotherapy. Despite the lack of firm evidence, it is possible, however, to establish certain principles that should guide management and to identify a few subtypes of low-grade glioma in adults where it is reasonably certain what should be done.

The main forms of treatment for these tumors are surgery and radiotherapy, and to a much lesser extent chemotherapy. Because of the uncertainties surrounding the best way to treat patients, it cannot be emphasized strongly enough that patients with these tumors should be treated jointly by neurosurgeons and neuro-oncologists working in close cooperation, although care must be taken to prevent the "specialist team" turning into an impersonal committee.

# Pathological Classification

## Varieties

The pathological classification of intrinsic cerebral tumors is various and, at times, confusing. A clear account is to be found in the standard work by Russell and Rubinstein [2]. We are concerned here primarily with the slow-growing gliomas of the cerebral hemispheres that are found in adults, so the list below will not, therefore, include the various astrocytomas found in children, such as optic pathway astrocytomas, brainstem gliomas and pilocytic cerebellar astrocytomas, some of which are truly benign in the sense of being curable by surgical resection. These essentially pediatric tumors can, however, occasionally be found in young adults.

Low-grade gliomas may be classified into the following categories:

Astrocytoma (grades I and II)
Oligodendroglioma
Mixed oligoastrocytoma

Miscellaneous, including ganglioglioma, pleomorphic xanthoastrocytoma and neurocytoma

## Presentation

In modern practice, the great majority of low-grade gliomas present with epilepsy. A small number of patients (1% in the author's own series of 160 patients with low-grade gliomas) will present with raised intracranial pressure or a focal neurological deficit. Most patients are relatively young: low-grade gliomas are found only occasionally in patients over the age of 40 years.

## Diagnostic Imaging

MRI scanning is the most sensitive means of detecting these tumors and showing the degree of infiltration into the surrounding brain. Good-quality CT (computed tomography) is less effective at delineating the extent of the tumor, and will completely miss some of the smaller tumors that are seen with MRI.

Low-grade gliomas in adults typically do not enhance. If a degree of enhancement is present, however, it is generally considered to mean that anaplastic change is present, that the grade of the tumor will be higher, and that the prognosis will be correspondingly worse than if there was no enhancement. There are some exceptions to this, such as pleomorphic xanthoastrocytomas and pediatric astrocytomas, which occasionally present in young adults and where enhancement is not necessarily an ominous finding. It is important to recognize that CT and MRI scanning are not always a reliable way of determining the histological grade of a tumor [4]. Interpretation of brain scans of patients who have undergone previous treatment can be particularly difficult, with post-operative changes causing enhancement that can mimic recurrent tumor, and radiotherapy producing white matter changes that are very similar to infiltrating tumor or cerebral edema caused by recurrent tumor.

The typical MRI findings for low-grade astrocytomas are of low-signal intensity on T1 spin-echo sequences, and of high-signal intensity on T2 and proton-density sequences, with varying degrees of white matter infiltration and edema around the central part of the tumor. On CT, the tumors appear as areas of low density, sometimes with patchy calcification, which is seen most commonly in oligodendrogliomas.

## Pathological Anatomy

The degree of infiltration of the surrounding brain by low-grade gliomas is very variable. Some tumors can appear to occupy much of a cerebral hemisphere, with the patient suffering surprisingly little, if any, neurological impairment (Fig. 9.1). In these cases the differential diagnosis from gliomatosis cerebri can be somewhat arbitrary. Other tumors (Fig. 9.2) can be relatively small and appear well circumscribed, although histologically all of these tumors are infiltrative to a greater or lesser extent. Most of these tumors do not infiltrate or cross the pia arachnoid so that on the scan, and at surgery,

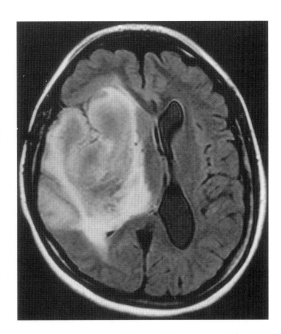

**Fig. 9.1.** Case HO. Inoperable low-grade astrocytoma (histologically verified).

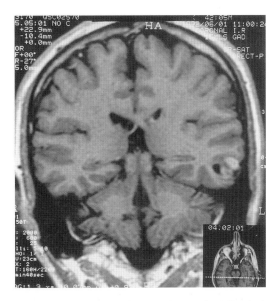

**Fig. 9.2.** Case MB. A small left temporal tumor that is histologically identical to Case HO.

one will find quite clear superficial edges to the tumor that are formed by the cerebral sulci. The infiltration occurs in the deep white matter beneath the cortex and it is the lack of a clear tumor–brain interface here that makes radical surgical resection difficult and often impossible. Radical resection can be made even more difficult by the fact that, as Skirboll et al.[5] have shown, tumor cells can infiltrate functioning brain, and histological studies have shown that the MRI scanning can underestimate the depth of tumor infiltration into the brain [6].

At surgery, with superficially placed tumors, one typically finds an area of the brain where the cerebral gyri are widened. Sometimes the surface of the abnormal area of the brain is paler and less vascular than that of the surrounding brain; sometimes it is more vascular. On opening the cortex, one usually finds that the white matter is firmer than normal, and sometimes slightly darker. The author will still often find it very difficult, after opening the dura, to know whether he has found the tumor or not. Usually it is fairly easy to be certain that one is in the central core of the tumor; the question of navigation, mapping and perioperative smear histology will be dealt with later. The problems arise, if one is aiming for radical resection, as one approaches the peripheral areas of the tumor, where it becomes impossible to know, by purely surgical appearances, whether the white matter is still infiltrated by tumor or not.

Although low-grade gliomas in adults can occur in any part of the brain, they are distinctly unusual in the posterior fossa, which is clearly in contrast to what is found in children. They can occur in any of the "lobes" of the cerebral hemispheres (which, it should be remembered, are relatively arbitrary anatomical boundaries), or deep in the basal ganglia. A few patterns of growth seem to be characteristic, such as the tumors that grow in the frontal lobe and root of the temporal lobe, so that they present on both sides of the Sylvian fissure.

# Management

The typical case of low-grade glioma is of a young adult who has had an epileptic fit, who has no neurological deficit, and in whom a brain scan has shown an intrinsic cerebral tumor without any contrast enhancement. The tumor may be remarkably large or relatively small. It may appear to be relatively well circumscribed, or it may be diffusely infiltrating. It may be very close to eloquent brain, or it may be located in the tip of one of the frontal, temporal or occipital lobes, or deep within the basal ganglia. It can be appreciated at once that there can be no single treatment policy for a tumor type that can be so variable. This variety of forms also explains why the neurosurgical literature is so unsatisfactory on the subject of low-grade gliomas, since few, if any, of the published papers stratify their results in accordance with the varied macroscopic anatomy.

The question that arises with this "typical" patient is whether any treatment should be offered at all, given the lack of evidence that treatment makes any significant difference to overall survival or median time to progression if patients with low-grade gliomas are taken as a whole. The central problem in the management of low-grade gliomas is whether radical or debulking surgery in patients without raised intracranial pressure makes any difference to long term prognosis. In other words, it is simply not known whether the extent of surgical resection has any impact on prognosis or not in these patients. A further problem is that there is no easy way of defining the extent of surgical resection; surgeons talk about "radical" or "subtotal" removal, or "debulking" of these tumors, but have no way of quantifying this. Post-operative MRI scanning clearly helps to some extent, but for the reasons mentioned earlier, these scans can be hard to interpret. Nevertheless, despite this central uncertainty, the neurosurgeon must make a decision on whether to operate or not, and if so, what form the operation should take.

For practical purposes, the management of low-grade gliomas can be divided into five groups. For the purposes of this discussion, "complete" resection is taken to mean "curative" resection, as shown by subsequent, long-term follow-up scanning, whereas "radical" resection only means that initial follow-up scanning shows no residual tumor. The groups are:

Large tumors in eloquent areas that, on the basis of the pre-operative scan, are too large for extensive resection to be possible without an unacceptably high risk of producing a major post-operative neurological deficit

Small tumors where, on the basis of the pre-operative scan, complete or radical resection is anticipated with little risk of neurological damage

Tumors where it is uncertain whether complete or radical resection can be achieved

Tumors that recur after treatment

Tumors that cause intractable epilepsy

## 1. Tumors that are Too Large for Complete Resection to be Possible Without Unacceptable Risk

Complete resection is clearly impossible in patients where the tumor is bilateral, having crossed the corpus callosum, or involves the basal ganglia and insular cortex. Early involvement of the corpus callosum is not, in itself, a complete contraindication to surgery, since it is possible to resect areas of the corpus callosum without major risk. However, the significance of corpus callosum involvement is that in most cases it is associated with bilateral hemispheric infiltration, and one of the fundamental rules of neurosurgery remains that bilateral hemispheric damage is associated with a high risk of major neurological deficit. In a very small proportion of these cases, at the time of presentation, there will be symptoms of raised intracranial pressure. In these cases standard debulking surgery is indicated. Since there is no evidence that debulking surgery prolongs survival in patients without raised intracranial pressure, some authors [7] have argued that there is little justification in carrying out such surgery in the absence of raised pressure. Others have argued, for instance Berger et al. [8], that aggressive debulking surgery delays recurrence when compared with more conservative resection, but no studies have shown any certain benefit in terms of long-term survival. It is an article of faith for some neurosurgeons that debulking surgery, sometimes described more impressively as "cytoreduction", is beneficial, but the fact remains that this is entirely unproven, and any theoretical benefits must also be balanced against the greater morbidity of aggressive surgery. Even with very large tumors several years can pass before raised pressure develops and palliative surgery becomes indicated. Since there is also no evidence [9] that radiotherapy prolongs life in this group of patients, there is little purpose in carrying out a biopsy (stereotactically or otherwise) unless there is doubt about the interpretation of the scan or unless the neurosurgeon's neuro-oncological colleagues strongly favor adjuvant treatment in such cases.

If it has been decided not to treat a patient in this group, and instead to follow up the patient with repeat scans, the tumor will, sooner or later, be shown to be growing larger, probably before the onset of the symptoms of raised intracranial pressure. A more rational approach might be to postpone repeating the scan until such symptoms have developed. However, most patients will wish to be followed up with scans, in the hope that they will not show any progression, and it is very difficult for the surgeon to refuse to organize follow-up scanning. However, once the scan shows progression – albeit asymptomatic – it is very difficult to continue to withhold treatment even though treatment is, by definition, palliative and there are no new symptoms to palliate.

There are two possible options. Firstly, further conservative treatment may be given with the blunt admission to the patient that there is no convincing evidence that treatment will make a significant difference. Secondly, treatment can be recommended in the hope that it will slow down the rate of progression, even though the evidence is lacking that such treatment works. In the author's experience, most patients will favor the latter policy.

Treatment can take the form of surgery and radiotherapy, or debulking surgery alone.

Biopsy will be required with either policy. Biopsy can be either closed or open, depending on the location of the tumor and the surgeon's preference. Different parts of the tumor can show different histological features and there is an argument either for multiple targets, if biopsied stereotactically, or for removing a reasonable volume of tumor if open biopsy is carried out. With large tumors it must be remembered that biopsy without debulking can precipitate post-operative cerebral herniation. Pre-operative steroids are essential and, on occasion, debulking surgery, even in the absence of symptoms of raised intracranial pressure, may need to be carried out as part of the biopsy. Treatment can also be confined to debulking surgery, and radiotherapy postponed until there is further evidence of progression, provided that histology shows that the tumor has not undergone malignant change. Once such malignant change has occurred, the tumor should be treated as a high-grade tumor, and palliative adjuvant treatment is then indicated in the great majority of cases.

*Illustrative Example: a 28-year-old woman with frequent focal epileptic fits affecting the left arm but no deficit (Fig. 9.3 and 9.4)*

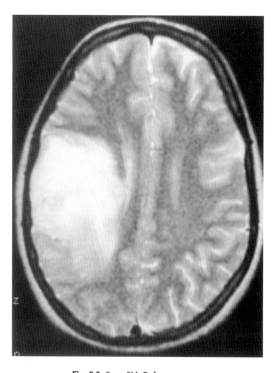

**Fig. 9.3.** Case CM. Before surgery.

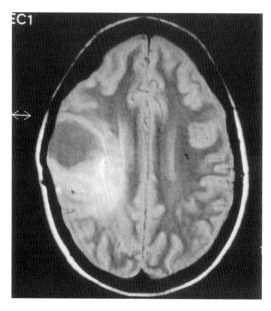

**Fig. 9.4.** Case CM. After partial resection.

The scan shows an extensive, infiltrating tumor involving both sides of the insular cortex.

A debulking operation under local anesthetic was attempted but abandoned after the patient developed severe weakness of the left arm. This did not get better and the epilepsy remained a major problem. The tumor was shown to be a low-grade astrocytoma. She died 6 years later from tumor progression.

Comment: This operation was carried out before the author's initial enthusiasm for radical surgery for large low-grade gliomas had been tempered by experience. In retrospect, it is easy to see that there was no prospect of obtaining sufficient tumor removal to influence the epilepsy and absolutely no question of "total" excision of the tumor. All that the operation achieved was to add weakness of her left arm to her epileptic fits.

## 2. Tumours where, on the Basis of the Pre-operative Scan, Complete Resection is Anticipated

These tumors are, unfortunately, in a distinct minority (probably no more than 5%). It is clear to all neurosurgeons that a few small, well-circumscribed, low-grade gliomas can be cured by radical surgery. (The relatively rare pleomorphic xanthoastrocytomas are usually cured by surgery alone but are clearly different from the majority of low-grade tumors.) The question of the suitability of a low-grade glioma for radical surgery is therefore a question of:

Tumor size and the degree of infiltration of the surrounding brain

The relationship of the tumor to eloquent structures (in other words, the risk of surgery producing a significant neurological deficit)

The surgeon's technique and experience.

*Illustrative Example: a 35-year-old army officer (Fig. 9.2 and 9.5) with a single epileptic fit*

The scan shows a small left inferior temporal tumor, presumed (and ultimately confirmed by surgery) to be a low-grade astrocytoma. An initial neurosurgical opinion advised against surgery on the grounds that it involved some risk of producing dysphasia, and there was no evidence that surgery would make any difference to the 10-year 80% mortality rate.

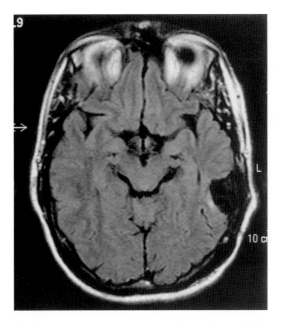

**Fig. 9.5.** Case MB 9 years after surgery. The small area of high signal on this FLAIR sequence has remained unchanged since surgery and presumably represents gliosis.

Using speech mapping with awake craniotomy and multiple marginal biopsies, what appeared to be complete removal was achieved without producing any neurological deficit. Ten years later, the patient remains free from fits, is off anticonvulsants with no evidence of recurrence on follow-up scanning, and is on active service in the army.

Comment: If the patient had not been operated upon and had been judged to have an effectively "inoperable brain tumor", he would have lost his job as well as remaining at risk of the tumor progressing. He would also have had the psychological burden of "living with" the tumor. Modern techniques have made resection reasonably safe although, from a single case such as this, one cannot know whether surgery has improved his chances of survival or not when compared with conservative treatment.

## 3. Tumors where it is Uncertain Whether Complete Resection can be Achieved

It is easy to justify an attempt at radical, curative resection of a small tumor, superficially placed in the tip of a lobe, without MRI evidence of extensive infiltration. The risks of such an operation are the risks of any craniotomy – that is, the risks of hemorrhage or infection – and these risks are almost certainly less than the risks of the tumor undergoing malignant change and proving fatal in the future. It can become a question of fine surgical judgement as to the point at which it becomes unrealistic to hope for total resection.

Radical resection depends upon:

Careful study of a pre-operative MRI scan, supplemented by functional MRI studies and neuronavigation if appropriate and available;

The use of intraoperative mapping methods combined with smear biopsy analysis (if the surgeon is lucky enough to work with a neuropathologist who is able to carry out smear analysis on many dozens of marginal biopsies as the resection proceeds). In a few centers, intraoperative MRI scanning is now available, but it is not yet clear if this makes a major difference to the surgery of these tumors.

Two principles must guide selection of patients for radical surgery of this sort. Firstly, there must be a realistic chance of "total" excision of the tumor. It will often not prove possible during the operation to achieve such a removal, but there must be a reasonable possibility of achieving this on the basis of examining the pre-operative MRI scan. Secondly, it is not acceptable to produce any degree of permanent neurological impairment since all of these patients are, by definition, in perfect condition and we know that the majority of them will eventually die from the tumor, despite treatment. That having been said, of course, there is bound to be some morbidity, although often temporary, especially when operating in the supplementary motor area. In the author's series of 130 "radical" operations for low-grade gliomas, there has been a 7% incidence of significant, permanent morbidity (although no mortality) and all in patients who ended up having only partial excision of their tumor. The morbidity, in short, probably conferred little benefit on the patients in terms of eventual outcome. Temporary neurological deficits, which resolved completely, occurred in 20% of patients.

By using neuronavigation, magnification, intraoperative mapping under local anesthetic

[9] and intraoperative histology, there can be no doubt that more low-grade gliomas are now suitable for an attempt at surgical cure than in the past. As discussed earlier, most of these tumors do not cross the pia arachnoid and hence are often well demarcated on the surface of the brain. The typical appearance of such a tumor is of an area of expanded, abnormally pale gyri, bounded by sulci. This superficial area can be identified in most cases by the experienced surgeon by eye alone, but others will find neuronavigation helpful. The area that is directly infiltrated is unlikely to be functional, but if eloquent speech or motor cortex is nearby, they should be identified by cortical mapping. The tumor can cause considerable distortion of the surrounding normal gyri, and the conventional anatomical and radiological landmarks for cortical localization no longer apply. In some cases it can be surprisingly difficult to know whether the tumor is in front of, or behind, the central sulcus. If tumors do not present on the cerebral surface, there can be considerable difficulties in finding them without navigation or ultrasound, but since they are more probably in the deep white matter, it is also less likely that they are suitable for an attempt at radical resection.

The reason why most low-grade gliomas are not curable by surgery is because they invade the deep white matter. It is impossible to establish any kind of surgical plane here. The marginal infiltrated areas of the brain adjacent to the central bulk of the tumor will look and feel no different from normal brain to the surgeon. Once one is operating in the deep white matter, there is also the risk of causing extensive neurological deficits from both undercutting the adjacent cerebral cortex and disrupting the association tracts. Neuronavigation will not help in the deep white matter as a result of both brain shift and distortion produced by surgery and the fact that MRI scanning often does not define the true boundaries of the tumor. The surgeon can only be guided by smear marginal biopsies (in some cases the author has sent more than 60 such biopsies during an operation) and by the patients themselves, who will need to be kept awake so that if any relatively deep resection is being carried out and a developing neurological deficit is identified early during resection, any further resection can then be abandoned.

Awake craniotomy allows the surgeon to operate with greater confidence close to eloquent areas of the brain, but "complete" removal of these tumors will often remain impossible. One difficulty with the awake-craniotomy technique is that patients can develop a degree of neurological deficit while the resection proceeds, which subsequently recovers. It can be a question of fine judgement as to when to abandon further resection as a deficit develops. It is only possible to carry out simple neurological testing during awake craniotomy – in particular of limb movements and speech, and sometimes of the visual fields. It is not possible to assess more subtle cognitive functions, but the patient's general alertness and responsiveness can serve as a guide to these to some extent. It is most important that the awake craniotomy is supervised by an anesthetist with experience in this area [9]. In skilled anesthetic hands it is remarkable how relaxed, pain free, cooperative and alert patients can be, despite being subjected to a very extensive craniotomy.

### Illustrative Example: a 26-year-old woman with a single generalized epileptic fit (Figs. 9.6, 9.7, 9.8)

The scan shows a large tumor arising in the region of the right primary sensory cortex. This was judged to be potentially resectable. Histology showed the tumor to be an oligodendroglioma, and she remains free from fits and without neurological deficit. Follow-up scanning shows persistent abnormality in the brain adjacent to the resection cavity. The abnormality has become a little smaller over time but it must remain likely that there is residual tumor here.

Comment: The very long natural history of oligodendrogliomas must be remembered when dealing with cases such as this. The author remains undecided as to what to recommend if further follow-up scans suggest tumor recurrence.

## 4. Tumours that Recur

The interpretation of post-operative scans can be very difficult. Flair MRI sequences are much more sensitive to both post-operative changes and recurrent tumor than are other sequences. Areas of signal change in the brain adjacent to the resection cavity may represent post-operative inflammatory effects or tumor

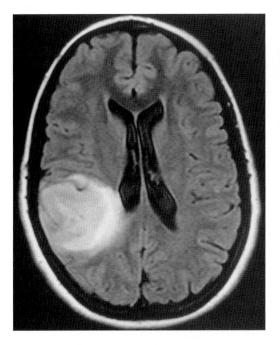

**Fig. 9.6.** Case LC before surgery.

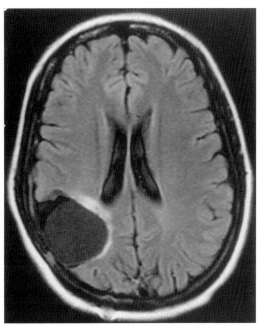

**Fig. 9.8.** Case LC three years after surgery.

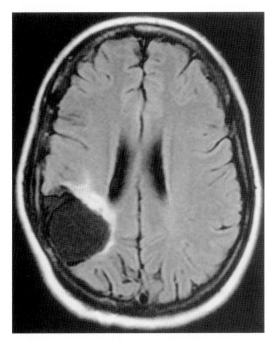

**Fig. 9.7.** Case LC 1 year after surgery.

recurrence. New contrast enhancement after surgery may reflect malignant change or simply post-operative effects. If there is any doubt, as there often is, about the interpretation, it is best to repeat the scan after a few months. Changes due to recurrent tumor will obviously tend to become more pronounced with time, and post-operative effects less pronounced. As with routine follow-up scanning of large, inoperable tumors, routine follow-up scanning of patients who have undergone what appeared to be "complete" resection will often cause great difficulties for the neurosurgeon and his or her patient when such scans show what is probably residual or recurrent tumor, which is not causing any symptoms.

In some patients it will be clear that the tumor has undergone malignant transformation and treatment is now as for a malignant glioma. Depending on the time interval since initial treatment and the extent of recurrence, further surgery may be indicated as well as adjuvant treatment. If the scans suggest malignant change, biopsy can be required to confirm this if adjuvant treatment is to be considered. If the follow-up scans show only slight progressive change over a number of years, it is reasonable to do nothing, although if the area of recurrence is well circumscribed and not very deep or eloquent, "second-look" surgery can be considered.

The question of how to treat possible or definite recurrence of low-grade gliomas is usually very difficult for both surgeon and patient. As mentioned above, it is most important that decisions about how to manage these cases are made jointly by neurosurgeons and neuro-oncologists working together.

## 5. Tumors that Cause Intractable Epilepsy

Provided that EEG studies have confirmed the tumor seen on the scan to be the epileptic focus, and provided that complete or near-complete resection of the tumor looks feasible, many patients can expect a significant improvement, with actual cure in some cases, of their epilepsy with surgery. The question of what constitutes "intractable" epilepsy can be difficult, as can the question of whether there are epileptic foci distant from the tumor. Simple, superficial tumors causing epilepsy can be dealt with on their merits, but other cases are probably best managed by surgeons with a particular interest in epilepsy, and are beyond the scope of this chapter.

## The Role of Radiotherapy and Chemotherapy

In the past, radiotherapy was used more widely for low-grade tumors than is currently the case. The EORTC controlled trial of adjuvant radiotherapy [10] showed no difference in survival between patients treated with surgery and patients treated with both surgery and postoperative radiotherapy. Whereas there is general agreement that radiotherapy should be used in patients whose tumor has undergone malignant change, its use in patients with low-grade tumors remains controversial. The long-term morbidity of radiotherapy remains a major concern in these patients, especially in view of the fact that so many of them, unlike patients with high-grade tumors, live for many years after treatment, and the known fact that the adverse effects of radiation increase over time. Cognitive impairment can be quite easily missed if not specifically looked for, or mistakenly attributed to the effects of the tumor itself. On the basis of what has been published to date, it is impossible

to quantify the nature or degree of these possible long-term adverse effects. In the short term, radiotherapy is well tolerated. Suffice it to say that, given the absence of any good evidence that radiotherapy improves survival in these cases, the author and his neuro-oncological colleagues do not routinely use radiotherapy in asymptomatic patients with low-grade gliomas.

Chemotherapy remains of uncertain value for low-grade astrocytomas that have not undergone anaplastic change. There is no clear evidence of efficacy in the literature and it is not widely used. With oligodendrogliomas [11,12], especially those with anaplastic change, there is an increasing body of evidence that chemotherapy has a role to play. At the present time, opinions vary as to whether it should be considered as first-line or second-line treatment for such tumors.

## Management of Oligodendrogliomas

The natural history of low-grade oligodendrogliomas appears to be considerably more indolent than that of astrocytomas, with a median overall survival time reported in one recent series [13] of 16.3 years. The question of whether to offer treatment to asymptomatic patients is therefore all the more important. In the patients reported by Olson et al., 36% of patients who had been treated with radiotherapy developed dementia, 20% treated with chemotherapy suffered toxicity, and 6% of those undergoing surgery suffered permanent neurological impairment. There is little reason to doubt that results in other centres will be similar. It seems reasonable to conclude that treatment should be postponed in these patients, unless the tumour appears amenable to complete and reasonably safe surgical resection, until tumour progression has been documented. Furthermore, there is little, if any, evidence that postponing treatment in this way has an adverse effect on outcome.

## Management of Gangliogliomas, Neurocytomas and Pleomorphic Xanthoastrocytomas

These rare tumors tend to have distinctive radiological appearances [14]. Complete resection and surgical cure is more often possible in these tumors than in the other gliomas, although recurrence can occur and the patients should be followed with regular scanning.

## Conclusions

Deciding on whether to operate on patients with low-grade gliomas is a particularly difficult area of neurosurgery although, from the purely technical point of view, the surgery itself is often relatively straightforward. It is easy to conclude that small, easily accessible tumors should be removed and that large, infiltrating tumors are best left alone unless they are causing raised intracranial pressure. The problems arise with the great majority of patients whose tumors fall between these two extremes. Using modern neurosurgical techniques, there can be no doubt that more tumors can now be totally excised than was the case in the past. Such patients, however, remain in a small minority. The majority of patients have tumors where there is little prospect of total removal and where is no clear evidence that partial removal improves outcome. It can be very difficult for both the surgeon and the patient to accept that nothing is to be done. Careful and sympathetic explanation is essential whatever treatment is recommended. If surgery is to be undertaken in those cases where total resection is clearly not going to be achieved, it is essential that surgical morbidity should be extremely low. On the other hand, the operation will become a meaningless charade if the morbidity is kept low by merely carrying out a limited biopsy, if it is already known from the pre-operative scan appearances that adjuvant treatment will not be recommended. There is no science in making decisions of this kind: instead the neurosurgeon must be guided by his experience (and, if necessary, by the greater experience of surgical colleagues), by discussion with his oncological colleagues and, above all, by honest and open discussion with the patients and their families.

Finally, it must be stressed that the neurosurgeon's responsibility to his patient does not end once an operation has been carried out, or if a decision has been made to defer treatment of a low-grade tumor, or if a tumor has been deemed inoperable. It is tempting for the surgeon to try to avoid the immense stress and anxiety that many people suffer when a diagnosis of this kind has been made, especially when they will have to live with the knowledge of the tumor, and the patient's probably impending death, for many years. Careful and sympathetic follow-up and explanation will often be just as important as the surgical or oncological treatment in determining the quality of the patient's life.

## Key Points

- *There are many varieties of low-grade glioma and few generalizations can be made as to how they are best treated other than that most patients will die of the disease within 10 years of diagnosis, whatever the treatment undertaken.*

- *There is no clear, trial-based evidence that can be used in deciding upon treatment and it is not known whether partial removal of tumors has any significant impact on prognosis.*

- *Small, well-circumscribed tumors can probably be cured by surgical resection, but this only applies to a minority of cases.*

- *Modern microscopic techniques, combined with intraoperative histology and cortical mapping under local anesthetic, increase the number of cases where curative resection is a possibility.*

- *Most patients present with epilepsy and will remain without any significant neurological deficit for several years before they eventually deteriorate. The risks of treatment, and its uncertain benefit in many cases, must be carefully balanced against the relatively benign short-term natural history.*

## References

1. Laws E, Taylor W, Clifton M, Okazaki H. Neurosurgical management of low-grade astrocytoma of the cerebral hemispheres. J Neurosurg 1984;61:665–73.
2. Bigner D, McLendon R, Bruner J. Russell and Rubinstein's pathology of tumors of the nervous system, 6th edn. London: Arnold, 1998.
3. Morantz R. Low grade astrocytomas. In: Kaye A, Laws E, editors. Brain tumours. Edinburgh: Churchill Livingstone, 1995;433–48.
4. Kondziolka D, Lunsford LD, Martinez AJ. Unreliability of contemporary neurodiagnostic imaging in evaluating

suspected adult supratentorial (low-grade) astrocytoma. J Neurosurg 1993;79:533–6.

5. Skirboll S, Ojeman G, Berger M, Lettich E, Winn H. Functional cortex and subcortical white matter located within gliomas. Neurosurgery 1996;38:678–85.

6. Lunsford LD, Martinez AJ, Latchaw RE. Magnetic resonance imaging does not define tumor boundaries. Acta Radiol Suppl 1986;369:154–6.

7. Recht L, Lew R, Smith TW. Suspected low-grade glioma: is deferring treatment safe? Ann Neurol 1992;31: 431–6.

8. Berger M, Deliganis B, Dobbins J, Keles G. The effect of extent of resection on recurrence in patients with low grade cerebral hemisphere gliomas. Cancer 1994;74: 1784–91.

9. Sarang A, Dinsmore J. Anaesthesia for awake craniotomy. Evolution of a technique that facilitates neurological testing. Br J Anaesth 2003;90:161–5.

10. Karim AB, Cornu P, Bleehen N et al. Immediate postoperative radiotherapy in low grade glioma improves progression free survival, but not overall survival: preliminary results of an EORTC/MRC randomised phase III study (abstract). Proc Am Soc Clin Oncol 1998;17:400a.

11. Cairncross G, Macdonald D, Ludwin S et al. Chemotherapy for anaplastic oligodendroglioma. J Clin Oncol 1994;12(10):2013–21.

12. Paleologos NA, G CJ. Treatment of oligodendroglioma: an update. Neuro-oncology 1999;1(1):61–8.

13. Olson JD, Riedel E, DeAngelis LM. Long-term outcome of low-grade oligodendroglioma and mixed glioma. Neurology 2000;54:1442–8.

14. Sanders WP, Christoforidis GA. Imaging of low-grade primary brain tumors. In: Rock JP et al., editors. The practical management of low grade primary brain tumours. 1999.

# 10

# Neurosurgical Management of High-grade Gliomas

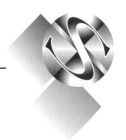

Robert C. Rostomily, Alexander M. Spence
and Daniel L. Silbergeld

## Summary

High-grade gliomas include malignant variants of tumors derived from astrocytic and oligodenropheral cell lines. These tumors demonstrate invasive behavior, are rapidly growing and are usually characterized by contrast enhancement and edema on MR or CT neuroimaging. Management includes either biopsy or surgical resection followed by radiotherapy in the majority of cases. Additional adjuvant chemotherapy is also a treatment consideration. Despite advances in management, the prognosis remains poor, with few patients surviving beyond 2–3 years.

## Introduction

The term "high-grade glioma" (HGG) refers to a histopathologically defined group of clinically aggressive glial neoplasms, which includes: glioblastoma multiforme (GBM), anaplastic astrocytoma (AA), anaplastic oligodendroglioma (AO), anaplastic oligoastrocytoma or "mixed" glioma, gliosarcoma and, possibly, the gemistocytic astrocytoma (GA). High-grade gliomas are the most common primary cerebral neoplasms in adults, with GBM and AA comprising the vast majority of these neoplasms. HGGs share common hallmarks of varying degrees of glial cell differentiation, an extremely poor prognosis for survival beyond 2–3 years, and a diffuse invasive growth pattern into surrounding brain. The designation HGG distinguishes these aggressive gliomas from their "low-grade" glioma (LGG) counterparts that confer median survival times of 6–10 years. Despite their similarities, the HGGs are biologically heterogeneous and differ significantly in their features of differentiation, presumed histogenesis, treatment responses and prognosis. This heterogeneity must be appreciated when considering management options for a particular patient with a HGG and in the interpretation of clinical trials.

Over the last 25 years, despite a plethora of novel treatment approaches, the prognosis for patients with HGGs has not significantly improved. Limitations imposed by tumor location, intrinsic biological features, and tumor growth patterns complicate the effective management of HGGs. It is now well recognized that HGG is a diffuse disease. While an extensive amount of research has recently targeted the study of HGG cell migration and invasion, we have yet to solve the clinical problem of loco-regional control of HGGs. Ultimately, significant improvement in outcome for HGG patients will require effective loco-regional tumor control, while cure will require novel strategies to address the diffuse invasive component of the tumor. The role of the neurosurgeon in the multidisciplinary management of HGG patients is continually evolving from simply providing tumor resection, to the design and delivery of intratumoral therapy, and adapting new technologies to improve surgical resection. This changing role underscores the need for neurosurgeons managing HGG patients to be versed not only in the technical aspects of HGG surgery but also in the biological principles that underlie these emerging treatments. This chapter reviews surgical management, patient selection and basic biological features of HGG relevant to its surgical management.

# Epidemiology

The overall incidence of HGGs in the USA is estimated at about 5/100,000 person-years, with approximately 13,000 new cases per year and 10,000 deaths. There is a direct correlation between age and higher tumor grade or aggressiveness, as well as mortality. Modest 2–4% increases in incidence have been shown in the last 10–20 years, with minimal improvements in 2-year GBM survival from 3 to 6% [1]. The relative incidence of the histological subtypes of HGG is difficult to determine accurately because rare entities such as gliosarcoma (GS) are either not reported separately or, in the case of more controversial diagnostic entities such as anaplastic oligoastrocytoma (AOA), are not uniformly diagnosed and reported. Nevertheless, the Central Brain Tumor Registry of the USA (CBTRUS) database (HYPERLINK http://www.cbtrus.org ) reports the incidence of GBM as 2.96/100,000 person-years, anaplastic astrocytoma (AA) as 0.49/100,000 person-years, anaplastic oligodendroglioma (AO) as 0.10/100,000 person-years, and malignant glioma NOS (not otherwise specified) as 0.35/100,000 person-years. Thus, in this database, GBM accounted for 76% of HGGs while AA and AO accounted for 13% and 2.6% of HGGs, respectively.

# Histogenesis and Histopathology

The precise histogenesis, or cell of origin, for adult HGGs is not known. Current paradigms invoke either the transformation of resident adult neural stem or glial progenitor cells or the de-differentiation of mature glial cells. The classification and grading of HGG is controversial and has undergone a number of modifications in the last few decades. The World Health Organization (WHO) classification system is currently the most widely used system and was born from an effort to provide a consensus for classifying and grading nervous system tumors [2]. In this chapter, we collectively refer to HGGs as those glial neoplasms that correspond to WHO grade III tumors, including AA, AO, AOA, and grade IV tumors, including GBM, giant-cell GBM, and GS. Of note, the gemistocytic astrocytoma is classified as a grade II tumor in the WHO classification; however, this tumor type has been associated with a more aggressive clinical course that is similar to grade III tumors, and thus these neoplasms are often also considered in the discussion of HGGs.

# Molecular Pathogenesis

Patterns of molecular genetic abnormalities have been associated with specific types of HGGs [3] (Fig. 10.1). The high frequency of genetic alterations that inactivate p53 and augment EGFR (epidermal growth factor receptor) activity and its downstream pathways, and their presence in the most common forms of HGG, have led to innovative therapeutic strategies that target these molecules and in some cases directly involve the neurosurgeon. These molecular genetic changes are presumed to underlie gliomagenesis and/or progression to HGG and have been most rigorously studied in glioblastoma. Secondary GBMs arise predominantly in younger patients from pre-existing lower grade tumors, while primary GBMs more commonly occur in older patients and are presumed to arise de novo from a target cell of origin. The former are more likely to have mutations that inactivate p53 function, while the latter typically have overactivation of EGFR-mediated pathways through various mechanisms such as gene amplification or mutation. In GBM, this latter abnormality is often due to the expression of a truncated, and constitutively activated, EGFR called "EGFRvIII", which is being investigated as a target for immunotherapy. In contrast, the molecular genetic changes that lead to the

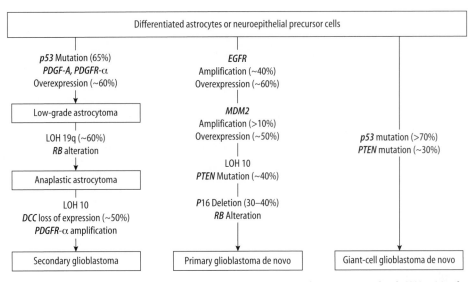

**Fig. 10.1.** Summary of distinct patterns of molecular genetic changes seen in HGGs that are associated with GBMs arising from lower grade lesions (secondary GBM) vs those arising de novo (primary GBM). Several of the molecular abnormalities noted in this figure have been used as targets for therapy that are delivered intraoperatively by the neurosurgeon (see text). (Courtesy of Kleihues et al. [3].)

formation of AO and AOA are not as well characterized as those that lead to the formation of AA and GBM. The recent description of allelic losses on chromosomes 19q and 1p in most low-grade oligodendrogliomas points to potential early events in their genesis, but candidate tumor suppressors for these loci have not been identified. In a subset of cases, the subsequent molecular changes associated with malignant progression to AO include allelic loss of 9p or homozygous deletion of the cell cycle inhibitor CDKN2A (p16INK4A) gene [4].

# HGG Biology

The unique biology of HGGs underlies their dismal prognosis and directly impacts the effectiveness and role of surgery in their management. Those aspects of HGG biology that impact surgical management, or provide targets for therapeutic intervention that potentially involve the neurosurgeon, are reviewed below.

## HGG Growth Patterns

HGGs can be modeled as containing distinct anatomical compartments: a central or bulk portion of tumor, which often contains a zone of central necrosis surrounded by regions of solid tumor, and a surrounding zone of infiltrating tumor with isolated migratory tumor cells. These compartments roughly correspond to areas of decreased signal on T1 images (necrosis), gadolinium enhancement (central or bulk tumor) and increased edema-associated T2 signal (infiltrative tumor cells) on MR images (Fig. 10.2). The central regions contribute to mass effect, generally take up intravenous contrast agents, and contain areas of both active metabolism and hypoxic zones that contribute to treatment resistance. The uptake of contrast agents indicates a disruption of the normal blood–brain barrier (BBB) in this tumor region, which is essential for the delivery of effective doses of most systemic chemotherapeutic agents. Although HGG is a diffuse disease process (see discussion below), approximately 80% of HGG tumor recurrences are detected within 2–3 cm of the original resection cavity [5, 6], and only with intense local therapy such as high-activity radiation implants have significant percentages of recurrences been reported outside this zone (45% in one study). Adding to these local problems of tumor control for HGGs is a poorly defined zone that encompasses bulk

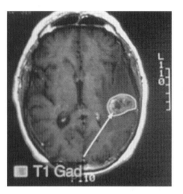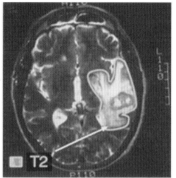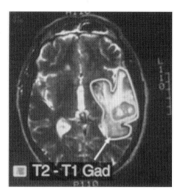

**Fig. 10.2.** An MR image of a glioblastoma demonstrating the different components of HGGs with central necrosis, surrounding solid tumor delineated by contrast-enhancing tissue and peripheral edema indicating a zone where infiltrative tumor cells reside. Gad, gadolinium.

tumor and is composed of infiltrative and diffuse tumor cells that reside amongst histologically normal brain where the BBB remains intact.

In 1938, Scherer carefully documented the diffusely invasive growth pattern of HGGs and correctly predicted that this biological property of HGGs would limit the ability to surgically cure these tumors [7]. Further confirmation of these studies came with the advent of CT and MR imaging. Histological analysis of stereotactic biopsies taken from radiographically defined regions of HGGs consistently demonstrates the presence of tumor cells beyond areas of contrast enhancement, with infiltration of tumor tissue and/or isolated tumor cells throughout areas of CT hypodensity and prolonged T2 signal on MR images. In a study by Kelly et al., only 18 out of 186 biopsy samples from regions of prolonged T2 signal had no evidence of isolated tumor cells or tissue [8]. Furthermore, isolated tumor cells can be detected histologically or cultured from HGG biopsy samples that are obtained from regions of radiographically *normal* brain [9].

Aside from limiting the ability to effectively resect HGGs, this invasive and diffuse growth pattern likely underlies the demonstration of functional cortex in areas of brain that are infiltrated or grossly involved by tumor [10]. In addition, the presence of an intact BBB in this region limits the ability to deliver many therapeutic agents that rely on its breakdown to achieve cytotoxic doses. While neurosurgical management is generally focused on maximal

resection of the central region of necrosis and solid or bulk tumor that contributes primarily to mass effect, emerging treatment modalities that address the invasive tumor component may require neurosurgical expertise as well (see below).

## Tumor Cell Invasiveness and Migration

As we achieve better local tumor control, effective therapy for HGGs will ultimately require treatment strategies to address the diffusely infiltrative component of HGGs. Accordingly, intense investigation has recently focused on the cellular and molecular biological characteristics underlying glioma tumor cell migration and invasion. Glioma tumor cell migration and invasion involve the coordination of various cellular processes, which include tumor cell adhesion to specific substrate(s), motility and protease-mediated degradation of extracellular matrix (ECM). Not surprisingly, important roles in this process have been attributed to: proteins that enhance motility (motogens), ECM components and adhesion molecules that provide anchors or permissive substrates for migration, cytoskeletal elements that provide the structural elements for locomotion, and proteases and their regulators that degrade non-permissive elements of the ECM and thus facilitate cellular migration.

Treatment strategies intended to limit tumor cell migration and invasion include agents such as marimistat, which inhibit matrix metallopro-teases elaborated by tumor cells that facilitate tumor cell migration by digesting ECM compo-nents. Another therapy has used injection of I-131-labeled antibodies into resection cavities after surgery to target the ECM protein tenascin, which is unique to the ECM of HGGs but not normal brain, and appears to promote prolifer-ation and angiogenesis as well as tumor cell migration. Other treatments specifically target-ing invasion that require neurosurgical inter-vention are likely to emerge in the future, such as the use of genetically engineered neural stem cells, which, in animal models, appear to "track down" isolated invasive tumor cells and facili-tate localized conversion of prodrugs into cytotoxic compounds [11].

## Treatment Resistance

Treatment resistance, a major contributing factor to the dismal prognosis for patients with HGGs, is the result of multiple mechanisms that include, among others, inactivation of drugs, molecular mechanisms of resistance to DNA damage and apoptosis, and attenuation of cyto-toxicity imposed by the microenvironment (e.g. hypoxia). Add to these mechanisms the limita-tions to delivery of therapy imposed by the dif-fusely invasive growth pattern of HGG tumor cells into brain regions with an intact BBB, and one can begin to understand the daunting problem of designing effective therapies. Through aggressive cytoreduction, the neuro-surgeon helps to eliminate a large portion of

hypoxic tissue, but the precise impact of cytore-duction on reducing resistance and improving efficacy in adjuvant treatment of residual disease is not known. Targeting one specific mechanism of resistance is unlikely to confer an appreciable improvement in tumor response and the neurosurgeon is likely to be called upon in the future to assist in delivering novel thera-pies aimed at overcoming multiple mechanisms of treatment resistance.

# Prognostic Factors

The prognosis of different subgroups of HGG patients is important to consider when selecting patients for surgery and resection versus biopsy. Prognostic factors are most often determined for overall patient survival, yet the length of an acceptable quality of life is ultimately the most relevant end-point. However, the paucity of prognostic data that specifically analyze quality-of-life issues precludes their general usefulness, and the ensuing discussion will focus on data related primarily to overall survival alone.

## Recursive Partition Analysis

Many studies have adopted the Radiation Therapy Oncology Group's prognostic stratifi-cation of HGG patients based on a recursive partitioning statistical analysis (RPA) of large numbers of patients enrolled into clinical trials [12]. Tables 10.1 and 10.2 outline these prog-nostic classes and the median survival for each

**Table 10.1.** RTOG malignant glioma RPA class definitions (courtesy of Curan et al. [12])

| Class | Definition |
|---|---|
| I | Age <50 years, anaplastic astrocytoma, and normal mental status |
| II | Age ≥ 50, KPS 70–100, anaplastic astrocytoma, and at least 3 months from time of first symptoms to start of treatment |
| III | Age <50 years, anaplastic astrocytoma and abnormal mental status |
| | Age <50 years, glioblastoma multiforme and KPS 90–100 |
| IV | Age <50 years, glioblastoma multiforme and KPS <90 |
| | Age ≥50 years, KPS 70–100, anaplastic astrocytoma, and 3 months or less from time of first symptoms to start of treatment |
| | Age >50 years, glioblastoma multiforme, surgical resection and good neurological function |
| V | Age ≥50 years, KPS 70–100, glioblastoma multiforme, either surgical resection and neurological function that inhibits the ability to work, or biopsy only followed by at least 54.4 Gγ of RT |
| | Age ≥50 years, KPS <70, normal mental status |
| VI | Age ≥50 years, KPS <70, abnormal mental status |
| | Age ≥50 years, KPS 70–100, glioblastoma multiforme, biopsy only, receiving less than 54.4 Gγ or radiation therapy |

RPA, recursive partition analysis; RTOG, Radiation Therapy Oncology Group; KPS, Kamowski Performance Status

**Table 10.2.** Survival for HGGs by RTOG RPA (courtesy of Curan et al. [12])

| RPA class | Median survival (months) | 2-year survival (%) |
|-----------|--------------------------|---------------------|
| I | 58.6 | 76 |
| II | 37.4 | 68 |
| III | 17.9 | 35 |
| IV | 11.1 | 15 |
| V | 8.9 | 6 |
| VI | 4.6 | 4 |

RPA, recursive partition analysis; RTOG, Radiation Therapy Oncology Group

RPA class, respectively. These studies confirmed prognostic factors found in most other studies, including age, Karnofsky performance status (KPS), histological grade, mental status, length and/or presence of neurological symptoms, surgical resection and adequate radiation. The predictors of outcome at the time of HGG recurrence have been evaluated in a large review of 375 patients enrolled on phase II treatment trials, which reported median survival for all recurrent HGGs of 30 weeks, with overall survival rates at 1 year of 47% and 21%, for AA and GBM patients respectively [13]. This study confirmed the prognostic significance of histology (AA vs GBM), KPS and prior intensive therapy, which were found in other previous studies [14]. The appropriate choice of surgical candidates and the aggressiveness of resection for primary and recurrent HGGs, discussed below, must account for these histological and clinical characteristics that dominate clinical outcome.

## Tumor Variables

Of all the tumor-related variables that have been analyzed for their prognostic significance, the histopathological grade, which integrates various specific histological features such as mitotic activity and anaplasia, shows the most profound influence on outcome. Other tumor variables, including tumor volume and location, molecular genetic alterations, gene expression patterns, and proliferation and apoptotic indices do not consistently show such an association with outcome. For example, while aberrant p53 function clearly plays an important role in gliomagenesis and malignant progression, the mutational status of p53 has not been convincingly shown to independently predict prognosis.

Similarly, indices of tumor proliferation or cell death (apoptosis) alone have not been shown to predict outcome consistently for patients with HGG. However, in a few studies attempting to estimate net cell production, apoptotic/proliferative ratios have shown predictive significance for outcome. Currently, the only example of a molecular genetic abnormality that has been consistently shown to correlate with survival and treatment response is the predictive value of 1p and 19q deletions for anaplastic oligodendroglioma, which, in the most favorable group, showed median survivals from diagnosis of greater than 123 months compared with 16 months for the least favorable group that lacked the 1p deletion (Fig. 10.3) [15]. It is likely that more general variables such as tumor grade and clinical status are better prognostic indicators than are individual tumor features, since they represent the biological summation of individual tumor and molecular variables. However, larger controlled studies may achieve statistical power to identify specific molecular features or profiles that reliably predict patient outcomes or even treatment response.

## Treatment Variables

### Radiation

Radiation therapy following biopsy or resection for HGGs is the most effective adjuvant treatment modality available. It is generally administered in 180 cGy fractions to a total dose of around 60 Gy when treating the bulk tumor plus a margin that encompasses the area of increased T2 signal. In a randomized trial of anaplastic glioma patients, the overall survival of patients treated with "best conventional care", BCNU alone, radiation alone, and radiation plus BCNU was 17 weeks, 18.5 weeks, 37.5 weeks and 40.5 weeks, respectively [16]. This beneficial effect of radiation on survival applies to other HGGs and GBM as well. The efficacy of radiation has been further validated for HGG by the demonstration of a dose–response relationship. Accordingly, external beam irradiation has become standard therapy for HGG patients after biopsy or resection. In addition, an objective radiographic response to radiation is also an independent predictor of prolonged overall survival for patients with GBM. Thus, the uniformity and adequacy of radiation treatment must

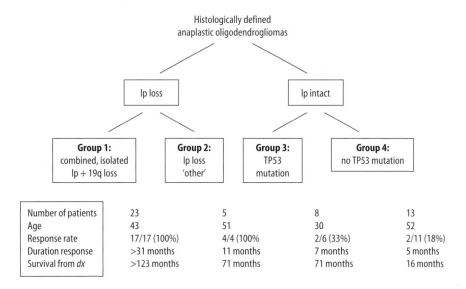

**Fig. 10.3.** Grouping of patients with anaplastic oligodendroglioma by molecular genetic profiles defines specific prognostic groups. Group 2 includes patients with 1p loss and either no 19q loss or "other" molecular genetic changes, including TP53 mutation, PTEN mutation, 10q loss, EGFR amplification or CDKN2A deletion. Group 4 patients have mutations including PTEN, 10q loss, EGFR amplification, CDKN2A deletion, or ring enhancement on CT. (Courtesy of Ino et al. [15].)

be determined when considering the prognostic impact of other treatment variables on outcome for HGGs.

## Chemotherapy

A multitude of cytotoxic and cytostatic chemotherapeutic regimens have been used for the treatment of HGGs and, with the exception of PCV therapy (procarbazine, CCNU & vincristine) for AO and AOA, the results have been disappointing. A complete review of the various chemotherapy protocols is beyond the scope of this chapter but a recent meta-analysis, which drew on data from 12 randomized trials of chemotherapy for adult HGGs, demonstrated an increase in 1-year survival from 40% to 46% and an overall 2-month increase in median survival [17]. An important exception is the demonstrated durable response and prolonged survival for AO and AOA associated with deletions of the 1p and 1p+19q chromosomes (see Fig. 10.3 and text above) [15].

## Surgical Resection

The impact of extent of surgical resection on survival for HGGs continues to be debated. Clearly, given the biological constraints noted above, a "complete" resection of an HGG is not possible. Extent of surgical resection is best defined based on volumetric analysis [18] of residual contrast-enhancing volume on MR or CT imaging obtained within 24–48 hours of surgery, although non-specific contrast enhancement can be seen after operation for non-neoplastic lesions as soon as 17 hours post-operatively [19]. While contrast enhancement is the most obvious and consistent radiographic indicator of HGG tissue, a small percentage of GBMs do not enhance, and 30–50% of non-GBM HGGs lack contrast enhancement on CT imaging. Conversely, up to 40% of non-enhancing gliomas are anaplastic.

The scientific analysis of cytoreductive surgery for HGG is further confounded by a lack of uniformity in defining and assessing extent of resection and use of subsequent treatment modalities that can prolong survival, and the variable and poorly understood interaction of the multiple patient, treatment and tumor factors that collectively determine patient survival. It is doubtful that a single study could be designed that would definitively address all of these confounding issues and clearly determine the impact of surgical resection on patient outcome. However, in the only study of its kind,

Keles et al. objectively quantified residual post-operative tumor volumes based on MRI, and showed that the volume of residual disease correlated with both time to progression and overall survival [20] (Fig. 10.4). The increasingly frequent demonstration of a significant impact for surgical resection in more recent studies may reflect the routine use of MR or CT imaging post-operatively to objectively quantify residual tumor. The determination of surgical impact on outcome is informative when a study accounts for established prognostic factors and objectively analyzes residual disease rather than percentage of resection or other subjective measures of resection not based on rigorous imaging data [21].

Two subgroups of HGG patients deserve additional mention: the elderly and non-GBM patients. The role of radical surgery for the elderly is controversial. While aggressive treatment strategies have been employed for the elderly (>65 or 70 years of age) and have been shown to provide meaningful periods of survival, the impact of surgical resection has not been adequately analyzed as an independent variable to more definitively define its impact on outcome. Evaluating the impact of surgical resection for grade III lesions is even more problematical than for grade IV lesions because they are more responsive to conventional therapy, display greater biological, clinical and radiological heterogeneity (e.g. less often

contrast enhance), are less common than grade IV tumors, and the analysis of their extent of resection is often embedded in generic studies of HGGs. Not surprisingly, studies evaluating the efficacy of resection for grade III HGGs have reported conflicting outcomes.

It is virtually inevitable that HGGs recur or, more correctly, progress. The role of re-operation at the time of recurrence and its impact on outcome have been evaluated in several studies that demonstrate, at best, modest impact on overall survival and, in some cases, prolonged good quality of life compared with patients treated without re-operation [14, 22]. In a recent large study of re-operation in patients enrolled in clinical trials, surgical patients had a median survival of 36 weeks compared with 23 weeks for non-operated patients [22], but the difference was partially attributed to selection bias. Other studies have shown no association between extent of resection and survival at recurrence, with median survival of 33 weeks for GBM patients and 79 weeks for AA patients [14].

If the utility of surgical resection is based primarily on cytoreduction, then it would be important to know what proportion of the tumor burden is represented by the enhancing portion of a tumor versus the diffusely infiltrative component. Accurate assessment of total tumor burden is not possible with current imaging techniques, and problematic even with detailed examination of pathological material.

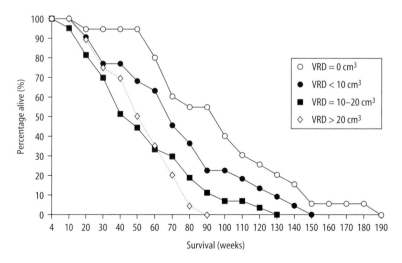

**Fig. 10.4.** Kaplan–Meier plots showing increasing survival with smaller post-operative tumor volumes in patients with GBM. VRD, post-operative tumor volume. (Courtesy of Keles et al. [20].)

One report estimates that the enhancing component represents as little as 50% of the total cell burden [23]. The fact that recent studies have been able to show any impact of surgical resection based on extent of removal of contrast-enhancing material suggests that this component of the tumor subserves an important biological function that is independent of tumor burden or volume. Recognizing that gross total resection improves outcome but that these benefits were negated by surgically induced neurological deterioration, Shinoda et al. developed a pre-operative MRI-based grading scheme that incorporates tumor size, location and proximity to eloquent cortex to select candidates suitable for gross total resection [24].

## Patient Evaluation

Pre-operative evaluation of patients with possible brain lesions requires a careful history and physical examination (including an accurate assessment of the patient's KPS) followed by radiological evaluation. The duration of pre-operative symptoms varies greatly, because some patients have harbored lower grade gliomas that have undergone malignant transformation, leading to longer histories than those with HGGs that arise de novo. Patients with HGG often present with headache (approximately 35%), new-onset seizures (approximately 20%), altered mental status (approximately 15%), or focal neurological signs and symptoms. Headaches associated with brain tumors vary in severity, location and quality. However, these headaches are usually different from previous headaches that the patient may have had, and because they may be secondary to elevated intracranial pressure (ICP), they are often associated with nausea and vomiting, and exacerbated by exercise and postural changes. Although drugs, alcohol and metabolic derangement may lead to seizures, new-seizure onset in adults is often associated with structural brain lesions, mandating a brain imaging study. Neurological signs and symptoms vary depending on tumor location and size. While large tumors in the frontal lobes may impart only subtle personality changes, small tumors in the brainstem or eloquent cortical regions may cause significant focal deficits. Patients with HGG rarely present with significant weight loss or pain (other than headache). These problems more often accompany systemic malignancies, which raises the diagnostic probability that the brain lesion may be metastatic or infectious.

Prior to contemplating any form of surgical intervention, the patient's overall medical status must be evaluated. Age, cardiopulmonary status, and medications that hamper coagulation (non-steroidal anti-inflammatory drugs, heparin, coumadin, etc.) may greatly impact the surgical strategy. Elderly patients, those with other life-shortening medical problems, and those with very low KPS may benefit more from biopsy than from an aggressive cytoreductive procedure.

The role of anti-epileptic drugs (AEDs) in patients with gliomas remains somewhat controversial. For those patients who have had seizures, it is clear that AEDs are indicated. Likewise, for patients who are to undergo cortical stimulation mapping during surgery, AEDs offer some protection from iatrogenic seizures. For patients who have never had seizures, the routine use of AEDs is arguable.

Corticosteroids are routinely administered to patients with HGG. Dexamethasone has become the steroid of choice owing to its high glucocorticoid effect and minimal mineralocorticoid effect. Steroids reduce peritumoral edema, often lowering ICP and reducing symptoms. These drugs may also impart some protection from surgical trauma when given prior to surgery. In contradistinction, steroids given following brain trauma do not improve neurological outcome and may increase infectious complications and peptic ulceration. It must be remembered that the normal daily steroid production is less than 1 mg of dexamethasone. Therefore, slow tapers of this medication, while indicated for persistent edema or evolution of neurological deficits, are not rational for hypothalamic-pituitary axis reasons. For HGG patients who are debilitated or elderly or have been on steroids for prolonged periods, dexamethasone should be replaced by prednisone and tapered carefully.

## Biopsy vs Resection

As discussed above, the three most important prognostic factors for patients with newly diagnosed HGG are age, KPS and tumor grade. Resection provides an accurate diagnosis, with a smaller chance of sampling error than biopsy. Resection can decrease mass effect, which can cause neurological impairment, steroid dependence and even death. However, the risks of open resection are higher than those of biopsy.

The best predictor of a specific post-operative neurological deficit is the presence of that deficit pre-operatively. Therefore, pre-operative neurological status is an important consideration for surgical strategy. The most important predictor of post-operative hemorrhage and clinically significant post-operative edema is residual tumor. Bilateral tumors and tumors that clearly extend into important functional areas may be best treated with biopsy and post-operative therapies. Patients with significant medical problems, the very elderly and those with a KPS of less than 60 should be offered biopsy. Furthermore, when the diagnosis of tumor vs other lesions (stroke, infection, demyelinating disease, multiple metastases, lymphoma, etc.) is in doubt, biopsy may be a better initial step.

# Anesthesia for Biopsy or Resection (see also chapter 4)

The anesthetic must be chosen to lower ICP and minimize seizure risk (especially during cortical stimulation mapping). The patient's hepatic, renal and cardiopulmonary status will also impact on the anesthetic chosen .

Volatile anesthetics are highly halogenated molecules with an unknown mechanism of action. The group includes halothane, enflurane, isoflurane, desflurane and sevoflurane. Halogenated anesthetics provide amnesia, analgesia, and muscle relaxation at higher dosage. The newer agents have a low solubility, permitting rapid adjustment of anesthetic depth and prompt awakening. Halogenated anesthetics decrease cerebral metabolic rate and oxygen consumption ($CMRO_2$) while increasing the CBF, hence producing a metabolic decoupling. They all preserve $CO_2$ reactivity. Volatile anesthetics can increase ICP, this effect being more prominent with halothane and desflurane, but this rise may be prevented by hyperventilation.

Nitrous oxide ($N_2O$) is a poorly soluble agent permitting rapid achievement of alveolar and brain partial pressure, and hence has a rapid onset and termination of action. It possesses weak amnestic properties, but provides prominent analgesia with no muscle relaxation. $N_2O$ increases ICP, this effect being completely reversed by hyperventilation. In addition, since $N_2O$ readily diffuses into sealed air pockets, it may cause a severe and rapid increase in ICP in the presence of a pneumocephalus. However, as shown by Domino et al. in craniotomies, it is usually not necessary to discontinue its use prior to dural closure [25]. $CO_2$ reactivity appears maintained when $N_2O$ is used alone or added to propofol, but may be reduced when used with isoflurane.

The site of action of barbiturates is located on the GABA receptor complex. Thiopental is a fast-onset short-acting drug, producing unconsciousness in 10–20 seconds. The short duration of action is explained by the rapid redistribution half-life of 7 minutes. Thiopental is principally used as an induction agent. Thiopental decreases $CMRO_2$ and CBF and can produce EEG suppression at clinical doses. It also decreases the intracranial pressure (ICP) of patients with intracranial hypertension to a greater extent than it decreases the mean arterial pressure (MAP), thus improving the cerebral perfusion pressure (CPP). $CO_2$ reactivity of brain vasculature is preserved with thiopental and does not change over time.

Like barbiturates, etomidate possesses a GABA-mimetic activity. Etomidate is a fast-onset drug producing loss of consciousness in 10 seconds. Etomidate is used as an induction drug, but it can also be used as an infusion. Etomidate decreases $CMRO_2$ by 45% and CBF by 35% and can produce a flat EEG. It decreases ICP, while increasing, or at least maintaining, the CPP. $CO_2$ reactivity of the cerebral vasculature is maintained with etomidate. The brain-protecting effect of etomidate was also shown to be a dose-dependent phenomenon with deleterious effect at higher doses, presumably because of the induction of spiking EEG activity without further depression of $CMRO_2$. In humans, a recent study showed that etomidate may even cause cerebral hypoxia at doses sufficient to induce burst-suppression. Although still widely used for neuroanesthesia, etomidate may not possess the brain-protecting virtues it was once thought to have.

Propofol is administered in an egg-oil-glycerol emulsion, and probably exerts its pharmacological effect by enhancing GABA-activated chloride channel. Propofol is a fast-onset, short-acting drug. Propofol decreases the CBF by 30% to 50%, with a 35% diminution of the $CMRO_2$, preserving $CO_2$ reactivity. Propofol decreases ICP with a concomitant decrease of MAP.

Narcotics currently used during anesthesia are synthetic phenylpiperidine derivatives and include fentanyl, sufentanil, alfentanil and remifentanil. They are pure opioid receptor agonists, and, unlike morphine, do not liberate histamine. These drugs are all ultrashort- to short-acting drugs. They are used as anesthetic adjuvant, but may be used as the main anesthetic agent. The effect of these drugs on cardiovascular and cerebral dynamics is quite variable. Remifentanil and fentanyl seem to have negligible effect on ICP, while sufentanil and alfentanil may increase it. Mainly because of their effect on MAP, they tend to decrease the CPP, sometimes below the range of autoregulation. Again, of the four drugs, fentanyl has the smallest effect on CPP. Sufentanil may even decrease CBF in a dose-dependent manner under anesthesia. Alfentanil seems to have negligible effects on both CBF and $CMRO_2$. Narcotics maintain $CO_2$ reactivity. Narcotics are not brain protectants.

## Intracranial Pressure Management

Several osmotic diuretic agents have been used to treat elevated ICP, including sucrose, albumin, urea and mannitol. Mannitol appears to be excluded from the CSF to a greater extent than other osmotic agents. Mannitol is a simple unbranched hydrocarbon with a half-life of approximately 0.25–1.7 hours. Its excretion is primarily renal, so its half-life may be extended in cases of impaired renal function. The recommended dose for mannitol is 0.25–2 g/kg intravenously every 4 hours, with a peak decrease in ICP approximately 15 minutes after administration. Use of a loop diuretic 15 minutes after the administration of mannitol has been shown to potentiate its effect. Like all osmotic diuretics, mannitol works primarily by shifting water from the brain parenchyma to the intravascular space, thereby decreasing the volume of the intracranial contents and reducing ICP. Additionally, mannitol reduces intracranial elastance. Mannitol may also affect the reactivity of

intracerebral capillaries, leading to an overall vasoconstrictive effect and decreased ICP. Finally, mannitol decreases the viscosity of whole blood, thereby decreasing intracerebral resistance. In combination with the increase in intravascular volume and cardiac output, this leads to increased CBF in the setting of decreased ICP, with an overall theoretical increase in CPP. These effects on ICP and CPP appear to be greatest in the setting of intact vascular autoregulation. The effectiveness of mannitol is also highly dependent on the intactness of, and osmotic gradient across, the BBB. Marked disruption of the BBB allows flow of mannitol into the brain parenchyma, thus antagonizing flow of blood into the intravascular compartment. In response to chronic osmotic therapy, the brain also accumulates "idiogenic osmoles", which act to sequester water in the brain compartment.

Barbiturates are a second-line agent for the management of elevated ICP. Their efficacy in this role remains controversial. The mechanism of action is believed to be their ability to modulate cerebral metabolism and therefore CBF. Barbiturates appear to act as cerebral vasoconstrictors, thus reducing intracerebral blood volume and lowering ICP. Barbiturates also appear to preferentially vasoconstrict normal cerebral blood vessels and increase CBF to relatively ischemic areas. Finally, barbiturates decrease $CMRO_2$, i.e. the cerebral metabolic rate and oxygen consumption. Decreases in $CMRO_2$ appear to result in decreased ICP. A burst-suppression EEG pattern (so-called "barbiturate coma") is often required to achieve a maximal decrease in $CMRO_2$. This effect, however, does not come without a significant price. Large doses of barbiturates may cause systemic hypotension and act as negative inotropes, both of which act to decrease cardiac output and, ultimately, CPP in the setting of elevated ICP. Pentobarbital is the most commonly used barbiturate for the management of ICP and has a half-life of 15–50 hours, which may be even further lengthened by the large doses required to achieve a barbiturate-induced coma. This effect is due to perturbation of hepatic-clearance mechanisms and also significantly affects the metabolism of other hepatically cleared drugs. Resolution of pentobarbital coma may take days after cessation of therapy. This side-effect profile mandates the use of frequent monitoring of drug levels, EEG, cardiac output and CBF.

Propofol is now frequently used in the ICU setting for ICP control. In the acute setting, and over relatively short periods of time (hours to days), the agent has an effective half-life of 2–4 minutes. The drug decreases CBF, ICP and $CMRO_2$ and induces less cardiac depression than barbiturates. Because of its short half-life, it has also shown utility for neuroleptic anesthesia. Propofol is also useful for sedation of agitated patients in whom serial neurological exams are necessary. Once the propofol infusion is stopped, within 10–20 minutes effective blood levels have dropped to near zero. Untoward side-effects include negative inotropy, respiratory depression and prolonged clearance after large doses.

## Stereotactic Biopsy

The sole goal of stereotactic biopsy of brain lesions is to obtain a diagnosis. Owing to HGG histological heterogeneity, undergrading of the tumor occurs at a rate of approximately 10%. Overall risks from biopsy include anesthesia, bleeding, infection, and obtaining non-diagnostic tissue. The reported complication rates vary from 1% to 5%, while mortality rates are reported as 0–3% [26]. Frameless sterotactic techniques provide the advantage of avoiding the discomfort of frame placement, but the disadvantage of some loss of accuracy. Typically, frame-based techniques offer accuracy within 5 mm.

When using general anesthesia, it is important to simulate the conditions at the time of the scan to maintain accuracy. Therefore, mannitol, hyperventilation and other methods for lowering ICP should not be used (unless they were also used during the time of scan acquisition). Following standard prepping and draping, a small incision is made. The entry site is chosen to provide the shortest, yet safest, course from the cortical surface to the lesion. Obvious regions to avoid include major blood vessels, the Sylvian fissure, and sulci. If the ventricle is entered, it is important not to remove CSF, as this may permit displacement of the target. A target site is chosen that will provide the most accurate diagnosis. Areas of enhancement and necrosis are more likely to yield the diagnosis of HGG. Following tissue acquisition, frozen-section pathology helps to ensure that tumor tissue has been obtained. If this is not the case, a second target site should be sampled. If bleeding occurs with the biopsy, instillation of 0.1–0.3 $cm^3$ of thrombin solution through the biopsy instrument may be helpful. However, significant hemorrhages may require open intervention. A post-operative CT scan is routinely obtained to verify the target site sampled and confirm that there has been no significant bleeding. It has been our practice to retain biopsy patients in the hospital overnight. Because the wound is small, radiotherapy may commence as soon as a final diagnosis has been provided by the pathologists.

## Open Surgical Resection

The objectives of HGG resection are accurate diagnosis, reduction of mass effect and reduction of the tumor burden. Risks from craniotomy for HGG resection vary, with reported morbidity rates ranging from 5% to 15%, and mortality from 1% to 5%. Techniques that minimize these problems and maximize resection will be discussed.

### Positioning and Flap Strategies

Patients should be positioned so that all pressure points are well padded, with the neck in a relatively neutral position to assure adequate jugular venous return. The tumor should be located at the highest point, with the patient in moderate reverse Trendelenburg position. Following adequate induction with general anesthesia (as discussed above), hyperventilation and administration of mannitol (1.0 g/kg under general anesthesia, 0.5 g/kg when the patient will undergo awake functional mapping) should commence.

The skin flap should be designed so that it is large enough to permit potential re-operation for recurrence if needed. Although the incision can be extended or "teed", it is best to plan ahead and avoid higher risk scalp flaps. The craniotomy should be large enough to permit adequate tumor exposure and access to potentially functional cortical regions that need to be identified with mapping techniques (see below).

## Intraoperative Navigation

Although many HGGs are easily differentiated from surrounding brain, others pose serious problems in this regard. Similarly, resection of tumors that cannot be seen on the cortical surface are best approached with some form(s) of intraoperative navigation (Fig. 10.5). Intraoperative ultrasound (IOUS), which is available at most centers, is helpful when the tumor is not iso-echoic with the brain (Fig. 10.5b). This is often problematic for infiltrating low-grade gliomas, but less often with HGG. IOUS can provide accurate data prior to resection, during resection and at the end of the resection (to determine the completeness of the resection). The accuracy of IOUS is not diminished by brain shifts that occur during resection and subsequent brain relaxation. Frame-based and frameless sterotactic systems are quite useful as well (Fig. 10.5c). They can be used in planning the scalp flap, the craniotomy and the resection. However, the accuracy of these systems relies on concordance between brain position and pre-operative imaging studies. Therefore, alterations in brain volume or shifts of the intracranial contents during resection may render these guidance systems less useful as the resection progresses. Intraoperative imaging systems allow the neurosurgical oncologist to bring the post-operative "gold standard" into the operation. Currently these systems are expensive, often cumbersome and prolong the surgery. However, they combine the advantages of IOUS and stereotaxy.

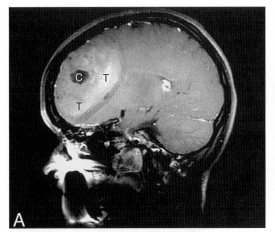

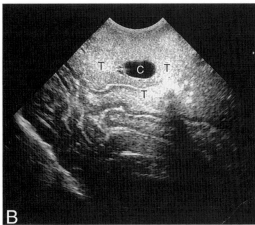

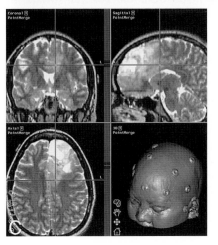

**Fig. 10.5. a** Sagittal MRI (T1-weighted with gadolinium) showing a large left frontal tumor (T) with a small central cystic component (C). **b** Intraoperative ultrasound image obtained in the transverse plane, demonstrating the tumor and tumor cyst. **c** Intraoperative MRI navigational system, demonstrating the posterior extent of the resection (at red crosshair).

# Functional Mapping

Identification of functional cortex, including Rolandic cortex and speech cortex, enables the surgeon to avoid these areas when formulating surgical strategy [27]. In addition to preservation of cerebral function during surgery, it is also possible with these techniques to achieve a greater extent of resection with increased safety. While somatosensory evoked potential (SSEP) and cortical stimulation mapping of motor cortex can be performed in patients under either general or local anesthesia, speech mapping requires the cooperation of an awake patient. Although resections in or near functional brain can be made safer by localizing important brain functions, there are a number of pitfalls that the surgeon must be aware of in order to avoid producing functional deficits.

## Localization of Somatosensory Cortex Using SSEPs

SSEP mapping to identify the primary somatosensory gyrus provides a quick, reliable means of Rolandic localization in both adult and pediatric populations [28]. SSEPs can be performed under general anesthesia or in awake patients. SSEP mapping has the advantage over stimulation mapping that seizures cannot be evoked because the cortex itself is not stimulated. When performed under general anesthesia, halogenated anesthetic agents should be avoided because they may increase the latency of the cortical SSEPs. High-dose barbiturate or propofol anesthesia may lead to burst-suppression activity, and is therefore contraindicated. Nitrous oxide combined with Pentothal or low-dose propofol provides excellent general anesthetics for these studies.

Techniques for intraoperative SSEP mapping are similar to those used for routine diagnostic studies (Fig. 10.6). A peripheral nerve is stimulated – most often the median nerve at the wrist due to the robust signal that can be recorded at the cortical surface. However, other nerves, such as the tibial nerve, can also be used. Stimulation is performed at a rate of 2–5 Hz with a 0.1–0.3 ms pulse duration, and the current adjusted to produce a minimal (not painful) twitch so that muscle activity can just be visualized. Stimulation can be accomplished with mechanical and thermal stimulation as well. The stimulus generates a signal that is transmitted via the spinothalamic pathways, to the medial lemniscus, then the thalamus, and finally to contralateral somatosensory cortex. Compared with scalp recordings, SSEP recordings made from the cortical surface have much higher voltages (10–100 mV). Recording typically uses a low, cut-off frequency of 1 Hz, a high-frequency filter of 3,000 Hz, and an analysis time of 100 ms. Usually, trials of 100–200 stimuli are needed to elicit well-defined responses from the somatosensory cortex. Cortical responses have a number of different components designated by their positive (P) or negative (N) polarity with respect to the reference electrode, followed by a number representing the typical latency (in ms) of the peaks. For instance, following median nerve stimulation, the contralateral somatosensory gyrus shows an initial N20 component followed by a P25 component.

Following craniotomy and durotomy, an array of electrodes is placed in the axial (transverse) plane on the cortical surface. An eight-contact electrode strip (1 cm center-to-center spacing) is quite adequate. The electrode contacts should extend over areas of the brain anterior and posterior to the presumed somatosensory gyrus. Alternatively, electrodes may be placed on the dura (this is especially helpful for re-operative and post-meningitis cases where the dura is adherent to the underlying cortex rather than directly on the cortical surface). If the craniotomy does not expose Rolandic cortex, an electrode strip can be slid beneath the edge of the craniotomy to reach distant cortical regions. A series of recordings are then made from the cortical surface by moving the electrode to different areas to verify localization of the somatosensory cortex.

## Cortical Stimulation Motor and Sensory Mapping

Functional localization by cortical stimulation mapping has been performed for over 40 years. Although this technique is reliable, it is often difficult to elicit responses in children or under general anesthesia. Stimulation mapping of somatosensory cortex requires an awake patient; however, motor cortex can be stimulated with the patient under general anesthesia. It is important to bear in mind during cortical stimulation that repetitive or prolonged stimulation at or

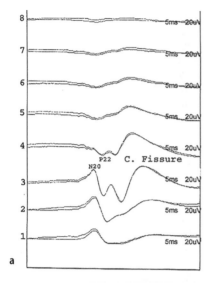

**Fig. 10.6. a** Bipolar montage from somatosensory evoked potential (SSEP) recording following stimulation of the right (contralateral) median nerve. The N20, denoting the primary somatosensory cortex is seen in channel "3". The P22, indicating motor cortex, is seen in channel "4". **b** Trans-dural SSEP electrode arrangement with an eight-contact electrode placed on the dura prior to durotomy. **c** SSEP recording directly from the cortical surface.

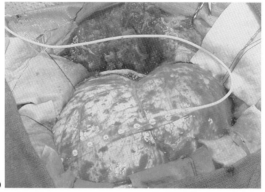

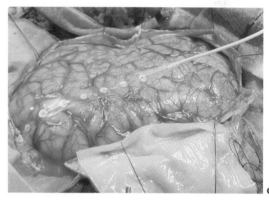

near the same site, or with higher currents, can elicit local or generalized seizure activity. Therefore, it is important to make sure that the patient has adequate serum anticonvulsant levels pre-operatively and that a short-acting intravenous anticonvulsant is readily available in the event that seizures are elicited.

A constant current, biphasic, square wave, 60 Hz, bipolar stimulator (Ojemann Stimulator, Radionics Sales Corp.; 5 mm between electrodes) set at 2–10 mA is used to elicit movement and/or sensation in the awake patient. Higher current settings may be necessary in younger children, in patients under general anesthesia, or when stimulating through the dura. It is best to start at lower current settings and gradually increase the current until sensation or movement is elicited, as this will help to avoid eliciting seizure activity.

Using this technique, the entire sensory and motor homunculi can be mapped. The technique can also be used to identify descending subcortical motor fibers when resections extend below the cortical surface, such as during supplementary motor area resections and insular resections. When performing subcortical motor mapping, the current needed to elicit movement is the same, or lower than, the current needed at the cortical surface. When the resection is very close to functional cortex, it is helpful to periodically repeat the stimulation mapping procedure to verify that cortical and subcortical functional regions are not damaged.

## Mapping of Language Cortex

In contrast to mapping Rolandic cortex, language cortex mapping depends on electrical blockade of cortical function rather than on eliciting function [29]. Most patients, even children as young as 10 years old, have little difficulty with the procedure, especially when propofol anesthesia is used during placement of the field block, cranial opening, the majority of the resection, and during closure. It is important to bear in mind that cortical stimulation mapping of language cortex is used to identify essential language cortex. This is distinctly different from involved language cortex, which is identified by functional imaging techniques such as positron emission tomography (PET) and functional magnetic resonance imaging (fMRI). Furthermore, the specific language task performed by the patient may lead to identification of different language sites.

It is first necessary to determine the after-discharge threshold so that depolarization is not propagated to nearby cortex, which may elicit local seizure phenomena or give false-negative or false-positive results. Therefore, electrocorticography (ECoG) must be performed during stimulation (Fig. 10.7). Using a U-shaped electrode holder, which is attached to the skull at the edge of the craniotomy (Grass model CE1), carbon-tip electrodes are placed over the exposed cortical surface and spaced approximately 10 mm apart. Bipolar stimulation, as described above, is then used, starting with a current of 2 mA. The current is gradually increased (0.5–1.0 mA increments) with successive stimulations until the after-discharge threshold is determined. The current used for language mapping is then set to 0.5–1.0mA below the after-discharge threshold.

Prior to mapping, 15–20 peri-Sylvian sites are selected and marked with small (5 × 5 mm)

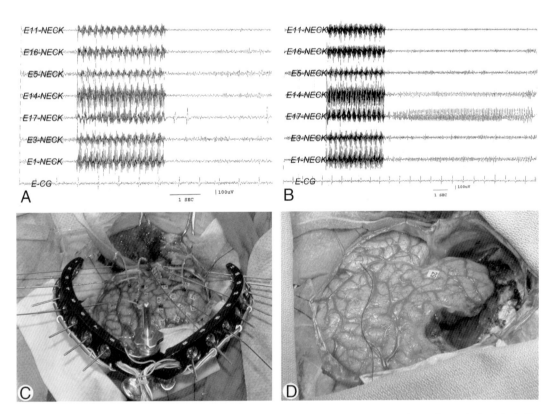

**Fig. 10.7. a** Intraoperative electrocorticogram showing three afterdischarges following cortical stimulation (in lead E17). The montage is referential to three neck electrodes (balanced neck reference, to minimize ECG interference). **b** A higher current than in a has produced a train of afterdischarges. **c** The cortical electrode arrangement is shown with numbered tickets on the left frontal lobe. **d** Ticket "29" shows the location of motor speech; the suture is on the central sulcus. The frontal lobe tumor resection can be seen.

numbered tags. Sites for stimulation mapping are randomly selected to cover all exposed cortex, including areas where essential language areas are likely to be located and those near or overlying the site of resection. Using a computer, the patient is shown images of simple objects. A new image is shown every 2–4 seconds (depending on the patient's verbal ability). Cortical stimulation is applied prior to the presentation of each image and continued until there is a correct response or the next image is presented. Each pre-selected site is stimulated three to four times, though never twice in succession. Sites where stimulation produces consistent speech arrest or anomia are considered essential to language function. Injury to essential language areas will lead to permanent difficulties.

It is important to remember that the topography of essential language varies from individual to individual. Furthermore, patients who are adept in more than one language will have separate essential language areas for each of their different languages. Standard anatomical temporal lobe resections (e.g. measured resections, resections anterior to the central sulcus, resections anterior to Labbé's vein) do not always spare essential language areas. Ojemann et al. [30] noted that subjects typically have two language areas: one in the posterior inferior frontal gyrus, and one in the posterior temporal lobe. However, individuals displayed a wide variety of language topography and some had three or more sites identified. The basal language area can probably be resected with relative impunity, indicating that, although this site is involved in language function, it is not essential.

As with the other types of mapping described above, language mapping can be performed through the dura or directly on the cortical surface. Furthermore, when the surgeon wishes to stimulate unexposed cortex, this can be accomplished by sliding a strip electrode beneath the edge of the bone flap and then utilizing a device that attaches to the electrode lead wire connection that permits direct bipolar stimulation [27]. When the resection is within 2 cm of the identified language area, it is best to have the patient continue object naming during the part of the resection that is close to the identified language site. The resection can then proceed slowly and be halted if naming errors occur.

## Pitfalls of Cortical Mapping

Although cortical mapping is an important tool, potential pitfalls must be recognized so as to use mapping safely and effectively [27]. Below are some of the major difficulties encountered. These have been separated into: (1) inability to identify functional cortex, and (2) injury to functional cortex once it has been identified.

### Inability to Identify Functional Cortex

In young patients, stimulation motor mapping is often not possible. SSEPs must be used to localize Rolandic cortex. Under general anesthesia, SSEPs and motor cortex localization may prove difficult. Nitrous/narcotic anesthesia is best for mapping. Inability to identify functional cortex does not prove that one is not in functional cortex. It may be indicative that there was a problem with mapping, not that resection is necessarily safe. During localization of speech cortex, ECoG must be used to determine the after-discharge threshold. This assures that there are no local seizures elicited by stimulation.

### Injury to Functional Cortex Following Mapping

There are often two or more essential speech areas within both the temporal and frontal lobes. Therefore, the entire region to be resected should be mapped (i.e. mapping should not be stopped simply because two speech areas have been identified). White matter underlying functional cortex can be injured. For Rolandic cortex, this can be avoided with subcortical mapping. For speech cortex, the patient should continue naming during resection of abutting cortex or white matter. Vascular injury in the neighborhood of functional cortex must be avoided. Lesional distortion of cortex superficially does not indicate that underlying white matter has (or has not) been displaced. Ascending or descending fibers may not travel perpendicular to the gyral crown.

# Intratumoral Therapies

Aside from the resection of tumor, neurosurgeons are becoming increasingly involved in the delivery of therapy at the time of resection or the delivery of intralesional therapy. While most of these neurosurgical-based therapies are experimental or undergoing evaluation in phase I or II clinical trials, a few have been approved for general use.

## Chemotherapy Impregnated Wafers

The implantation of degradable wafers impregnated with BCNU (Gliadel) has been used extensively at the time of re-operation for recurrent HGGs, and recently has been approved by the FDA for use at the time of initial surgery. In a large phase III trial enrolling 222 patients with recurrent HGGs, the use of Gliadel provided a statistically significant prolongation of survival of 8 weeks (from 23 to 31 weeks) for all HGG patients as well as for the GBM subgroup [31]. A recent multicenter prospective trial evaluated the use of Gliadel at initial surgery and reported median survival times of 13.9 vs 11.6 months for HGG patients receiving Gliadel vs placebo, with median survival of 13.5 vs 11.4 months in the GBM vs placebo group [32].

Complications associated with the use of Gliadel include infection, cerebral edema, wound-healing problems and CSF leak, particularly in patients with recurrent HGG. Careful attention to tissue handling and dural closure, with use of dural patches, helps to reduce these complications.

## Brachytherapy

Brachytherapy for HGGs includes the temporary use of high-activity implants and permanent placement of lower-activity sources. Early reports on the use of brachytherapy with temporary high-activity implants were encouraging, but subsequent re-evaluation showed that much of the treatment effect was due to selection bias [33]. Subsequent randomized prospective trials of interstitial, high-activity, temporary I-125 implants, used as a boost at the time of initial treatment, have reported contradictory results. Permanent low-activity I-125 implants placed at initial operation have produced promising results but require additional validation.

Similar brachytherapy strategies using either high-activity I-125 temporary, or low-activity I-125 permanent, implants have been used for HGGs at the time of recurrence. While the efficacy of these approaches is not clearly established, one study reported the survival of patients receiving permanent implants was almost two-fold longer than a comparable group of historical controls treated aggressively with surgery and chemotherapy. One consideration in their use is that treatment-related morbidity appears to be less for permanent low-activity implants than for temporary high-activity implants. One difficulty with any brachytherapy approach is achieving uniform dose distributions to all involved regions of tumor. Dose heterogeneity can lead to under-treated (cold spots) or over-treated areas (hot spots) at risk for rapid progression or radiation injury and necrosis, respectively. While the use of stereotactic radiation techniques provides boosts with more defined dosimetry, it is often difficult to shape the radiation field to the irregular growth patterns of most HGGs.

# Future Directions

A host of novel experimental therapies, including gene-based therapy and immunotherapy, have emerged based on our continually evolving understanding of HGG biology. The delivery of many of these newer therapies involves the technical expertise of the neurosurgeon [34]. The following examples of emerging therapeutic approaches emphasize how targeting specific aspects of glioma tumor biology translates into new treatment strategies, and how the delivery of these agents – often with novel techniques – is likely to further involve the neurosurgeon in the future treatment of HGG.

Immunotherapy approaches include the use of antibodies conjugated to radioactive compounds, or toxins directed against tumor-specific antigens (such as transferrin receptors, EGFRvIII, tenascin, and VEGF receptors). Tumor vaccines are being developed, and other means to boost inherent immune responses to tumor antigens, such as dendritic cell therapies, are being actively pursued. Gene therapy encompasses a multitude of different approaches as well. Early clinical trials of gene therapy used the local administration into glioma resection beds of retroviruses engineered with bacterial enzymes (thymidine kinase) capable of converting prodrugs (ganciclovir) into cytotoxic metabolites. Other, newer, gene-based therapies under development include: gene replacement (e.g. p53), production of dominant-negative receptors (e.g. to VEGF receptor) to disrupt signaling pathways, antisense oligonucleotides to knock down expression of specific genes, and administration of cytolytic viral vectors. These approaches are theoretically attractive because they target specific molecular aspects of glial tumors and may reduce toxicity, but none has proven to be particularly efficacious. Thus, their integration into standard therapy will require further investigation.

One of the major impediments to successful treatment of HGGs is the inability to deliver cytotoxic drug concentrations to bulk tumor or to access the diffusely invasive tumor cells that reside within regions of an intact BBB. Not surprisingly, concurrent with the development of new treatment approaches described above has been the introduction of novel techniques for delivery of these therapies and others, which attempt to overcome these limitations. These new approaches to delivery include the use of convection-enhanced delivery and osmotic or pharmacological opening of the BBB and intralesional delivery of high-dose chemotherapy. Convection-enhanced delivery uses intracerebral catheters to infuse therapeutic agents through the brain by bulk flow, such that therapy can be delivered to large areas of brain without reliance on a disrupted BBB. Disruption of the BBB itself by administration of osmotic agents or with drugs that specifically reduce endothelial-cell-tight junctions, such as the bradykinin agonist RMP-7, can be used to achieve higher drug levels within bulk tumor and surrounding diffusely invaded brain tissue with a normally intact BBB. The use of direct intralesional injection of therapeutic agents is also under investigation in an attempt to provide local cytotoxic therapy with minimal systemic toxicity [34].

Perhaps the most intriguing new method for delivery of therapy involves the use of genetically engineered neural stem cells (NSCs). In animal models, NSCs injected intracranially or even intravascularly migrate into the brain and appear to have a unique tropism for isolated invasive tumor cells. NSCs engineered to produce the enzyme cytosine deaminase were shown to be capable of converting systemically administered prodrug 5-FC into the cytotoxic metabolite 5-FU, which led to a significant reduction of implanted brain tumor size in animals [11].

## Key Points

- *High-grade gliomas are the most common primary cerebral neoplasms in adults and the majority of these tumors are glioblastoma multiforme and anaplastic astrocytoma.*
- *High-grade gliomas can either arise de novo or arise from malignant degeneration of low grade gliomas.*
- *Treatment of high-grade gliomas includes confirmatory biopsy or surgical resection followed by radiation therapy. Chemotherapy can also be considered.*
- *Important predictors of survival include age, histological grade, Karnofsky performance status and adequacy of treatment.*
- *Despite advances in imaging, surgical techniques to maximize resection, and chemotherapy and radiation therapy techniques, the prognosis for survival beyond 2–3 years remains poor.*

## References

1. Legler JM, Ries LA, Smith MA, Warren JL, Heineman EF, Kaplan RS et al. Cancer surveillance series (corrected): brain and other central nervous system cancers: recent trends in incidence and mortality. J Natl Cancer Inst 1999;91(16):1382–90.
2. Kleihues P, Louis DN, Scheithauer BW, Rorke LB, Reifenberger G, Burger PC et al. The WHO classification of tumors of the nervous system. J Neuropathol Exp Neurol 2002;61(3):215–25;discussion:226–9.
3. Kleihues, P, Ohgaki H. Primary and secondary glioblastomas: from concept to clinical diagnosis. Neuro-oncol 1999;1(1):44–51.
4. Bigner SH, Matthews MR, Rasheed BK, Wiltshire RN, Friedman HS, Friedman AH et al. Molecular genetic aspects of oligodendrogliomas including analysis by comparative genomic hybridization. Am J Pathol 1999;155(2):375–86.
5. Chan JL, Lee SW, Fraass BA, Normolle DP, Greenberg HS, Junck LR et al. Survival and failure patterns of high-grade gliomas after three-dimensional conformal radiotherapy. J Clin Oncol 2002;20(6):1635–42.
6. Halligan JB, Stelzer KJ, Rostomily RC, Spence AM, Griffin TW, Berger MS et al. Operation and permanent low activity 125I brachytherapy for recurrent high-grade astrocytomas. Int J Radiat Oncol Biol Phys 1996;35(3):541–7.
7. Scherer HJ. Structural development in gliomas. Am J Cancer 1938;34(3):333–51.

8. Kelly PJ, Daumas-Duport C, Kispert DB, Kall BA, Scheithauer BW, Illig JJ. Imaging-based stereotaxic serial biopsies in untreated intracranial glial neoplasms. J Neurosurg 1987;66(6):865–74.

9. Silbergeld DL, Chicoine MR. Isolation and characterization of human malignant glioma cells from histologically normal brain. J Neurosurg 1997;86(3):525–31.

10. Ojemann JG, Miller JW, Silbergeld DL. Preserved function in brain invaded by tumor. Neurosurgery 1996;39(2):253–8;discussion:258–9.

11. Aboody KS, Brown A, Rainov NG, Bower KA, Liu S, Yang W et al. From the cover: neural stem cells display extensive tropism for pathology in adult brain: evidence from intracranial gliomas. Proc Natl Acad Sci USA 2000;97(23):12846–51.

12. Curran WJ Jr, Scott CB, Horton J, Nelson JS, Weinstein AS, Fischbach AJ et al. Recursive partitioning analysis of prognostic factors in three Radiation Therapy Oncology Group malignant glioma trials. J Natl Cancer Inst 1993;85(9):704–10.

13. Wong ET, Hess KR, Gleason MJ, Jaeckle KA, Kyritsis AP, Prados MD et al. Outcomes and prognostic factors in recurrent glioma patients enrolled onto phase II clinical trials. J Clin Oncol 1999;17(8):2572.

14. Rostomily RC, Spence AM, Duong D, McCormick K, Bland M, Berger MS et al. Multimodality management of recurrent adult malignant gliomas: results of a phase II multiagent chemotherapy study and analysis of cytoreductive surgery. Neurosurgery 1994;35(3): 378–88;discussion:388.

15. Ino Y, Betensky RA, Zlatescu MC, Sasaki H, Macdonald DR, Stemmer-Rachamimov AO et al. Molecular subtypes of anaplastic oligodendroglioma: implications for patient management at diagnosis. Clin Cancer Res 2001;7(4):839–45.

16. Walker MD, Alexander E Jr, Hunt WE, MacCarty CS, Mahaley MS Jr, Mealey J Jr et al. Evaluation of BCNU and/or radiotherapy in the treatment of anaplastic gliomas. A cooperative clinical trial. J Neurosurg 1978;49(3):333–43.

17. Stewart LA. Chemotherapy in adult high-grade glioma: a systematic review and meta-analysis of individual patient data from 12 randomised trials. Lancet 2002;359(9311):1011–18.

18. Duong DH, Rostomily RC, Haynor DR, Keles GE, Berger MS. Measurement of tumor resection volumes from computerized images. Technical note. J Neurosurg 1992;77(1):151–4.

19. Henegar MM, Moran CJ, Silbergeld DL. Early post-operative magnetic resonance imaging following nonneoplastic cortical resection. J Neurosurg 1996;84(2):174–9.

20. Keles GE, Anderson B, and Berger MS. The effect of extent of resection on time to tumor progression and survival in patients with glioblastoma multiforme of the cerebral hemisphere. Surg Neurol 1999;52(4):371–9.

21. Silbergeld DL, Rostomily RC. Resection of glioblastoma. J Neurosurg 2002;96(4):809;discussion:810.

22. Barker FG Jr, Chang SM, Gutin PH, Malec MK, McDermott MW, Prados MD et al. Survival and functional status after resection of recurrent glioblastoma multiforme. Neurosurgery 1998;42(4):709–20; discussion:720–3.

23. Alvord EC Jr. Simple model of recurrent gliomas. J Neurosurg 1991;75(2):337–8.

24. Shinoda J, Sakai N, Murase S, Yano H, Matsuhisa T, Funakoshi T. Selection of eligible patients with supratentorial glioblastoma multiforme for gross total resection. J Neurooncol 2001;52(2):161–71.

25. Domino KB, Hemstad JR, Lam AM, Laohaprasit V, Mayberg TA, Harrison SD et al. Effect of nitrous oxide on intracranial pressure after cranial-dural closure in patients undergoing craniotomy. Anesthesiology 1992;77(3):421–5.

26. Field M, Witham TF, Flickinger JC, Kondziolka D, Lunsford LD. Comprehensive assessment of hemorrhage risks and outcomes after stereotactic brain biopsy. J Neurosurg 2001;94(4):545–51.

27. Silbergeld DL. Cortical mapping. In: Luders HO and Comair YG, editors. Epilepsy surgery. Philadelphia: Lippincott Williams & Wilkins, 2002; 633–5.

28. Silbergeld DL, Miller JW. Intraoperative cerebral mapping and monitoring. Contemp Neurosurg 1996;18(11): 1–6.

29. Silbergeld DL, Ojemann GA. The tailored temporal lobectomy. Neurosurg Clin N Am 1993;4(2):273–81.

30. Ojemann G, Ojemann J, Lettich E, Berger M. Cortical language localization in left, dominant hemisphere. An electrical stimulation mapping investigation in 117 patients. J Neurosurg 1989;71(3):316–26.

31. Brem H, Piantadosi S, Burger PC, Walker M, Selker R, Vick NA et al. Placebo-controlled trial of safety and efficacy of intraoperative controlled delivery by biodegradable polymers of chemotherapy for recurrent gliomas. The Polymer-brain Tumor Treatment Group. Lancet 1995;345(8956):1008–12.

32. Westphal M, Hilt D, Bortey E, Delavault P, Olivares R, Warnke P et al. A phase 3 trial of local chemotherapy with biodegradable carmustine (BCNU) wafers (Gliadel wafers) in patients with primary malignant glioma. Neuro-oncol 2003;5(2):79–88.

33. Florell RC, Macdonald DR, Irish WD, Bernstein M, Leibel SA, Gutin PH et al. Selection bias, survival, and brachytherapy for glioma. J Neurosurg 1992;76(2): 179–83.

34. Broaddus WC, Gillies GT, Kucharczyk J. Minimally invasive procedures. Advances in image-guided delivery of drug and cell therapies into the central nervous system. Neuroimaging Clin N Am 2001;11(4):727–35.

# 11

## Sellar and Parasellar Tumors

Richard J. Stacey and Michael P. Powell

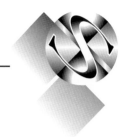

## Summary

Pituitary adenomas are by far the most common tumours of the sellar region, comprising 90 to 95% of all such tumours. Meningiomas, craniopharyngiomas(particularly in children), Rathke's cleft cysts and aneurysms are the most likely differential diagnoses. The majority of pituitary tumours are asymptomatic, discovered as "incidentalomas" in the course of investigation for other conditions. The rest, along with other sellar lesions, present with symptoms of endocrine dysfunction, mass effect on surrounding structures, commonly the optic nerves or chiasm, or headache. Apart from Prolactin secreting tumours, which respond to dopamine agonists, the mainstay of treatment is surgery, with or without radiotherapy. Prior to surgery, even as an emergency, all sellar tumour patients should have thyroid function tests, Prolactin levels and adequate imaging. Any patient with a tumour with suprasellar extension should undergo formal visual field assessment. MRI scanning is the imaging modality of choice, with a CT scan for sphenoid septal anatomy if a transphenoidal approach is to be undertaken.

## Introduction

### Embryology of the Sellar Region

Holding the key position at the center of the skull, the sella turcica ("Turkish saddle") is used as a reference point for many lesions, which may be described as sellar, suprasellar or parasellar. The close proximity of many important structures explains the often striking and characteristic clinical presentation of pathology in this compact region.

The cartilaginous neurocranium is the basal region of the developing skull. In its earliest stage of development, it exists as a narrow condensation of mesenchyme forming a plate that links the anterior rim of the foramen magnum with the most anterior part of the skull. Central to the development of this region is the formation of the body of the sphenoid bone. Subsequently, cartilaginous plates develop on either side of the developing sphenoid body to form the wings and complete the development of the middle cranial fossa.

The greater wings of the sphenoid form the majority of the middle cranial fossa. The lesser wings start at the anterior clinoid processes, passing laterally to become the sphenoid ridge of the pterion. Between the two is the superior orbital fissure. By the middle of the third month of gestation, the skull base is a unified mass of cartilage known as the "chondrocranium".

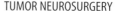

Subsequent ossification takes place in several centers.

The sella develops as a depression in the body of the sphenoid and is lined with dura and houses the pituitary gland. It is roofed over by the diaphragma, which transmits the infundibulum or pituitary stalk. On either side of the sphenoid bone the cavernous sinuses, made from folded dura, transmit the carotid artery, the maxillary division of the trigeminal nerve, and cranial nerves III, IV and VI.

The cavernous sinuses receive blood from the petrosal and sphenoparietal sinuses in addition to local veins draining the sella. They also interconnect with each other, which explains why petrosal venous sampling seldom localizes the side of a pituitary microadenoma. The posterior articulation of the sphenoid body is with the clivus at the spheno-occipital synchondrosis. Above the sella are situated the optic nerves, chiasm, third ventricle and hypothalamus.

## Lesions of the Sellar Region

There are numerous diagnostic possibilities for any lesion in the sellar region (Table 11.1) but the astute clinician or radiologist is aware that there is a high statistical chance of any lesion in the area being a pituitary adenoma. Adenomas in their various forms make up 90–95% of most series. Meningiomas, craniopharyngiomas, Rathke's cleft cysts and internal carotid artery aneurysms make up the commonest of the less frequent lesions. Of the remainder, because their frequency of presentation is considerably less than 1%, it is sufficient to be aware of their existence.

## Pituitary Adenomas

### Incidence

The majority of pituitary tumors are asymptomatic, as shown by the discrepancy between the reported prevalence of 200 per million and the post-mortem findings of pituitary tumors in 10–27% of the population [1].

### Pathophysiology

The anterior portion (adenohypophysis) of the pituitary gland is thought to develop from endothelium lining the primitive buccal cavity (stomatodeum) passing cranially as Rathke's

**Table 11.1.** Differential diagnosis of neoplasms and "tumor-like" lesions of the sellar region

**Tumors of adenohypophyseal origin**
*Pituitary adenoma*
*Pituitary carcinoma*
**Tumors of neurohypophyseal origin**
Granular cell tumor
Astrocytoma of posterior lobe and/or stalk (rare)
**Tumors of non-pituitary origin**
*Craniopharyngioma*
Germ cell tumors
Gliomas (hypothalamic, optic nerve/chiasm, infundibulum)
*Meningioma*
*Hemangiopericytoma*
Chordoma
Hemangioblastoma
Lipoma
Giant cell tumor of bone
Chondroma
Fibrous dysplasia
Sarcoma (chondrosarcoma, osteosarcoma, fibrosarcoma)
Post-irradiation sarcomas
Paraganglioma
Schwannoma
Glomangioma
Esthesioneuroblastoma
Primary lymphoma
Melanoma
**Cysts, hamartomas and malformations**
*Rathke's cleft cyst*
Arachnoid cyst
Epidermoid cyst
Dermoid cyst
Gangliocytoma
**Metastatic tumors**
Carcinoma
Plasmacytoma
Lymphoma
Leukemia
**Inflammatory conditions**
Infection/abscess
Mucocele
*Lymphocytic hypophysitis*
Sarcoidosis
Langerhans' cell histiocytosis
Giant cell granuloma
**Vascular lesions**
Internal carotid artery aneurysms
Cavernous angioma

*NB. Lesions in italics are discussed in the text.*

pouch. This joins a downward projection of the hypothalamus (neurohypophysis), destined to form the posterior lobe and pituitary stalk. This composite gland is distinct and separate from the primitive stomatodeum by the seventh week of gestation and further develops under the influence of the hypothalamus through a series of permissive and specific trans-acting proteins. It is fully functioning by the time of birth but retains considerable plasticity throughout life. Occasionally, cystic remnants of embryological development persist within the pituitary as Rathke's cleft cysts.

The majority of pituitary tumors are benign epithelial neoplasms that develop from adeno-hypophyseal parenchyma and, as such, resemble normal pituitary histology. In addition to the clinically relevant hormones produced by the pituitary, a number of additional peptides and hypothalamic hormones are known to be produced. These include, amongst many, vasoactive intestinal polypeptide, growth-hormone-releasing hormone (GHRH), somato-statin, substance P and renin. Such findings attest to the functional complexity of the gland.

In addition to the hormone-producing cells, apparently functionally inert or "null" cells are also found in the parenchyma, which also give rise to adenomas. These cells may produce either no hormone or an imperfect form with no biological activity. Multiple-hormone gene and gene receptor products are commonly seen in adenomas; for example, growth hormone (GH) gene expression occurs in 50% of prolactinomas and 30% of corticotrophic adenomas. This functional diversity may explain the occasional response of mixed somatotroph and lactotroph adenomas to dopamine receptor agonists.

The pathogenesis of pituitary adenomas is likely to be multifactorial. As with other neoplasms, the potential mechanisms of oncogenesis fall into three groups:

- Abnormalities of genes regulating growth and development
- Abnormalities of tumor-suppressor genes
- Alterations in the genes controlling programmed cell death

## Classification of Pituitary Tumors (Table 11.2)

The new World Health Organization classification divides pituitary tumors simplistically into

**Table 11.2.** Simplified classification of pituitary adenomas

| |
|---|
| GH cell adenoma |
| PRL cell adenoma |
| Mixed GH cell / PRL cell adenoma |
| Mammosomatotroph cell adenoma |
| ACTH cell adenoma |
| FSH/LH cell adenoma |
| TSH cell adenoma |
| Null cell adenoma |
| Pluri-hormonal adenoma |
| Unclassified adenoma |

pituitary adenomas and carcinomas, and the traditional categorization of pituitary adenomas by their tinctorial properties has been abandoned. Ultrastructural appearance, in particular the size of the cytoplasmic granules, also aids in the diagnosis of these tumors. The latter system, however, requires pituitary adenomas to be extensively examined by multiple modalities in specialist centers [2].

The majority of adrenocorticotrophic hormone (ACTH)-producing tumors are microscopic. GH, prolactin (PRL) and ACTH-containing tumors correlate well with endocrinological behavior, whereas the others do not. Pituitary adenomas are also subdivided by virtue of their size into those less than 1 cm in diameter (microadenomas) and those greater than 1 cm (macroadenomas). These divisions usually correlate with presentation – microadenomas presenting with endocrinological manifestations and macroadenomas with compressive effects – although GH-secreting tumors and prolactinomas in males, in particular, may reach substantial size before diagnosis.

## Presentation

Pituitary tumors and most other sellar lesions present in four general ways:

- *Endocrinological dysfunction.* This may result from overproduction of the six pituitary hormones: PL, GH, ACTH or, rarely, thyroid-stimulating hormone (TSH) and gonadotrophins, but may also result from underproduction syndromes, such as Addisonian crisis or secondary amenorrheas. Specific endocrinopathy will be covered for each tumor type in turn (see below).

- *Mass effect on adjacent structures* (Fig. 11.1a and b). Tumors usually compress the optic nerves and chiasm, but occasionally they compress the third nerve, particularly in apoplexy [3] (Fig. 11.2). They may also very occasionally cause hydrocephalus by blocking CSF outflow in the third ventricle.
- *Headache.* This may possibly occur as a result of compression or stretching of the dural lining of the sella or of the diaphragmata, which are innervated by branches of the trigeminal nerve. It is this sudden stimulus that is believed to cause the pain of pituitary apoplexy, which may be so severe as to mimic subarachnoid hemorrhage.
- *Incidental finding.* Tumors may be found during investigation for some other condition. They are now officially known as the "incidentalomas".

Endocrine and visual symptoms are the most common forms of presentation, with headache and incidentalomas being infrequent.

## Visual Manifestations

The classic bitemporal field loss is found in chiasmatic compression. Early compression may lead to upper quadrantic defects. This results from inferior chiasmal fiber compression. The

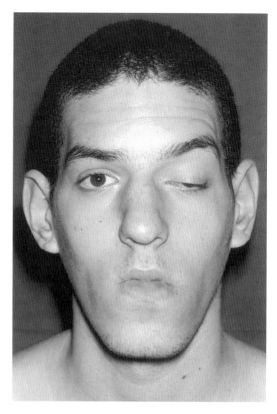

**Fig. 11.2.** A young man with acromegaly and pituitary apoplexy. The apoplexy has resulted in a left oculomotor nerve palsy.

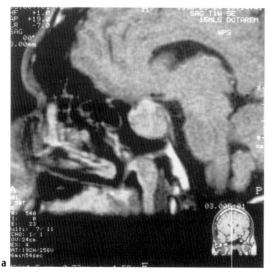
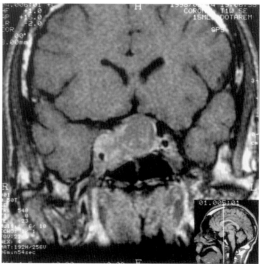

**Fig. 11.1. a–b** A large pituitary tumor compressing surrounding structures. **a** Sagittal MRI. **b** Coronal MRI.

reverse may occur in lesions compressing the chiasm from above, such as craniopharyngioma. Field loss often begins unilaterally when the intracranial optic nerve is compressed close to its junction with the chiasm. Decussating fibers from the nasal retina of the other eye loop forwards into the optic nerve for a short distance before turning through 180° and passing backwards into the optic tract. Early additional involvement of such decussating fibers is signaled by a small contralateral upper temporal or "junctional" defect. Patients frequently complain of bumping into objects on one or both sides of the contracted visual field, reflecting both unilateral and bitemporal field loss. The affected field is described as absent, or blank, rather than black (blackness is usually a symptom of retinal rather than optic fiber disease). Central vision may be affected by direct compression of the intracranial optic nerve. This may present as a blurring of vision or scotomatous central field defects. This is more common in individuals with a "post-fixed" chiasm – an anatomical variation where the chiasm is situated further back, thus exposing more optic nerve to the compressive effects of an expanding adenoma. If compression has been longstanding, fundoscopy may reveal optic atrophy. Diplopia usually signals lateral compression of the nerves in and around the cavernous sinus either by gradual lateral extension or apoplexy. Optic tract compression in a "pre-fixed" chiasm (the opposite of a post-fixed chiasm) is rare and may produce an homonymous field pattern that may be incongruous.

## Visual Testing

All patients with suprasellar extension should have formal eye assessment. This will include:

- *Acuity*, using the Snellen chart.
- *Fields*. For reproducibility, the automated Humphrey field analyzer is the most popular, although in the hands of the expert, the Goldman perimeter is the most accurate and will overcome difficulties of interpretation from true ocular disease.
- *Color vision*, particularly temporal desaturation to red, which will give information on early anterior pathway pathology.

# Individual Pituitary Tumor Types, and Related Hormones

## Growth-hormone-producing Adenomas

### Incidence

This group of tumors includes the somatotroph adenomas, the mammosomatotroph adenomas and the mixed somatotroph–lactotroph adenomas. The prevalence of acromegaly is 30–50 per million and the incidence is five per million.

### Clinical Features

Growth hormone, a 191 amino acid protein, is released from the anterior pituitary gland under the stimulatory influence of GHRH. Its release is inhibited by somatostatin, which, in turn, is stimulated by hyperglycaemia. This is useful clinically as somatostatin analogues can be used to suppress GH production and the glucose tolerance test can be used to assess response to surgery (see below). In excess, it causes acromegaly, gigantism or both. Gigantism results from growth hormone excess before epiphyseal closure and frequently it is accompanied by the soft tissue thickening characteristics of acromegaly (Fig. 11.2).

Acromegaly is insidious in onset. The diagnosis may be made coincidentally or because of complications such as carpal tunnel syndrome, diabetes mellitus, hypertension, hypopituitarism or sleep apnea. Chronic hypertension can lead to cerebrovascular disease, coronary artery disease and congestive cardiac failure. Patients with acromegaly also have a higher incidence of malignancy, including colonic polyps, colonic carcinomas and breast carcinoma, than the general population.

Some acromegalic patients have an associated hyperprolactinemia. This has led to the discovery of the mixed monomorphous mammosomatotroph adenomas and the bimorphous somatotroph–lactotroph adenomas mentioned above.

### Histology

Grossly the more common macroadenomas are frequently well demarcated. Microadenomas are confined to one of the lateral wings – the principal site of GH-producing cells in the normal gland. Larger tumors often spread outside the sella and invade neighboring tissues. GH levels correlate with tumor size. Mammosomatotroph adenomas are composed of a single cell type that is capable of producing GH and PRL. Mixed lactotroph and somatotroph tumors consist of different, coexisting tumor colonies.

### Biochemical Investigations

The biochemical diagnosis is based on the demonstration of a random GH of more than 10 mU/l (5.0 ng/ml), failure of suppression to less than 2.0 mU/l (1.0 ng/ml) following an oral glucose load of 75 g, and an elevated insulin-like growth factor 1 (IGF-1). Very rarely, acromegaly may be due to ectopic GHRH production. Circulating GHRH levels should thus be examined in the case of an acromegalic in whom imaging has failed to demonstrate a pituitary adenoma. Because GH is released in bursts and has a half-life of less than 1 hour, single estimations can be misleading. For this reason some authorities are switching to IGF-1 (somatomedin), with its longer half-life, as a more accurate indication of GH exposure. PRL measurements should always be taken in order to detect cases of mammosomatotroph adenomas, which co-secrete prolactin and which may be sensitive to dopamine agonists such as bromocriptine.

### Radiological Investigations

As with most pituitary tumors, MRI is now the investigation of choice. It has excellent spatial resolution and also has the advantage of being able to image in any plane with the acquisition of three-dimensional data sets. These may be used for volumetric analysis and navigational purposes and may be supplemented with MR angiography to assess major vascular relations. The pituitary has no blood–brain barrier, and when gadolinium is given there is an orderly sequence of enhancement of the gland. Within seconds, the infundibulum and posterior pituitary enhance owing to their direct arterial supply. The anterior gland, supplied by the slower portal system, then begins to enhance. Signal intensity becomes homogeneous after about 90s. This is followed by slow washout, which is faster from the posterior pituitary. The cavernous sinuses enhance early, outlining the non-enhancing cranial nerves III and V.

Plain X-rays, in addition to documenting fossa erosion, can give important information about sphenoid pneumatization and septation. This may be of vital importance in transsphenoidal surgery, particularly in adhering to the midline and avoiding lateral structures such as the carotid arteries.

### Medical Treatment

The mainstay of treatment is surgery with or without radiotherapy. However, in cases of co-secretion of GH and PRL, 20% will respond to treatment with dopamine agonists. Treatment with the inhibitory somatostatin analogues has been shown to decrease GH secretion. However, its use has been restricted by expense, need for parenteral administration, and tendency to cause cholelithiasis.

## Prolactin-secreting Tumors

### Incidence

Over half of hormone-producing (functioning) tumors secrete the 198 amino acid lactotroph PRL, the only hormone under inhibitory control by dopamine from the hypothalamus. The clinical syndrome characterized by amenorrhea and galactorrhea was first described by Chiari and colleagues in 1855. PRL was not discovered as a human hormone until 1971.

### Clinical Features

Ninety percent of such tumors are in females with secondary amenorrhea as the common presenting feature. Galactorrhea is not always present, perhaps because a permissive level of estrogen may be required for milk production. In men, impotence with decreased sperm count is the endocrinological equivalent. Women, possibly owing to a greater awareness of the effects of hypersecretion, tend to present at a younger age with microadenomas, while men present later in life with visual field disturbances.

Because of the inhibitory control of the hypothalamus, any mass lesion in this area may produce relative hyperprolactinemia. This is termed the "stalk effect". Generally, when this occurs, the levels are under 3000 mU/l (200 ng/ml). Many physiological events can cause hyperprolactinemia: pregnancy, lactation, stress, physical activity and nipple stimulation. Pharmacological agents such as dopamine receptor agonists (phenothiazines, metoclopramide), tricyclic antidepressants, reserpine and cimetidine may cause increased levels, as may the systemic disorders, hypothyroidism and chronic renal failure.

### Histology

Although lactotroph adenomas are recognized as having two variants that are analogous to the two types of somatotroph adenomas (densely and sparsely granulated), sparsely granulated tumors make up the vast majority.

### Biochemical Investigations

The diagnosis is made by single blood level measurement and the serum level correlates well with tumor size.

### Radiological Investigations

As with all pituitary adenomas, good-quality MRI supplemented with plain films is usually sufficient.

### Medical Treatment

First-line treatment of prolactinomas is medical. Dopamine agonists such as bromocriptine and cabergoline will reduce prolactin levels to normal in 85% and 92% respectively and will lead to concomitant shrinkage even in giant tumors, causing visual symptoms. Surgery should be reserved for the dopamine-agonist-intolerant or -resistant patient. Radiotherapy has a disappointing track record in the control of hyperprolactinemia. In patients wishing to conceive, bromocriptine should be continued until a positive pregnancy test, and then stopped. There is no evidence to suggest that bromocriptine is teratogenic. The risk of tumor enlargement in symptomatic patients during pregnancy is 2–5% for treated microadenoma and up to 37% for macroadenoma. Experience would suggest that tumors of less than 5 mm are unlikely to cause problems during pregnancy.

## ACTH-producing Tumors

### Incidence

ACTH-secreting pituitary tumors are relatively rare, making up only 4% of functioning tumors. It is a dangerous condition with a poor 5-year survival rate if untreated. There is a high female to male ratio of 8:1.

### Clinical Features

Lesions associated with excess circulating cortisol produce the manifestations of Cushing's syndrome. This can be due to lesions of the adrenal cortex, to extrapituitary, "ectopic" production of ACTH by neoplasms, to excessive corticotrophin-releasing hormone (CRH) production, and to pituitary-dependent ACTH excess. The latter, termed "Cushing's disease", was recognized and described by Harvey Cushing in 1932. The syndrome is characterized by centripetal obesity, plethoric moon-shaped facies, hirsutism, acne, diabetes, hypertension, muscle weakness, bruising, mental disorders, amenorrhea and osteoporosis, all due to glucocorticoid hypersecretion. Hyperpigmentation is associated with ectopic ACTH production and, in severe cases, with pituitary-dependent ACTH excess. This is because the pro-hormone from which ACTH is eventually cleaved (proopiomelanocortin) also contains the amino acid sequences for melanocyte-stimulating hormone. Left untreated, Cushing's disease leads to severe complications.

### Histology

The most common cause of pituitary-dependent Cushing's disease is a basophilic microadenoma.

### Biochemical Investigations

Loss of diurnal rhythm of plasma (or salivary) cortisol, with increased excretion of urinary free cortisol and lack of overnight suppression of cortisol in response to a low dose (1 mg) of dexamethasone, confirms cortisol overproduction. A combined low-dose and high-dose (8 mg) suppression test usually distinguishes between Cushing's disease and adrenal overproduction. In the former, suppression occurs, but not usually in the case of adrenal adenoma or ectopic production of ACTH. This is because the pituitary adenoma cells still have some susceptibility to negative feedback.

The presence of detectable levels of ACTH suggests ACTH-dependent disease – either pituitary or ectopic. In ectopic ACTH secretion, usually from an oat-cell carcinoma of the bronchus, very high levels of ACTH, pigmentation and hypokalemic alkalosis are found.

If an adenoma is not detected on imaging, then inferior petrosal sinus sampling after CRH injection is justified. With such sampling, peripheral blood ratios of more than 2.0 in the basal state and more than 3.0 following CRH injection are strongly suggestive of a pituitary origin. It does not guarantee the side of the gland where the occult microadenoma may be located because of trans-cavernous sinus veins that allow mixing of the blood from each side. CRH testing can be helpful in differential diagnosis, where a 100 g injection of CRH-41 will produce a normal or exaggerated response in Cushing's disease, but will make no difference in cases of ectopic ACTH secretion and adrenal adenoma.

### Radiological Investigations

As with the other pituitary tumors, good-quality MRI and plain films usually suffice, supplemented by petrosal sampling if required.

### Medical Treatment

The definitive treatment for Cushing's disease is surgery. For those in whom surgery is not possible or has failed, radiotherapy is usually given. This may be accompanied by adrenalectomy and steroid replacement. Adrenalectomy carries a 20% risk of Nelson's syndrome (pituitary hyperplasia and autonomous production of ACTH) and thus medical rather than surgical adrenalectomy is usually the first choice. The 11β-hydroxylase inhibitor metyrapone is the most commonly used agent. Ketoconazole, which inhibits steroid production and release of ACTH, may also be used, or mitotane, which destroys adrenal tissue. All of these agents have potentially serious side-effects, particularly ketoconazole and mitotane, which my cause liver damage and hypercholesterolemia respectively. Another group of agents acts centrally by enhancing the activity of endogenous inhibitors, or by antagonizing endogenous ACTH stimulators. The most commonly used agents are bromocriptine (dopamine agonist), cyproheptadine (a serotinin antagonist) and the GABA transaminase inhibitor sodium valproate. Responses to these agents are unpredictable and idiosyncratic.

## Glycoprotein-secreting Tumors (TSH, FSH and LH)

These hormones are composed of alpha- and beta-chains and differ according to the structure of the latter.

### Thyroid-stimulating Hormone (TSH) Adenomas

These are the least common of the overproduction syndromes. There have been only two cases in over 1,000 on the National Hospital pituitary database.

*Clinical Features* The diagnosis is made on raised TSH in the presence of hyperthyroidism. Pituitary-dependent TSH excess may also be associated with hypothyroidism. These patients have longstanding primary hypothyroidism, which induces hypersecretion of TSH, thyrotroph hyperplasia and even adenoma.

*Histology* Thyrotroph adenomas are usually large chromophobe tumors with a sinusoidal architecture.

*Treatment* This is by surgical excision.

### Gonadotrophic Adenomas

Although a number of "non-functioning" tumors have gonadotroph expression on immunostaining, the tumors may release only the alpha subunit or have lost the ability to release the hormone. Although it has been suggested that they may be more common in hypogonadal individuals, there is no increase in frequency in menopausal women. Most authorities consider them to be clinically non-functioning tumors.

*Clinical Features* Although patients with gonadotroph adenomas occasionally present with signs or symptoms of gonadal dysfunction, most present with features of chiasmal compression. Clinically diagnosed gonadotroph tumors occur mainly in middle-aged males. In young women, gonadotrophin-secreting adenomas may masquerade as primary ovarian failure because chronically elevated serum gonadotrophins reversibly inhibit ovarian function.

*Histology* Gonadotroph adenomas are usually chromophobic tumors with trabecular or papillary architecture and pseudo-rosette formation around blood vessels.

*Treatment* The treatment is surgical.

## Clinically Non-functioning Adenomas

Approximately 25% of pituitary adenomas are clinically non-functioning. Although their presentation is usually visual, they may present with panhypopituitarism or apoplexy. Many of these adenomas may produce excess amounts of the clinically silent alpha subunit unaccompanied by the specific beta unit. Stalk compression may produce a moderate rise in PRL.

Since the tumors are invariably macroadenomas, the most important investigations are of thyroid function and prolactin levels (see below) and visual field and acuity estimation. The treatment is surgical.

## Null Cell Adenomas

As their name suggests, these tumors have no specific markers to enable characterization of their cytodifferentiation. Patients are usually older than 40 years and treatment is surgical.

## Posterior Pituitary Hormones

ADH overproduction (SIADH) and lack of ADH (diabetes insipidus) are occasionally seen in large pituitary tumors. Diabetes insipidus in the setting of pituitary disease is, however, more usually associated with an inflammatory or infiltrative condition such as lymphocytic hypophysitis or histiocytosis.

## Pituitary Carcinomas

### Incidence

Primary pituitary carcinoma is extremely rare. Metastatic pituitary deposits, for example from the breast, although rare, are the more common type.

### Clinical Presentation

The clinical presentation is usually similar to that of a pituitary adenoma. Although pituitary carcinomas can be associated with acromegaly, hyperprolactinemia or Cushing's disease, they usually present as a pituitary mass.

### Investigations

In addition to standard imaging, further investigations should be directed at potential sources of primary tumors such as the breast or lung.

### Treatment

This is by surgery to the sella region and other sites, as appropriate, usually followed by radiotherapy.

## Pre-operative Investigations and Work-up

Ideally, all pituitary tumors should be managed in specialist centers [4]. In an emergency there are three important tests without which no pituitary surgery should take place. These are:

- *Thyroid function.* Operations on the myxedematous patient severely threaten cardiac function, and also make interpretation of investigation difficult.
- *Prolactin levels.* In macroadenomas with severe visual loss, even short-term dopamine agonist treatment can quickly restore vision, and although tumor shrinkage can lag behind, a better result than with surgery is usually obtained with patience.
- *Adequate imaging.* This should include details of the sphenoid septation if transsphenoidal surgery is to be attempted.

Cortisol cover is recommended for all large tumors for safety, as loss of ACTH output is dangerous and may occur postoperatively. Successful surgery for Cushing's tumors demands replacement.

Hydrocortisone 100 mg given with the induction of anesthesia is sufficient.

### Surgical Aims

Each tumor poses a different problem. Surgery can achieve:

- *Total tumor removal.* This is demanded for true endocrine cure in functioning tumors. Endocrine remission may result from near total removal. For macroadenomas, total tumor removal is probably infrequent.
- *Decompression of the optic chiasm and nerves.* It is surprising how sensitive the chiasm is to small increases in tumor size, but the net result is that vision can recover even when a comparatively small amount of the tumor has been removed.

- *Tumor debulking*. Large invasive tumors are probably best debulked prior to radiotherapy in order to reduce tumor mass.
- *Biopsy*. When radiological diagnosis is uncertain, this may be required to clarify subsequent management.

## Surgical Approach

The transsphenoidal approaches are the only rational approaches for microadenomas and usually suffice for tumors with suprasellar extension. They include:

- sub-labial trans-septal approach, as described by Cushing and, later, Hardy
- direct trans-nasal apparoach
- endonasal approach. This approach utilizes elements of both of the above. It was first described by Landolt.
- trans-ethmoidal approach. This approach remains popular in the UK with some otolaryngologists.
- endoscope-assisted surgery.

Transcranial approaches are required for those tumors with complex suprasellar extension, and for those rare tumors with normal fossae but suprasellar extension.

# Early Postoperative Management

As the majority of patients will have undergone transsphenoidal surgery, greater detail will be given to these patients [4]. The same principles apply to cranial surgery patients.

## General Considerations

Functioning and non-functioning tumors both require rigorous fluid balance, which includes the measurement of urine specific gravity (SG). As a rule, any patient able to concentrate to specific gravity (SG) 1005–1010 does not have diabetes insipidus (DI). DI seldom occurs in the first few hours but should be suspected if the patient is producing more than 1 litre of urine in 4 hours and the serum sodium is above 145 mmol/l. Urinary flow rates alone are insufficient to diagnose the condition, and a number of common perioperative events can produce a relative diuresis. The diagnosis is made on a combination of increased plasma osmolarity

>300 mOsmol/kg, hypotonic urine <300 mOsmol/kg and a urine flow of >2 ml/kg/h. If the patient is conscious and has a normal thirst mechanism, DI is seldom dangerous, whereas treatment with DDAVP can lead to hypotonic plasma with all the attendant problems of confusion, epilepsy and even death.

## Nasal Packs

These may be removed early. In our unit, they are removed on the first postoperative day.

## Antibiotic Prophylaxis

Since two leading authorities with thousands of cases between them do not use them at all, we suggest using the standard local protocol for normal cranial surgery.

## Complications

In experienced hands, there should be few complications. Many series have no mortality and many of the complications are both minor and transient. One example, in a series of 67 patients operated on for large tumors causing visual loss, had as complications: five transient CSF leaks, four cases of DI (only one of which persisted for over 3 months), one minor cardiopulmonary event and a period of postoperative confusion. The most serious complications were in three patients who suffered sellar hematomas, one causing temporary worsening of vision and requiring second transsphenoidal surgery.

## CSF leaks

Once again, in experienced hands these are relatively rare, even in macroadenoma series. Generally they are dealt with packing and if profuse, a lumbar drain. There continues considerable debate with regard to the need for packing. We use it in cases of obvious leak when fat or fascia lata suffices. For persistent leaks a lumbar drain may be used. It can usually be switched off in 36–48 hours.

## Cortisol Replacement

From the postoperative high of 100 mg hydrocortisone twice a day, this may be reduced to 20 mg in the morning and 10 mg in the mid afternoon within 48 hours, and to 15 mg and 5 mg at discharge.

## Hyponatremia

This may occasionally occur spontaneously with inappropriate secretion of ADH (SIADH) caused by the non-specific release of ADH from degenerating posterior pituitary neurosecretory terminals 7–14 days following surgery. The condition is managed by fluid restriction.

## Specific Postoperative Investigations

### Acromegaly

Reduction of growth hormone levels results in an early cessation of sweating. Diabetes mellitus becomes easier to control and many patients can be managed on diet or oral hypoglycemic alone. On the second day, it is useful to carry out a glucose tolerance test with GH levels (i.e. before discharge). GH will fall to below 2 mIU/l, and ideally below 0.5 mIU/l if cured. If the patient is not "cured", early re-exploration is often worthwhile.

Expected cure rates vary between 60% and 80%. If surgery fails, the patient will need to have GH hypersecretion controlled by somatostatin analogues and undergo pituitary irradiation.

### Cushing's Tumors

A patient cured of their disease will become dependent on cortisol replacement. If hydrocortisone is not given during the procedure, the cortisol level can be checked the following day, about 24 hours later. If the surgery is successful, cortisol levels will have fallen to below 50, but replacement must start immediately. Surgical failure warrants prompt re-exploration, particularly if an adenoma was found at the first exploration. Most experienced authors in large series report a cure rate of better than 70%. Failed surgical treatment of Cushing's disease requires radiotherapy. Currently, the fashion for bilateral adrenalectomy may be waning in favor of controlling the cortisol hypersecretion with ketoconazole.

### Prolactinomas

A single postoperative estimation is sufficient to estimate the success of the procedure. Female patients may regain their menstrual cycle when the level remains a little above normal. Surgical cure rates in prolactinoma series vary between 50–70%. Cure rates for invasive tumours are lower than 20%, with drug treatment and radiotherapy usually required at some stage following surgery.

## Long-term Management

This is directed at assessing vision, controlling residual effects of the tumor on endocrine function, and assessing the need for radiation therapy:

Vision is usually improved in about three-quarters of patients [5]. The degree of improvement is related to the severity of the visual loss and, to a lesser extent, the length of the history (as this is notoriously unreliable).

Endocrine function is maintained in the majority (80%) of patients with normal function at the time of surgery, whereas, if this is lost altogether and the patient has panhypopituitarism at the time of surgery, function is not regained.

Because of the ease of imaging, most clinics decide on the need for radiotherapy based on the postoperative MRI approximately 2 months following surgery, when the effects of the surgery in the fossa and sphenoid have lessened. Significant residual tumor usually needs radiotherapy, whereas an empty fossa can be watched. Likewise, most clinicians prefer to leave young patients for as long as possible as radiotherapy leads to pituitary failure in 12–15 years.

### Radiotherapy

Conventional radiotherapy will stabilize the majority of large tumors and allow a certain amount of shrinkage. In acromegaly, GH levels usually start to fall within 2–3 years but may only approach normality at 5–8 years. A recent Cushing's series suggests that the response in ACTH-secreting tumors may be better.

Currently, there is a strong pressure to change to conformal techniques – the gamma knife and stereotactic linear accelerator methods (LINAC) – particularly the single dose regimens. The attraction of these techniques is their ability to deliver a higher radiation dose to the tumor, with much greater sparing of normal tissue. Although there is intense interest, their indications, efficacy and complication rates are, to a certain extent, unknown.

# Rathke's Cleft Cysts

## Incidence

Rathke's cleft cysts (RCCs) are clinically significant but uncommon lesions. They are less common than pituitary tumors. Occasionally they coexist. However, the vast majority must be asymptomatic since they are encountered in 12–33% of normal pituitary glands in routine autopsies [6]. The first symptomatic RCC was reported by Goldzeiher in 1913. By 1977, only 34 cases had been reported. By 1992, this number had more than doubled to 87 cases of histologically confirmed RCC [7]. This recent increase is attributed to the widespread use of MRI.

## Pathophysiology

The origin of Rathke's cleft cysts lies in the embryological development of the pituitary gland. During development, a small diverticulum lined with endodermal epithelium – Rathke's pouch – grows from the roof of the primitive buccal cavity or stomatodeum. Simultaneously a small ectodermal process – the infundibulum – grows downwards from the floor of the diencephalon. During the second month of development Rathke's cleft lies in contact with the anterior surface of the infundibulum, and its connection with the oral cavity disappears. Rathke's pouch now flattens itself around the anterior and lateral surface of the infundibulum, forming the pars anterior, pars tuberalis (around the infundibulum) and pars intermedia. These embryological distinctions are rarely seen clinically. The cystic center of Rathke's cleft normally now disappears. It is the persistence and growth of this vesicular space, probably by epithelial proliferation and accumulation of secretions, that give rise to Rathke's cleft cysts. Other theories of RCC formation postulate origin from neuroepithelial tissues or from anterior pituitary cells by reverse metaplasia. The relatively common finding of squamous epithelium in portions of the cyst lining has led to the hypothesis of origin from squamous rests along the craniopharyngeal canal (or hypophyseal-pharyngeal duct). This is a theory that might explain a possible common origin of a spectrum of cystic sellar lesions ranging from RCCs to craniopharyngiomas.

## Presentation and Clinical Features

The three main presenting features are similar to pituitary adenomas: endocrine disturbance, headache and visual impairment. In a recent large series of over 28 RCCs [1], the mean age at presentation was 45 years. Clinically, endocrine disturbance was the most common presentation (50%), including amenorrhea (37.5% of female patients), growth retardation, impotence and DI. Biochemically, hypopituitarism, hyperprolactinemia and gonadotrophin deficiencies were the common endocrine findings. Headache was a major feature in 32.1% and visual disturbance in14.3%. Patterns of visual disturbance included central field loss as well as the peripheral field loss expected in sellar region lesions. Four patients had pre-operative DI, a feature that, in the authors' opinion, excludes pituitary adenoma.

## Diagnosis

As with other sellar lesions, in addition to the clinical and biochemical features, the mainstay of diagnosis is imaging. CT characteristics include well-defined, homogeneous, non-enhancing sellar lesions without calcification and usually with suprasellar extension. These features, however, are not always specific and can be seen in other sellar lesions such as cystic pituitary adenomas, craniopharyngiomas, epidermoids and arachnoid cysts. The MRI features are also variable, possibly in keeping with the cyst contents, reflecting the number and activity of secretory cells in the wall. Given the variable imaging, the most difficult differential diagnosis remains that between RCCs and craniopharyngiomas. Some would say that the latter is suspected in pre-operative DI, calcification of the cyst wall, and possibly in cases of recurrence, reflecting the behavior of true craniopharyngiomas.

## Treatment

The treatment for symptomatic RCCs is surgical. The pre-operative investigations and precautions are similar to those for surgery on pituitary adenomas. The majority can be adequately dealt with via the transsphenoidal route. In this technique the anterior portion of the cyst wall is removed. The remaining cavity is then left to drain into the sphenoid sinus to avoid recurrence. Symptomatic recurrence can be dealt with via a repeat transsphenoidal approach or by using the trans-glabella approach via the frontal sinus.

## Postoperative Adjuvant Therapy

Since RCCs are not neoplastic, there is no proven case for either radio- or chemotherapy. Most cases of recurrence are effectively dealt with by repeat surgery.

## Outcomes

In our series, recovery of visual acuity and field was seen in 66.6% and 68% of eyes respectively. Postoperative PRL levels declined to normal or near normal in 62.5%, and 20% of those with low pre-operative gonadotrophin levels achieved normal levels after surgery.

# Meningiomas

## Incidence

The first description of a meningioma was given by a Swiss physician, Felix Plater, in 1664. The first series of "fongueuses de la dure-mère"[8] was described by Antoine Louis in 1774. The term "meningioma" was coined by Cushing in 1922 [9]. Meningiomas comprise 15% of intracranial tumors. They occur predominantly in the fifth and sixth decades, with a peak at around 45 years, and 90% are intracranial. They are more common in females than in males, and, in the case of intracranial tumors, by a ratio of 3:2. Meningiomas are rare tumors in children. Meningiomas of the sellar region comprise approximately 15% of the intracranial total, occurring on the tuberculum sella or planum sphenoidale (suprasellar meningiomas), on the medial sphenoid wing and cavernous sinus (parasellar meningiomas) or, very rarely, within the sella turcica itself. Occasionally they arise from the optic nerve sheath and expand in a dumb-bell fashion, passing from the orbit through the optic canal.

## Presentation and Clinical Features of the Sellar Region Meningiomas

Although meningiomas may present with hemorrhage and epilepsy, most exert local pressure effects, and this is especially true of sellar-region tumors.

*Tuberculum sellae (suprasellar) meningiomas* arise from the meninges of the anterior clinoid or tuberculum sellae. They displace the optic nerves and chiasm upwards or backwards. They present with visual failure involving a central scotoma in conjunction with an asymmetrical bitemporal field loss. Some degree of optic atrophy is usually present and this, in conjunction with lack of papilledema or anosmia, helps to distinguish this tumor from an olfactory groove meningioma. Backward growth of the tumor may impinge upon the hypothalamic-pituitary axis and produce endocrinological deficits.

*Cavernous sinus (parasellar) meningiomas* present with retro-orbital pain and sixth cranial nerve palsy. The other cranial nerves in the area – III and IV – may also be affected. The first and second division of the fifth cranial nerve may also be involved.

*Anterior clinoid and medial third sphenoid wing (parasellar) meningiomas* generally present with progressive loss of vision and optic atrophy on examination. There is unilateral loss of acuity due to optic nerve compression; this may be seen in conjunction with an incongruous field loss resulting from an element of chiasmal compression. Tumors growing "en plaque" may invade the cavernous sinus and produce the features mentioned above.

## Diagnosis

CT at the base of the skull can be misleading owing to the superimposition of skull density over tumor density and because of artifact. This is particularly true for sellar region tumors. MRI is superior and has the advantage of allowing multiplanar viewing in relation to local structures such as the optic apparatus. MRA and MRV sequences help to assess vascular involvement. This is particularly helpful in sellar region tumors to determine the position of the carotid artery and tributaries in relation to the tumor. Conventional angiography, particularly if pre-operative embolization is envisaged, gives more detailed information and is still the "gold standard".

## Treatment

The mainstay of treatment of symptomatic meningiomas is surgery with as complete a resection as possible. In the case of tumors of the sellar region, careful pre-operative planning is essential to assess the extent of possible resection and likelihood of damage to neighboring structures. This is particularly important in the case of cavernous sinus meningiomas, where several questions remain unanswered. Are cavernous sinus meningiomas curable and is the cranial nerve morbidity associated with resection acceptable? Surgeons base these decisions on the degree of involvement of the internal carotid artery. Many authors believe that tumors completely encircling and compressing the artery or invading the cavernous sinus cannot be totally resected without unacceptable morbidity. In such cases a subtotal resection, with or without radiotherapy, may be an effective short-term strategy.

## Surgery

### Tuberculum Sellae (Suprasellar) Meningiomas

The standard approach is via a frontotemporal or pterional craniotomy, with adequate anterior exposure to allow sufficient subfrontal exposure to gain access to the tumor along the upper part of the sphenoid wing. The side chosen is usually determined by the side on which the optic nerve is most compromised. Another approach, recently adopted in the authors' unit, is via a direct trans-glabella route passing through the frontal sinus. This involves minimal retraction and direct access and is uncomplicated provided that the sinus is adequately repaired. Olfactory tracts are preserved. (This is also suitable for the resection of olfactory groove meningiomas.) The blood supply comes mainly from meningeal vessels over the tuberculum, with little from the carotid. These tuberculum vessels should be taken first as the tumor is undermined. Internal decompression is performed prior to dissection from the vessels and optic apparatus.

### Cavernous Sinus and Medial Sphenoid (Parasellar) Meningiomas

The approach for cavernous sinus and medial sphenoid meningiomas is similar to the frontotemporal approach described above, sometimes with orbitozygomatic extension, particularly if the orbit has been invaded. Complete removal of cavernous sinus meningiomas is not usually possible without considerable morbidity. Rather, an aggressive internal decompression is performed in preparation for postoperative radiotherapy should this prove necessary. Medial sphenoid wing meningiomas are more amenable to surgical removal.

## Radiotherapy

Reports of tumor response to standard external beam radiotherapy are variable except in the case of malignant tumors and hemangiopericytomas, where there does appear to be some benefit. Recently, attention has been focused on conformal techniques such as stereotactically directed gamma rays ("gamma knife") or X-rays. The object of these techniques is to prevent disease progression while preserving neurological function. Encouraging results have recently been published with progression control in more than 80% [11]. However, the results of studies with longer follow-up times are awaited.

## Chemotherapy

Although both estrogen and progesterone receptors have been found in meningiomas, to date attempted hormonal manipulation has met with little success. The observation that hydroxy urea inhibits the growth of meningioma cells in cell culture has led to its use in the treatment of unresectable and recurrent meningiomas of the skull base. In a small study of four patients, three of whom had cavernous sinus meningiomas, the results are encouraging, showing marked regression in three subjects and failure of recurrence of a malignant meningioma in the fourth [12]. The results of larger studies are awaited.

## Recurrence

When assessed radiologically, more than 50% of recurrences occur within 5 years and 80% within 10 years. The most important factor in tumor recurrence is the amount of meningioma left behind. Simpson [13] related the recurrence rates to the extent of resection and devised a grading system based upon this (Table 11.3).

**Table 11.3.** Five-year recurrence rate for meningioma based on the extent of tumor resection

| Grade | Description | Recurrence rate at 5 years (%) |
|---|---|---|
| 1 | Complete macroscopic tumor removal with excision of involved dura and bone | 9 |
| 2 | Complete macroscopic tumor removal with coagulation of dura/bone | 19 |
| 3 | Complete macroscopic tumor removal but no treatment of involved dura and bone | 29 |
| 4 | Intracranial tumor left in situ | 44 |
| 5 | Tumor decompression only | – |

# Hemangiopericytoma

## Incidence and Epidemiology

This rare tumor was formerly regarded as a variant of meningioma [14]. However, it has more aggressive behavior and a tendency to recurrence and extraneural metastases.

Unlike meningioma, it occurs more commonly in males.

## Pathology

Its macroscopic appearance is that of a red, solitary, firm nodule. It is usually vascular, with a tendency to hemorrhage when cut. Microscopically it is highly cellular, with dense reticulin deposits broken at intervals by "staghorn" vascular spaces. Mitoses are present but, unlike meningiomas, whorls and psammoma bodies are not typical. These features, plus its aggressive behavior, have led it to be classified with the mesenchymal non-meningothelial tumors, such as chondrosarcomas.

## Presentation And Clinical Features

Hemangiopericytomas of the sellar region usually present as a suprasellar space-occupying lesion often producing a field defect. Preoperatively they may be mistaken for a pituitary tumor or a suprasellar meningioma. Rarely and confusingly, like the meningiomas, these lesions may also be seen in the ventricular system [15].

## Treatment

The diagnosis is not usually made before surgery, but may be suspected at operation owing to its firm consistency and excessive hemorrhage. When the diagnosis is suspected clinically, the lesion is usually approached transcranially. Due to its aggressive behaviour, total excision and radiotherapy is the treatment of choice.

# Craniopharyngioma

## Incidence and Epidemiology

Craniopharyngiomas comprise approximately 2.5–4% of all intracranial tumors. Although half of these occur in adults, they account for a greater percentage of childhood tumors (5–13%) and are responsible for 54% of sellar region pathology in children. There appears to be a bimodal age distribution, with peaks occurring at ages 5–10 and 55–65 years. There are important differences in clinical presentation, pathology and outcome between children and adults. They remain, whatever the age group, a continuing challenge for the neurosurgeon, endocrinologist and radiotherapist.

## Pathophysiology

In common with other sellar region lesions generally and with Rathke's cleft cysts in particular, it seems likely that the origin of these lesions lies, at least in part, in disordered embryogenesis. In 1899, Mott and Barret [16] were the first to appreciate that these sellar and parasellar epithelial tumors might arise from the hypophyseal duct or Rathke's pouch. Subsequently, craniopharyngiomas have been discovered along the path of development of Rathke's pouch from the pharynx to the sella. However, the pathology of RCCs and craniopharyngiomas differs and this might reflect the differing ability of squamous cell rests to undergo neoplastic change and form a craniopharyngioma or to persist as a simple cyst. The pathology is further complicated by the observation that certain craniopharyngiomas, particularly those presenting in childhood, resemble both adamantinomas or tooth bud tumors of the jaw and odontogenic cysts [17]. This raises the possibility of two separate tumor types, with the adult craniopharyngioma arising from squamous metaplasia of pituitary cells later in life. This would help to explain the differences seen in clinical presentation and response to treatment.

Most craniopharyngiomas appear near the infundibular stalk, distorting the surrounding anatomy and eventually obliterating the suprasellar cisterns.

Morphologically these lesions vary from predominantly solid to cystic. Mixed solid and cystic lesions are more common in pediatric series. Predominantly cystic tumors are more common across the age range, with predominantly solid lesions in only 10% of pediatric tumors. Cyst walls may be thin or thick structures impregnated with calcium deposits, and cyst fluid is dark green and laden with birefringent cholesterol crystals. Calcification is found in half of adult tumors and virtually all childhood tumors. Often there is a florid glial reaction around the craniopharyngioma, which is most marked around papillary-like tumor projections into the hypothalamus, making manipulation dangerous. Craniopharyngiomas are often adherent to major vessels, the chiasm and hypothalamus. This may preclude total removal.

## Presentation and Clinical Features

The clinical presentation varies between children and adults. Craniopharyngiomas are slow-growing tumors and hence may reach considerable size before diagnosis. Children will often tolerate marked visual deterioration and hydrocephalus before they complain. Nonspecific symptoms such as poor school performance, poor memory (hypothalamic compression) and disruptive behavior may go unnoticed. The endocrine features are manifest in short stature, delayed puberty, hyperphagia and obesity (this may be a prominent postoperative feature), and other behavioral problems. DI is less common. Adults present mainly with varying degrees of visual failure. Hydrocephalus at presentation is relatively rare, but neurobehavioral syndromes unrelated to hydrocephalus are relatively common, including confusion, dementia and hypersomnia. The most common endocrinopathy in adults is gonadal failure, presenting as secondary amenorrhea in women and loss of libido in males.

## Diagnosis

With its high resolution and multiplanar capabilities, MRI in conjunction with MRA is usually the investigation of choice, particularly when looking at the relationship to surrounding anatomy. This is important in deciding upon an operative approach. Evaluation of endocrine function – particularly cortisol, thyroid function and fluid balance – is, of course, mandatory, as is visual assessment.

## Treatment

Total resection can be achieved and offers the best chance of cure, but the degree of tumor removal must be tempered by the degree of difficulty envisaged pre-operatively and encountered intraoperatively if formidable postoperative problems are to be avoided. There is a considerable variation between the surgical "hawks" and "doves" in this difficult disease.

Radiological risk factors include involvement of structures above the chiasm, such as the hypothalamus, as well as extensive lateral spread, particularly through the cavernous sinus and surrounding the carotid arteries. The overall management of the pediatric disease has been reviewed in the excellent paper from the Hospital for Sick Children, Great Ormond St, London [18].

## Surgical Approach

Symptomatic hydrocephalus must be controlled and this may require a biventricular shunt if the tumor blocks both foramina of Monro.

When choosing a surgical approach (Table 11.4), there are several factors to consider: firstly the size, secondly whether or not it is cystic, and thirdly, the relationship to surrounding structures, namely the hypothalamus, third ventricle, optic pathways, pituitary and stalk, vessels, brainstem, dura and CSF pathways. In cranial approaches, the position of the chiasm, which is often pre-fixed, and the shape and laterality of the tumor must also be taken into consideration.

If the lesion is confined to the sella, or has moderate suprasellar extension but remains mainly midline, then a transsphenoidal approach may be attempted, particularly if cystic. Equally a subfrontal or pterional approach may be used (with or without orbitozygomatic extension), particularly if there is lateral extension.

In a cooperative study involving 415 patients [19], subfrontal routes were used in 46%, pterional in 27%, transsphenoidal in 8%,

**Table 11.4.** Operative approaches for craniopharyngioma

| Approach | Advantages | Disadvantages |
|---|---|---|
| **Extra-axial** | | |
| Subfrontal | Good visualization of optic nerves and chiasm Below circle of Willis | Poor visualization of third ventricle mass |
| Pterional | Below circle of Willis Shortest distance to parasellar region Good visualization of retrosellar region | Unilateral Poor view of contralateral optic nerve |
| Lamina terminalis | Access to mass in anterior third ventricle | Risk of hypothalamic damage |
| **Trans-axial** | | |
| Transsphenoidal | No craniotomy Direct sella view and decompression of inferior surface of chiasm | Unable to see supra and parasellar regions Possible pituitary damage |
| Transcallosal | Direct approach good third ventricle view | Divides corpus callosum Risk of fornix damage Poor view of sella |
| Transcortical | Good view of ventricular system Risk of postop seizures Poor sella view | Requires hydrocephalus |

transventricular in 3%, subtemporal in 2.6% and transcallosal in 0.7%. Anterior approaches allow opening of the lamina terminalis and possible removal of tumors situated wholly or partly within the third ventricle. Transcallosal and transventricular approaches also give good ventricular access, but limited suprasellar access. Some surgeons attempt to solve this with a simultaneous and additional pterional craniotomy. We have also used a trans-glabella approach.

## Postoperative Morbidity

Most patients experience anterior and posterior pituitary endocrine deficits postoperatively, with less than 10% having normal endocrine function. Growth hormone deficiency is usually present, as is DI. Hyperphagia and obesity also occur and are attributed to hypothalamic damage. Choux cites the predictive factors in postoperative morbidity as: age less than 5 years, severe hydrocephalus, pre-operative hypothalamic disturbance, large tumors over 3.5 cm and intraoperative complications [19].

## Surgical Results

Although total surgical excision gives the best chance for longevity, it can only be achieved in a limited number of cases. Choux quotes 25% in his large cooperative study. However, these results must be set against the appreciable recurrence rate in those having "total" excision of 19.1%.

## Other Treatments

### Conventional Irradiation

The role of radiation in these tumors remains controversial. The majority of tumors respond and shrink to some extent. Views differ as to the long-term effectiveness in a disease in which the behavior is, in any case, notoriously difficult to predict [20]. Although efficacious, its consequences may be severe, particularly in children.

### Stereotactic Radiotherapy

Although its use is becoming more widespread and with some encouraging results [21], the results of large series with longer follow-up are awaited.

### Intracavity Brachytherapy and Chemotherapy

Beta emitters have mainly been used, such as gold-198 and yttrium-90. These are implanted stereotactically. Some success is claimed, particularly in the reduction in size of cystic lesions. The cytotoxic bleomycin has also been introduced into cystic craniopharyngiomas via an Ommaya reservoir. This has also produced favorable results, but has yet to become a definitive treatment.

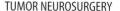

# Key Points

- *The majority of sellar and parasellar tumors are pituitary adenomas or meningiomas.*
- *Pituitary tumors usually present with endocrine or visual disturbances, or both.*
- *A PRL estimation is essential prior to surgery since prolactinomas can usually be treated medically.*
- *Sellar region meningiomas present with local pressure effects, and surgical resection is the treatment of choice.*
- *Craniopharyngiomas and Rathke's cleft cysts probably have a common embryological origin.*

# References

1. Kontogeorgos G, Kovacs K, Horvath E, Sheithauer BW. Multiple adenomas of the human pituitary: a retrospective autopsy study with clinical implications. J Neurosurg 1991;74:243–7.
2. Wass JAH et al. Pituitary tumours: recommendations for service provision and guidelines for management of patients. J R Coll Physicians Lond 1997;31:628–36.
3. Thompson D, Powell MP, Foster O. Atypical presentation of vascular events in pituitary tumours: "non-apoplectic" pituitary apoplexy. J Neurol Neurosurg Psychiatry 1994;57:1441–2.
4. Powell MP, Lightman SL. The management of pituitary tumours; a handbook. London: Churchill Livingstone, 1996.
5. Powell MP. The recovery of vision following transsphenoidal surgery for pituitary adenomas. Br J Neurosurg 1995;6:367–73.
6. El-Mahady, W Powell M. Transsphenoidal management of 28 symptomatic Rathke's cleft cysts, with special reference to visual and hormonal recovery. Neurosurgery 1998;42(1):7–17.
7. Ross DA, Norman D, Wilson CB. Radiologic characteristics and results of surgical management of Rathke's cleft cysts in 43 patients. Neurosurgery 1992;30:173–9.
8. Louis A. Memoire sur les tumours fongueuses de la dure-mère. Memoires de l'Academie Royale de Chirurgie (Paris), 1774;5:1–59.
9. Cushing H. The meningiomas (dural endotheliomas): their source and favoured seats of origin. Brain 1922;45:282–316.
10. Gordon DE, Olson C. Meningiomas and fibroblastic neoplasia in calves induced with bovine papilloma virus. Cancer Res 1993;28:2423–31.
11. Hakim R, AlexanderE, Loeffler JS et al. Results of linear accelerator based radiosurgery for intracranial meningiomas. Neurosurgery 1998;42:3.
12. Schrell UHM, Rittig MG, Anders M, Koch UH et al. Hydroxyurea for treatment of unresectable and recurrent meningiomas. Decrease in the size of meningiomas in patients treated with hydroxyurea. J Neurosurg 1997;86:840–44.
13. Simpson D. The recurrence of intracranial meningiomas after surgical removal. J Neurol Neurosurg Psychiatry 1957;20:22–39.
14. Kleihues P, Burger PC, Scheithauer BW. The new WHO classification of brain tumours. Brain Pathol 1993; 3:255–68.
15. Abrahams JM, Forman MS, Lavi E, Goldberg H, Flamm ES. Haemangiopericytoma of the third ventricle. Case report. J Neurosurg 1999(Feb);90(2):359–62.
16. Mott FW, Barret JOW. Three cases of tumours of the third ventricle. Arch Neurol (London) 1899;1:417–40.
17. Bernstein ML, Buchino JJ. The histological similarity between craniopharyngeoma and odontogenic lesions: a reappraisal. Oral Surg 1983;56:502–11.
18. De Ville CJ, Grant DB, Kendall BE, Neville BGR, Stanhope R, Watkins KE et al. Management of childhood craniopharyngeoma: can the morbidity of radical surgery be predicted? J Neurosurg 1996;85:73–81.
19. Choux M, Lena G. In: Surgery of the third ventricle, 2nd edn. Appuzo M, editor. William & Williams: Baltimore, 1998.
20. Wara WM, Sneed PK, Larson DA. The role of radiation therapy in the treatment of craniopharyngeoma. Pediatr Neurosurg 1994;(suppl 1):98–100.
21. Kobyashi T, Tanaka T, Kida Y. Stereotactic radiosurgery of craniopharyngiomas. Pediatric Neurosurg 1994; (suppl 1):69–74.

# 12

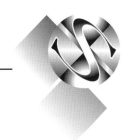

# Meningiomas

James J. Evans, Joung H. Lee, John Suh
and Mladen Golubic

## Summary

The epidemiology, pathology, natural history, and recurrence of meningiomas are reviewed, as are treatment options and their indications. Several important surgical concepts are presented, with an emphasis on general principles that apply to resection of meningiomas at most intracranial locations. The role of therapeutic radiation – including gamma-knife radiosurgery, linear accelerator radiosurgery and intensity-modulated radiation therapy – is discussed. A review of current understanding of meningioma tumor biology is presented, as is the possible direction of future therapy.

## Introduction

Surgical management of patients with meningiomas is arguably the most rewarding, challenging and, at times, daunting task for a neurosurgeon: rewarding because of the benign nature of most meningiomas, leading to a possibility of providing cure following total removal; challenging because of the tumor's common sites of involvement in proximity to critical neurovascular structures and/or along the skull base, making surgery difficult and highly risky; daunting because of the associated risks of surgery, the tumor's tendency to recur following incomplete (and at times complete) removal, and its frequent involvement of the surrounding skull-base bone, dura and neurovasculature, making complete removal often impossible.

The term "meningioma" was introduced by Cushing in 1922 to clarify the hitherto confusing and numerous histopathological nomenclatures used to describe the tumor. These names have included: "fongueuses de la dure-mère" (Louis 1774), "epithelial cancer" (Bennett 1858), "tumeurs fibro-plastiques" (Lebert 1854), "cylindroma" (Billroth 1856), "epithelioma" (Bouchard 1864), "sarkome der dura mater" (Virchow 1863), "endothelioma" (Golgi 1869), "villous arachnoid tumor" (Cleland 1864), "arachnoid fibroblastoma" (Mallory 1920) and "meningeal fibroblastoma" (Penfield 1932). Whereas the previous names were descriptive based on the tumor's varying appearances, or based on its presumed histogenesis, the new term "meningioma" was used to simply convey the meningeal involvement. The first report of this fascinating tumor dates back to 1614, and it is credited to Felix Plater of Switzerland. Although there are earlier reports of partial or failed removal of meningiomas, W.W. Keen is credited with the first successful surgical resection of a meningioma in the USA, in 1887.

Surgery continues to be the treatment of choice for most patients with meningiomas. Recent advances in neuroimaging, anesthesia, microsurgery, surgical instrumentation, radiation oncology and skull-base techniques have improved the overall surgical management of patients with meningiomas and their outcome. However, we are still far from providing optimal care to all patients with meningiomas. Ultimately, the future of meningioma treatment will likely evolve through detailed elucidation of tumorigenic mechanisms at the subcellular level coupled with further advances in molecular therapy that will rely upon the re-classification of these tumors based on their genetic profile yet to be determined.

Comprehensive coverage of meningiomas in a single chapter is utterly impossible. Therefore, in this limited space, the epidemiology, pathology, natural history and recurrence of meningiomas are briefly discussed. Then, treatment options, together with their indications, are briefly outlined. Several important surgical concepts are presented, with an emphasis on general principles that apply to resection of meningiomas at most intracranial locations. The role of therapeutic radiation, including various techniques utilized for treatment of meningiomas such as conventional radiation, gamma-knife and linear accelerator radiosurgery, and intensity-modulated radiation therapy, are delineated. Finally, a review of the current understanding of meningioma tumor biology is presented. Possible directions for future therapy implicated by this basic scientific knowledge are also postulated.

# Epidemiology

## Incidence

Meningiomas account for 15–20% of all intracranial neoplasms, second only to the incidence of primary gliomas [1,2]. Excluding autopsy data, one study concluded that the most common intracranial tumors are gliomas (43%), meningiomas (21%) and pituitary adenomas (17%) [3]. It should be noted that these incidence data represent only those patients with meningiomas that cause neurological symptoms leading to clinical diagnosis and treatment. With recent advances in neuroimaging, many asymptomatic meningiomas are being detected today, raising the true incidence significantly higher than was previously reported. When autopsy data are included, the proportion of meningiomas among common intracranial tumors changes to 40% for meningiomas, 35% for gliomas, and 17% for pituitary adenomas [3]. The incidence of clinically significant meningiomas is approximately 2.3/100,000 population, and about 5.5/100,000 population when autopsy data are included [3]. Such discrepancy between these incidence rates underscores the fact that the majority of meningiomas actually remain asymptomatic and undetected during life. In fact, Nakasu et al. [4] noted that incidental meningiomas are found in as many as 2.3% of autopsy specimens, and that, among people over the age of 60 years undergoing autopsy, 3% are found to have an incidental meningioma.

The male:female ratio ranges from 1:1.4 to 1:2.1 depending on the series, but it is widely accepted to be approximately 1:2. [1,2]. This finding, however, is not necessarily true among blacks, who have been reported to have a fairly even distribution between males and females [5]. The peak age of clinical presentation for all patients with meningiomas is in the sixth decade.

The intracranial distribution of primary meningiomas has been reported by many authors [1,6]. These reports may vary, depending on the type of neuroimaging used and whether autopsy data are included. DeMonte and Al-Mefty [2] summarized the overall intracranial distribution of meningiomas by combining several large reported series, and concluded the following: parasagittal/falcine 25%, convexity 19%, sphenoid ridge 17%, suprasellar (tuberculum) 9%, posterior fossa 8%, olfactory groove 8%, middle fossa/Meckel's cave 4%, tentorial 3%, peri-torcular 3%, lateral ventricle 1–2%, foramen magnum 1–2%, orbit/optic nerve sheath 1–2%.

Meningiomas occur in children, yet they are exceedingly rare, accounting for only 1–4% of all brain tumors in patients less than 18 years old [7]. Furthermore, pediatric meningiomas account for only 1.5–1.8% of all intracranial meningiomas [8]. In children, the male:female ratio is nearly equal or with a slight male predominance [7]. Intraventricular meningiomas are more common in children than in adults, and make up 11% and 3.9% of all meningiomas in these groups, respectively [6]. In addition to this predilection for unusual locations, children are also more likely than adults to harbor aggressive forms of meningiomas, such as atypical and anaplastic variants. A recent paper, however, suggests that malignant meningiomas in young patients may not be quite as frequent as was previously thought [9]. Meningioangiomatosis, a reactive perivascular proliferation of fibroblasts and meningothelial cells which can trap islands of gliotic cortex, is occasionally associated with meningiomas in younger patients, and may be mistaken for brain invasion [9].

The association of meningiomas and head injury has been addressed by many authors, although the reports are mainly anecdotal [1]. In a rather large review, Inskip et al. [10] did not find a significant increase in the incidence rate of meningiomas, gliomas or neurilemmomas in association with head trauma. It is more likely that a portion of the many asymptomatic meningiomas in the general population is simply detected incidentally by routine neuroimaging following head trauma.

Unlike trauma, radiation as a cause of meningioma development has been well documented [1]. In such cases, the meningiomas must meet certain criteria to be considered radiation-induced, such as the tumor location in the field of radiation, pathology distinct from the original neoplasm or condition under treatment, and occurrence after an appropriately long "latent period" following the radiation exposure [1]. Meningiomas have been reported following low-dose radiation exposure for tinea capitis and following high-dose radiation treatment for other central nervous system (CNS) or head and neck neoplasms. The male:female ratio seems to be more equal for radiation-induced meningiomas, in contrast to the female predominance for sporadic intracranial meningiomas in the general population.

Multiple meningiomas are rare. Only 1–9% of all intracranial meningioma patients have multiple lesions [11]. The patient age and tumor locations do not differ significantly from those with single meningiomas, yet there is a distinction among patients with familial syndromes such as neurofibromatosis (NF) who are prone to developing multiple meningiomas at a much younger age. Intracranial meningiomas are far more common in NF-2 than in NF-1, but they have been reported in both syndromes. It is questionable, however, whether meningiomas occur at a greater rate in NF-1 than in the general population. In NF-2, it has been estimated that 50% of all patients develop meningiomas, and 30% of these patients have multiple meningiomas.

Malignant (i.e. anaplastic) meningiomas account for only approximately 1–3% of all meningiomas. One large series of 936 primary intracranial meningiomas revealed that 94.3% were grade I (benign), 4.7% were grade II (atypical) and 1.0% were grade III (anaplastic). Additionally, anaplastic meningiomas occurred in 12% of males and in only 4% of females in that study. The precise definition of "malignant meningioma", however, has recently been a source of debate. Perry et al. found that frank anaplasia and high mitotic activity (20 or more mitoses per high-powered field) were most closely associated with malignant meningiomas. Extracranial metastases from meningiomas have also been considered to be one of the strong indicators of malignancy and have been shown to occur in 11–23% of patients with frankly anaplastic meningiomas. Interestingly, brain invasion, a traditional criterion of malignant meningiomas, has recently been considered as a diagnostic feature that is more common in atypical meningiomas than in anaplastic types.

Spinal meningiomas occur approximately one-tenth as frequently as intracranial meningiomas. Of all intradural extramedullary spinal tumors, meningiomas account for 25% and are second only to schwannomas, which account for nearly 30%. The peak age of presentation for spinal meningiomas occurs between the 5th and 7th decades, but they may be found in patients of any age. The male:female ratio ranges from 1:3 to 1:6, and 80% of all spinal meningiomas are found in the thoracic region [12].

Ectopic meningiomas are exceedingly rare and likely arise from rests of arachnoid tissue trapped in ectopic locations during development. These must be distinguished from the equally rare extracranial metastases of malignant meningiomas that occur in less than 0.1% of all meningiomas. Primary cutaneous meningiomas are the most common and typically occur in the scalp of frontal and occipital regions. Other reported locations of primary ectopic meningiomas include: paranasal sinuses, eyelids, parotid gland, temporalis muscle, temporal bone and zygoma, as well as some distant sites, such as the lungs, mediastinum and adrenal gland.

Lastly, meningiomas have been found in association with several other types of cancer. Due to the fact that meningiomas are relatively common tumors, and mostly benign with many years' survival, a chance of incidental association with other tumors is possible. However, there have been reports of some tumors that seem to have a "more-than-chance" association with meningiomas. Fox [13] compiled several reported series for a total of 52 cases of (non-NF, non-radiation-induced) meningiomas associated with gliomas of various grades, some of which were juxtaposed and some located at distant intracranial sites. Whether there is some common genetic or environmental factor involved in the concurrent development of meningiomas and gliomas, or whether they are entirely coincidental, remains unclear.

There has also been an association between meningiomas and breast cancer, as suggested by several authors. Studies of hormonal receptors as the link have not been conclusive, although meningiomas have been reported to have an increased incidence and growth rate in women during pregnancy, possibly supporting a hormonal role. Other molecular analyses have placed emphasis on the loss of heterozygosity of the long arm of chromosome 22 and have indicated that a tumor suppressor gene associated with breast cancer may exist at the chromosome locus 22q13 [14]. Interestingly, 22q13 is just slightly distal to the NF-2 tumor suppressor gene locus (22q12) implicated in NF-2-associated meningiomas and in about 50% of sporadic meningiomas.

# Pathology

## Cellular Origin

John Cleland, an anatomy professor in Glasgow in 1864, made an initial observation of two tumors that seemed to take their origin from the arachnoid, not the dura mater [6]. Schmidt, in 1902, and subsequently Cushing & Weed, in 1915, reported similar findings that these tumors seemed to arise from the arachnoid.

Currently, it is thought that meningiomas originate from specialized cells of the arachnoid granulations, called "arachnoid cap cells", but other possibilities include arachnoidal fibroblasts, or meningoblasts that are theoreti-

cal precursor cells of the meninges. Whether arachnoid cap cells are derived from the neural crest or the mesoderm remains unclear as cap cells may exhibit both mesenchymal and epithelial characteristics. Factors supporting the origin of meningiomas from arachnoid cap cells, particularly for the meningothelial variety, include histological and ultrastructural similarities between the tumor and cap cells. These include: the formation of whorls by the cells in-vivo and in-vitro, complex intertwining cell processes, the presence of intracellular junctions, named desmosomes, and an abundance of intracellular intermediate filaments that stain positive for vimentin. Fibroblastic and transitional benign varieties may have additional features that are similar to the fibroblasts found in deeper layers of the arachnoid adjacent to the subarachnoid space.

# Classification

It is beyond the scope of this chapter to discuss in detail all the pathological subtypes of meningiomas. Instead, a summary of the latest World Health Organization 2000 classification of meningiomas is presented: grade I (low risk of recurrence and aggressive growth) includes meningothelial, fibrous (fibroblastic), transitional (mixed), psammomatous, angiomatous, microcystic, secretory, lymphoplasmacyte-rich and metaplastic meningiomas; grade II (greater likelihood of recurrence and/or aggressive behavior) includes atypical, clear cell and chordoid meningiomas; grade III includes rhabdoid, papillary and anaplastic (malignant) meningiomas, as well as any subtype named above that has a high proliferation index and/or brain invasion.

# Natural History

## Understanding the Natural History

Understanding of the natural history of any disease is critical as it forms the basis for treatment. In the case of meningiomas, the natural history has not been well established owing to the fact that most meningioma patients in the past presented with sizable tumors that caused neurological symptoms and deficits, requiring surgical removal. When patients were unable to undergo surgery because of their advanced age, failing health or "inoperable" tumor location, most were treated with radiation and/or not amenable to a long-term "natural" follow-up. Therefore, data on patients diagnosed with a meningioma that were followed clinically, without surgical or radiation treatment, have been very limited and mainly anecdotal.

Autopsy data have revealed that there are a significant number of meningiomas that remain asymptomatic and are undetected during life [3,4]. With recent advances and availability of neuroimaging, asymptomatic meningiomas have been increasingly diagnosed over the past two decades, providing an ample opportunity now to study and understand better the natural history of meningiomas. Patients with asymptomatic meningiomas may not, however, represent a cross-section of all meningioma patients because of a possible selection bias toward tumors that have an inherently more benign course. Nevertheless, important information that is currently unavailable may be derived from such studies. Olivero et al. reported 45 females and 15 males, aged 38–84, who were diagnosed with asymptomatic meningiomas. Forty-five of their patients underwent serial clinical and imaging follow-up. Thirty-five patients (78%) had no change in the tumor size (average follow-up 29 months; range 3–72 months), while 10 patients (22%) showed tumor growth (average follow-up 47 months; range 6 months to 15 years). Among the latter group, tumor growth ranged from 0.2 cm/180 months to 1.0 cm/12 months (average growth rate of 0.24 cm/year). Kuratsu et al. [15] reported on 196 asymptomatic meningiomas out of a total of 504 meningiomas diagnosed in a 6-year period. Sixty-three of the asymptomatic meningiomas were followed conservatively with serial imaging studies. Two-thirds of their patients had no change in the tumor size (average follow-up 36.6 months; range 12–96 months), while one-third of them revealed tumor growth (average follow-up 27.8 months; range 12–87 months). Rates of tumor growth were not included in their report. Although the overall incidence of asymptomatic meningiomas was significantly higher among patients older than 70 years compared with younger patients, there were no significant differences in age, sex or initial tumor size between the group with meningiomas that progressed and the group that did not. Conclusions from both of these studies, in addition to the possible selection bias mentioned above, are certainly limited owing to the short length of follow-up. An update of these cohorts in future years is essential and will be more revealing.

## Growth Estimates

Another method of approximating the "natural history" of meningiomas is to estimate the mean doubling time of tumor volume (Td). Jaaskelainen et al. [16] determined the Td in a series of 43 patients with meningiomas by following them for recurrence after resection. Individual and mean Tds for their patients were determined by measuring tumor volume on serial imaging studies. They found that the Td was 415 days (range 138–1045) for benign meningiomas, 178 days (range 34–551) for atypical meningiomas, and 205 days (range 30–472) for anaplastic meningiomas. However, these average estimates are derived from wide-ranging values, and significant overlaps exist among the different groups.

By using bromodeoxyuridine (BUdR) labeling and tumor Td determinations, Cho et al. [17] found Tds ranging from 8 to 440 days in eight tumor samples (two benign, four malignant, two hemangiopericytomas). This group also noted a close inverse correlation between the BUdR labeling index and the tumor doubling time. The implications of these findings were that BUdR labeling may supplement histopathological information in estimating prognosis and may be used to calculate the Td before actual recurrence of the tumor. Clearly, such information would be valuable when formulating plans for any additional treatment of residual tumor following subtotal resection or recurrent meningiomas after complete resection.

Although the Td and BUdR studies have provided some insight toward the growth rates of meningiomas, in clinical practice they require at least an operative biopsy to determine the histology and the BUdR labeling index. A novel approach from Shino et al. [18] was to correlate the MIB-1 staining index (SI) with proton magnetic resonance spectroscopy (MRS) data. They reported that "a significant linear correlation was observed between the increased choline:creatine ratio and the MIB-1 SI" and that a high lactate and/or methylene signal suggested a tumor of higher grade. In this manner, proton MRS data may serve in the future as a non-invasive way of predicting the proliferative rate or malignant potential of meningiomas. Further refinement and availability of MRS will be necessary for this technique to be of value in estimating the growth rate, tumor grade or recurrence in clinical practice.

## Recurrence

Recurrence of meningiomas after seemingly complete resection, as well as progression after subtotal resection, has been studied for many decades. In a seminal paper by Simpson [19] in 1957, the rate of recurrence was stratified according to the extent of tumor resection and removal or coagulation of the associated dura: grade I – complete surgical resection of the tumor and its dural attachment; grade II – complete surgical resection of the tumor with coagulation of its dural attachment; grade III – complete surgical resection of the tumor without coagulation of its dural attachment; grade IV – partial tumor removal, leaving the dura in situ; and grade V – simple decompression with or without biopsy. In Simpson's series of 265 meningiomas, 55 (21%) had recurrence. The rates of tumor recurrence according to the extent of resection were: grade I, 9%; grade II, 19%; grade III, 29%; grade IV, 44%. Other studies appearing subsequently, with at least 10 years' follow-up, found similar recurrence rates, which depended on the extent of resection. Using Simpson's classification, Melamed et al. [20] reported recurrence rates of: grade I, 8%; grade II, 15%; grade IV, 29%; and grade V, 33%. Similarly, Chan et al. [21] reported recurrence rates as: grade I, 11%; grade II, 22%; grade IV, 33%; and grade V, 100%. Both of these studies confirmed Simpson's initial finding that the extent of meningioma resection is the single most important prognostic factor for tumor recurrence in benign meningiomas [20,21].

In a study of 225 patients, Mirimanoff et al. [22] reported a recurrence-free rate after total resection of 93%, 80% and 68% at 5, 10 and 15 years, respectively. After subtotal resection, however, the progression-free rates were 63%, 45% and 9% at the same time intervals,

respectively. They also evaluated tumor location as a factor for recurrence and found that 96% of their convexity meningiomas were totally resected, with a 3% recurrence rate at 5 years. Fifty-eight percent of the parasellar meningiomas in their study were totally excised, with a 5-year recurrence rate of 19%, while only 28% of the sphenoid ridge meningiomas were totally excised, with a 5-year recurrence rate of 34% [22]. Kallio et al. [23] analyzed the surgical outcome of their series of 935 patients in terms of relative survival rate (RSR) following resection. RSR was defined as the ratio of the observed to the expected survival rate (SR). The expected SR was considered to be that for a population identical to the patient group, except for the meningioma. They found no difference between the observed and expected SR of their patients following resection at 3 months (91%) and at 1 year (89%). At 15 years' follow-up, they found a cumulative observed SR of 63%, which was 78% of the expected SR. The RSR was largely dependent on the degree of resection: the RSR at 15 years was 84% following a complete resection (Simpson grades I & II) and 50% following an incomplete resection (Simpson grades III–V) [23]. Overall, several studies have reached the similar conclusions that surgical outcome and recurrence of meningiomas are dependent on the degree of resection. The degree of resection is, in turn, dependent on the tumor location and, therefore, the accessibility of the tumor and the involved dura and bone [22].

Jaaskelainen observed that the following three factors were significantly associated with meningioma recurrence: (1) coagulation of the involved dura instead of removal, (2) attachment of the tumor to bone, and (3) the soft consistency of the tumor. If none of these criteria were present, the recurrence rate at 20 years was 11%, while if one or two of these criteria were present, the recurrence rates were 15–24% and 34–56%, respectively. Although the histological criteria for grading meningiomas have evolved in recent years, Jaaskelainen et al. [24] reported in 1986 that the 5-year recurrence rates following complete resection were 3% for benign, 38% for atypical, and 78% for anaplastic meningiomas. Pathological features associated with a significantly higher rate of recurrence include histological anaplasia, (20 mitoses per 10 high-powered fields, nuclear atypia, and papillary or rhabdoid cellular features. Kakinuma et al. [25] evaluated 182 meningiomas and found that the Ki-67 SI for recurrent meningiomas (14.78 ± 3.17%) was significantly higher than for non-recurrent meningiomas (4.71 ± 1.96%). Similarly, May et al. [26] noted that a proliferative index of (19% on flow cytometry was associated with meningioma recurrence.

Several authors have attempted to find neuroradiological characteristics that can predict recurrence. Mantle et al. [27] reported that the chance of brain invasion and recurrence increased by 20% with each centimeter of brain edema surrounding the meningioma on computed tomography (CT) scanning. Nakasu et al. showed that the "lobulated" or "mushrooming" appearances of meningiomas noted on pre-operative imaging studies correlated with an increased Ki-67 SI and a higher recurrence rate for these tumors. Lobulated tumors showed higher SI (2.85 ± 3.68%) than round tumors (1.06 ± 0.67%). Three of three "mushrooming" type of tumors and seven of 22 (32%) "lobulated" tumors recurred, while only five of 74 (7%) "round" meningiomas recurred following the similar extent of resection for all three groups. The median interval for recurrence was 10 months for "mushrooming" tumors, 82 months for the "lobulated" ones, and 111 months for "round" meningiomas [28].

# Management

## Pre-operative Evaluation

Patients with meningiomas are often referred to the neurosurgeon after a primary care physician or neurologist has obtained a CT scan of the head for a variety of neurological symptoms. The radiological appearance of meningiomas with this modality of imaging has been well described. Meningiomas are typically isodense on CT before contrast and homogeneously hyperdense following intravenous iodinated contrast. In addition to being inexpensive and convenient, CT offers the advantages of determining the extent of hyperostosis and the degree of tumor calcification, both of which add to the diagnostic accuracy and help the surgeon with surgical planning.

It is, however, becoming more frequent that the initial head scan performed is magnetic resonance imaging (MRI), due to its increasing availability and decreasing cost. MRI is proven to be the gold standard neuroimaging method of detection for meningiomas. MRI with and without gadolinium contrast is necessary to precisely delineate the full extent of the tumor, particularly in the case of skull base tumors that can involve critical neurovascular structures (such as the optic nerve(s) and major intracranial vessels). On T1-weighted MRI, the majority of meningiomas are isointense, while the remainder is slightly hyperintense to grey matter. Contrast-enhanced T1-weighted images reveal dramatic and usually homogeneous enhancement of meningiomas and, often, their associated "dural-tail". On T2-weighted sequences, nearly 50% of all meningiomas are hyperintense, while the other half are isointense to grey matter. T2-weighted sequence is also highly sensitive in delineating the extent of peritumoral edema. Furthermore, utilization of MRI allows the opportunity to obtain MR-angiography (MRA) and/or MR-venography (MRV) in order to better visualize the extent of vascular involvement, particularly the patency of dural sinuses and the encasement of major arteries. Moreover, the contrast-enhanced MRI is essential in detecting any residual or recurrent tumor following surgery.

For large meningiomas, cerebral angiography may be helpful to determine precisely the extent of involvement of the intracranial arteries and their branches, in addition to providing further information regarding the venous anatomy. Also, large tumors may have significant arterial supply from the external carotid and middle meningeal arteries that may be safely embolized during the angiogram. Many posterior fossa meningiomas are fed by vessels not amenable to catheterization or successful embolization. However, in rare instances of successful embolization of deep-seated, large posterior fossa meningiomas, surgery is dramatically facilitated by embolization. Therefore, in the authors' practice, all supratentorial meningiomas larger than 4–5 cm and infratentorial meningiomas larger than 3–4 cm are routinely evaluated for possible embolization.

When the internal carotid artery (ICA) is noted to be completely encased and/or narrowed by the tumor on pre-operative MRI, ipsilateral ICA test balloon occlusion (TBO) may be performed. Such information is helpful as it allows the surgeon to plan the extent of resection around the ICA. For patients passing the TBO, an aggressive tumor resection may be pursued, and in the rare event of intraoperative ICA injury, the surgeon has the options of direct ICA repair, bypass or ICA sacrifice. If a patient does not pass the TBO, however, tumor resection around the ICA may be more conservative in order to prevent a devastating stroke. Alternatively, an arterial bypass may be performed in preparation for an aggressive tumor resection.

New modalities for imaging meningiomas are emerging. Although MRI is very sensitive and the radiological features of meningiomas have been well described, it can lack specificity and a tissue biopsy, at least, is required for definitive diagnosis. There are numerous reports of other lesions that have mimicked meningiomas on imaging, such as lymphoma, plasmacytoma, primary CNS sarcoidosis and metastases from breast, renal and prostate carcinomas. Highly specific neuroimaging is desirable to definitively diagnose meningiomas, or any other CNS lesions, non-invasively. One example of an advance in this area is MRS, which measures tissue levels of compounds such as choline, phosphocreatine/creatine and N-acetylaspartate. The goal of much ongoing research is to find distinct patterns of these compounds that will provide the ability to non-invasively discern the pathology and the histological grade of a neoplasm. Such information may facilitate therapeutic decisions and prognostic determinations prior to resection, or in place of biopsy.

Another type of imaging – octreotide single-photon emission computed tomography (SPECT) – has proven to be very sensitive for detecting meningiomas. Although virtually all meningiomas have octreotide-binding somatostatin receptors, it must be noted that this technique is not specific for meningiomas alone, as other primary and metastatic CNS tumors often express somatostatin receptors. The non-invasive diagnostic specificity for meningiomas is improved when octreotide-SPECT is used in combination with other neuroimaging modalities. Due to its extreme sensitivity, however, octreotide–SPECT is particularly useful for detecting the recurrence of a meningioma following resection. Some centers are even exploring the utility of combining the information from octreotide-SPECT with F-2-fluoro-2-

deoxyglucose positron emission tomograhy (FDG-PET) scanning in an attempt to predict non-invasively which tumors will behave more aggressively, but definitive results are forthcoming.

## Pre-operative Medical Therapy

Symptomatic patients with a significant amount of peritumoral edema seen on T2-weighted MRI are started on dexamethasone as an outpatient, and surgery is planned within the following 1–2 weeks. Anticonvulsants are started pre-operatively only for patients who present with seizures. Otherwise, a loading dose of phenytoin is given at induction of anesthesia and then therapeutic levels are maintained postoperatively for 1–6 weeks, depending on the tumor size, brain manipulation required during surgery, and the extent of perioperative swelling.

## Treatment Options

In general, management options include observation, surgery, radiation alone, or as an adjuvant therapy following surgery. To date, no definitively effective chemotherapeutic agent has been identified or developed. As meningiomas are mostly benign and slowly progressive tumors, emergency intervention is usually not required. Final treatment plans must be individualized for each patient based on the age, overall condition of the patient, tumor location and size, neurological symptoms and deficits caused by the tumor, and the patient's personal wish after a thorough discussion of all available options.

## Observation

Surgery is not necessary for every patient with a meningioma. Observation alone, with periodic (usually yearly) follow-up neurological and MR evaluations, is reasonable for elderly patients, especially if they have minimal or no symptoms caused by the tumor. As people are living healthier and longer lives today, the age at which a person is considered "elderly" is debatable. The patient's absolute age is no longer important in the decision-making process in the management of meningiomas; however, it may be reasonable to consider those with less than

10–15 years of remaining life expectancy to be "elderly". In addition, observation may be an appropriate option for the following people regardless of their age: (1) patients with certain skull base meningiomas with minimal or no symptoms (e.g. cavernous sinus meningioma causing mild facial tingling or numbness), (2) patients with incidental small tumors with no surrounding edema, and (3) patients who insist on non-intervention after a thorough discussion of all treatment options. However, these patients must be compliant with the necessary radiographic and neurological follow-up evaluations.

As with other brain tumors, the risks of surgery may vary in direct proportion to the tumor size, while the chances of total resection vary inversely in proportion to the size of meningiomas of most locations. For example, it is quite obvious that removal of small parasagittal tumors without any involvement of the sagittal sinus would be immensely easier compared to the removal of larger ones which commonly invade the sagittal sinus. The same may be said of small clinoidal or tuberculum sella meningiomas before causing optic nerve and ICA involvement, or petrous meningiomas prior to reaching a large size that would encase the basilar artery and compress the brainstem and cranial nerves. Therefore, the initial recommendation of observation must be decided upon carefully, especially in younger patients, taking into consideration the increased potential risks posed in the future by further growth in the tumor size and involvement of nearby critical neurovascular structures.

# Surgery

## General Principles

Surgery is the treatment of choice for most patients with meningiomas. In patients with benign meningiomas, which comprise approximately 94% of all meningiomas [24], the tumor location largely dictates the extent of resection, which, in turn, determines the tumor recurrence and, ultimately, the patient's survival [2,19,22,24]. Primary goals of surgery include: (1) total resection of the tumor and the involved surrounding bone and dura when possible, and (2) reversal or improvement in neurological

deficits/symptoms caused by the tumor. In meningiomas of certain locations, such as the cavernous sinus or petroclival regions where complete resection is not always possible, additional surgical goals may include confirmation of diagnosis and tumor reduction (to less than 3 cm maximum diameter) in preparation for radiosurgery. Given the benign nature of meningiomas and the established efficacy of adjuvant radiation, the goal of total removal must be balanced by the physician's basic credo to "do no harm". When total removal carries a significant risk of morbidity, a small piece of tumor may be left, with further plans of observation followed by re-operation or radiation when the tumor is noted to be growing or causing new symptoms (Fig. 12.1).

## Surgical Technique

Meningiomas of different locations require varying surgical approaches that are primarily dictated by anatomical considerations inherent to each particular location. Surgical procedures of many different anatomical regions are discussed in several other chapters in this book. Furthermore, an abundance of excellent descriptions of "standard" techniques and approaches for meningioma surgery is available [2]. This chapter is written not to replace, but to supplement, those previous important writings on the topic. Several key concepts and principles deemed important are reiterated, and new insights and lessons learned by the senior author, based on his personal surgical experience with over 600 meningioma patients, are summarized and presented.

Surgical approaches may vary in meningioma surgery depending on the tumor location and size and the surgeon's personal experience and preference. However, the following basic principles hold for meningioma surgery of most locations:

- Optimal patient positioning, incision and exposure
- Early tumor devascularization
- Internal decompression or extracapsular dissection
- Early localization and preservation of adherent or adjacent neurovasculature
- Removal of involved bone and dura

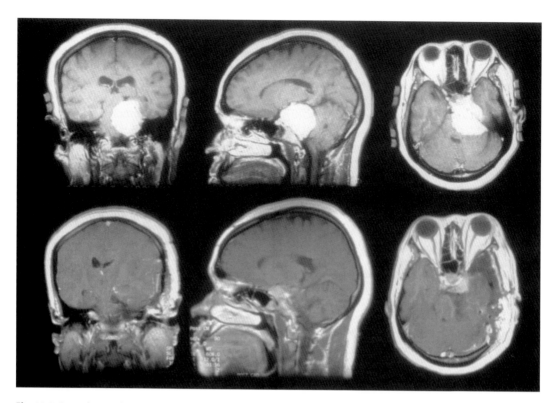

**Fig. 12.1.** Coronal, sagittal and axial gadolinium-enhanced T1-weighted MR images of a 36-year-old female patient who presented with unsteady gait and cerebellar ataxia (upper left, upper middle and upper right). This large tumor, involving both the petroclival and cavernous sinus regions, was resected in two-staged operations. A small tumor nodule adherent on the intracavernous ICA was left (lower left, lower middle and lower right). Post-operatively, she developed hearing loss and mild hypesthesia in the left V2 and V3 distributions, but her extraocular motility was normal with resolution of her presenting unsteadiness and ataxia. This residual tumor is being observed closely, with plans of gamma knife radiosurgical intervention in the event that the tumor progresses in the future.

## Positioning, Incision and Exposure

The patient positioning, appropriate incision placement, and selection of the optimal approach for tumor exposure are the critical elements of successful meningioma surgery. The patient is positioned in such a way that the patient's safety is maximized. Moreover, the ideal position must allow for an approach that provides complete exposure of the tumor and the involved surrounding bone and dura. At the same time, maximal brain relaxation must be achieved by use of gravity and uncompromised venous drainage. The head should be no lower than the level of the heart, regardless of the position selected, and undue severe neck rotation or flexion must be avoided. In addition, surgeon's comfort for the duration of surgery must be maintained. The sitting position, preferred by some neurosurgeons for tumors of the pineal and select posterior fossa locations, places the patient at a higher risk of developing air embolism and the surgeon at an increased level of discomfort. When considering the sitting position for the aforementioned lesions, pre-operative sagittal MRI should be reviewed carefully to appreciate the relative size of the posterior fossa and the steepness of the tentorial angle. Patients with a small posterior fossa usually have a low-lying posterior tentorial attachment because of the inferior location of the torcular and inion. This anatomical variation leads to a very steep, nearly vertical tentorial angle, making the infratentorial/supracerebellar approach with the patient seated extremely difficult. Other approaches to be considered in this situation include the transoccipital/transtentorial approach with the patient in the prone position, or the infratentorial/supracerebellar approach with the patient in the modified park-bench (the "Concorde") position (Fig. 12.2).

For superficial tumors (e.g. convexity or parasagittal), the planned scalp flap should contain the tumor in the center, and the patient is positioned so that the tumor is at the highest point. Importantly, the incision must be planned to avoid any visible cosmetic defect or significant compromise to the scalp vascular supply. If a horseshoe-shaped incision is planned, the depth must not exceed the width of the flap. Again, for superficial tumors, the size

of the scalp and bone flaps must be sufficiently large so as to allow for maximal exposure of the tumor, the involved bone and dura, as well as the limits of the dural tail as noted on pre-operative MRI scans. With the availability of frameless stereotactic image-guidance systems, the exact extent of the tumor and the dural tail may be fully delineated before surgery. This aids in optimal positioning and placement of incision and craniotomy.

An optimal approach should provide the shortest and most direct route to the tumor without "sacrificing" any normal brain tissue or creating undue brain damage by retraction. The need for retraction is minimized by taking advantage of gravity. For example, for surgery

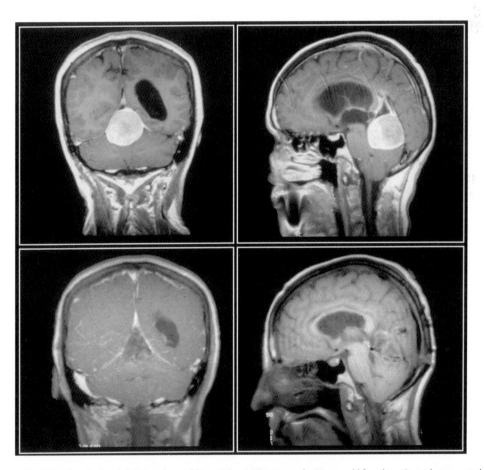

**Fig. 12.2.** Coronal and sagittal gadolinium-enhanced T1-weighted MR images of a 55-year-old female patient who presented with headache and unsteady gait (upper left and upper right). Because of the small posterior fossa and the near-vertical tentorial angle noted on the sagittal MRI (upper right), the tumor was approached via the occipital interhemispheric/transtentorial route with the patient in the prone position. Following total resection (lower left and lower right), her presenting symptoms resolved completely.

of an olfactory groove meningioma the head can be slightly hyperextended, and for a cerebello-pontine-angle lesion the patient may be placed in the lateral position. For large, deep, falcine tumors, the patient's head may be placed with the side of the tumor down and the direction of the sagittal sinus parallel to the operating room floor. In all of these examples, the brain falls away from the tumor and its attachment. In deep-seated tumors, brain retraction may be minimized by use of cerebrospinal fluid (CSF) drainage via either a ventricular drain (in patients with obstructive hydrocephalus) or a lumbar drain. Furthermore, many of the skull base approaches developed over the last two decades, which convert the deep basal meningiomas to more superficial "convexity" lesions by reducing the working distance to the tumor, may reduce the need for brain retraction.

An optimal surgical approach also facilitates surgery by maximizing exposure of the tumor and surrounding structures, thereby minimizing risks of injury to the adjacent neurovascular structures. For example, in surgery of large clinoidal or suprasellar meningiomas, complete removal of the anterior clinoid process (ACP) provides improved access and exposure of the regions surrounding the optic nerve, optic chiasm, ICA and sella. Additionally, by opening the optic sheath as an extension of the dural incision following anterior clinoidectomy, the optic nerve can be decompressed and visualized early, and mobilized safely during surgery, thereby reducing the risk of intraoperative injury to the nerve [29]. This maneuver also expands operative windows, particularly the optico-carotid triangle, facilitating access to tumors in the suprasellar and subchiasmatic regions.

In most situations, there exist a number of options in selecting the patient's position, surgical approach and exposure. The final selection must be based on what is best for the patient and the surgeon, based on the surgeon's knowledge, past experience and preference.

## Tumor Devascularization

Many meningiomas can be quite vascular. In addition to utilization of pre-operative embolization when appropriate, early operative devascularization of the tumor reduces blood loss and makes surgery easier. In superficial

tumors, upon dural exposure prior to opening the dura, extra time should be expended to coagulate all the dural feeding vessels – most commonly the branches or the main trunk of the middle meningeal artery. In olfactory groove meningiomas, bifrontal craniotomy, preferred by many surgeons, provides early access to the main tumor feeders, i.e. ethmoidal arteries, as they enter the medial anterior fossa floor. In large sphenoid wing meningiomas, which receive significant transdural blood supply, utilizing the extradural skull base technique of orbitosphenoid bone removal obliterates many dural feeders prior to dural opening. Similarly, in petroclival meningiomas, the transpetrosal approach allows the exposed petrous dura and tentorium to be aggressively coagulated and may significantly devascularize the tumor. In falcine or tentorial meningiomas, wide exposure and coagulation of the surrounding falx and tentorium reduce tumor vascularity. Yasargil advocates initial transtumoral devascularization of basal meningiomas by working through a small "window" created in the tumor to reach the blood supply coming through the base. However, this technique may not be suitable for an inexperienced surgeon as there may be a significant risk of injury to unexposed neurovascular structures that may be located on the other side of the tumor.

## Internal Decompression and Extracapsular Dissection

Although small meningiomas may be removed "en bloc", internal decompression is a key initial step in actual tumor removal for most meningiomas following adequate exposure and initial devascularization. Internal debulking is carried out until a thin rim of exposed portion of the tumor is remaining. This internal debulking minimizes brain retraction and facilitates extracapsular dissection. Following initial internal decompression, extracapsular dissection is initiated by identifying a layer of arachnoid (maintained in most meningiomas) at the brain–tumor interface. As surgery progresses, rather than increasing brain retraction to expose more of the tumor hidden under the brain, the thinned capsule is pulled towards the center of decompression. Cottonoid patties are placed in the brain–tumor interface as the capsule is being pulled away from the brain, while maintaining the arachnoidal layer intact between the brain and the tumor. As patties are being placed sequentially around the tumor, they are used to gently strip the arachnoid from the tumor capsule, covering the brain and arachnoid together, thereby protecting the brain from surgical trauma. As the remaining tumor capsule is brought into the surgeon's view, any adjacent cranial nerves are carefully dissected, and exposed blood vessels on the capsule surface are thoroughly inspected. Only tumor-feeding vessels are obliterated, preserving and dissecting free those transit vessels that are either passing through the depth of tumor or adherent to the tumor surface. Portions of tumor capsule thus devascularized and completely dissected from the surrounding neurovasculature are further removed in segments. These alternating sequential steps of internal decompression, extracapsular dissection and removal of devascularized capsule are repeated until the entire tumor is removed.

For meningiomas in the clival, petroclival or cerebellopontine-angle regions, the surgeon must analyze the pre-operative MRI scan carefully. First, evidence of surrounding edema in the brainstem noted on T2-weighted scan must be appreciated prior to surgery as this indicates disruption of the arachnoidal layer and the blood–brain barrier. This implies that the surgical plane between the brainstem and tumor may have been obliterated and, therefore, that aggressive resection off the brainstem should be avoided. Second, the basilar artery location in relation to the tumor and brainstem must be noted. Although rare, if the tumor is located between the brainstem and basilar artery or completely encases the artery, this indicates that all the perforating branches of the basilar artery are stretched and course through the tumor. In this situation, an attempt at aggressive tumor removal is likely to result in a brainstem infarct. When the basilar artery is abutting directly on the brainstem, aggressive tumor removal off the brainstem is possible.

During extracapsular dissection, as a rule, no artery or arterial branch is sacrificed except when the vessel is definitely confirmed to be a tumor feeder. Commonly, loops of vessels may be encased by the tumor or may course onto the capsule surface and become adherent. In these situations, the surgeon may initially misinterpret these vessels as tumor feeders. Before con-

cluding that a vessel is a tumor feeder and therefore amenable to obliteration, the afferent and efferent course of the vessel must be fully appreciated. It is very rare for meningiomas to have feeders directly from main intracranial arterial trunks. Therefore, no vessels coming directly off the ICA (in tuberculum sella or clinoidal tumors), basilar artery (in petroclival- and cerebellopontine-angle tumors) or vertebral artery (in foramen magnum meningiomas) should be coagulated. If any appreciable vasospasm occurs while dissecting tumor off arteries, small pieces of gelfoam soaked in papaverine applied directly onto the vessel readily reverse the spasm.

In removing the tumor from cranial nerves, especially the optic nerve, fine vessels feeding the nerves must be preserved. The optic chiasm and intradural optic nerve have main feeders on the inferior surface, and therefore removal of large tumors involving the subchiasmatic and suboptic space must be done carefully so as to preserve these fine vessels. Again, the preserved arachnoid around the cranial nerves facilitates tumor removal and reduces risks of intraoperative neurovascular injury.

## Early Localization and Preservation of Adjacent Neurovasculature

Whenever possible, any adjacent or nearby normal neurovasculature (e.g. a cranial nerve or a vessel) should be identified and dissection carried out following this structure into the tumor. For example, in large clinoidal tumors encasing the optic nerve and the ICA, the conventional technique for removal has been first to identify the distal middle cerebral artery branches, and follow these vessels proximally toward the ICA with further tumor removal and dissection. However, until the ICA, and eventually the intradural optic nerve, are located, surgery progresses slowly. More importantly, the risk of intraoperative neurovascular injury persists during surgery as the exact location of the optic nerve and ICA remains unknown to the surgeon, and the optic nerve remains compressed. During this time, any minor surgical trauma caused by retraction, dissection or tumor manipulation may exacerbate compression of the optic nerve, especially against the falciform ligament. To circumvent these critical problems, the optic nerve can be exposed and simultaneously decompressed early in the surgery by unroofing the optic canal, followed by anterior clinoidectomy and opening of the optic sheath [29] (Figs 12.3, 12.4, 12.5). The location of the optic canal, and therefore the intracanalicular segment of the optic nerve, is fairly constant; only the intradural cisternal segment of the optic nerve varies in location, depending on how the tumor causes nerve displacement during its growth. The exposed optic nerve can then be followed from the optic canal proximally, toward the tumor in the intradural location. As tumor resection progresses further, the ICA can be readily found adjacent to the exposed distal intradural segment of the optic nerve. Complete optic sheath opening, along the length of the nerve within the optic canal to the anulus of Zinn, relieves any focal circumferential pressure on the optic nerve contributed by the falciform ligament. Optic nerve decompression thus achieved also leads to reduced intraoperative injury to the nerve, because the force of retraction is then dispersed over a much larger surface area. Moreover, if the tumor eventually recurs, the patient's impending visual deterioration may be delayed as the optic nerve is already decompressed from the surrounding falciform ligament and optic canal. In the senior author's personal experience utilizing the described technique in eight patients presenting with pre-operative visual deterioration from large clinoidal meningiomas, six patients (75%) experienced significant improvement in their vision postoperatively [29].

Whenever possible, no cortical vein or dural sinus is "sacrificed". Although the anterior third of the sagittal sinus is traditionally said to be amenable to obliteration without any significant sequelae, there is a risk of developing significant venous infarcts. Therefore, even in large olfactory groove or planum sphenoidale tumors, rather than routine anterior sagittal sinus obliteration following a bifrontal craniotomy, either a unilateral pterional or a bilateral interhemispheric approach with preservation of sagittal sinus is used whenever possible in the authors' practice. In parasagittal meningiomas, the tumor is removed aggressively, along with the involved segment of sagittal sinus, only when the sinus is completely occluded by the tumor. Otherwise, every effort is made to preserve the sagittal sinus integrity and patency while removing as much tumor as possible. Nearby prominent cortical veins, especially in the posterior two-thirds along the sinus, are preserved as well.

## Removal of the Involved Bone and Dura

Following complete tumor removal, the site of tumor origin is carefully inspected. If possible, the involved dura and bone are removed. In tumors of basal locations, the involved bone is drilled using a small diamond burr, which is also quite effective in achieving hemostasis from tumor feeders arising directly from the base of the skull. Involved bone adjacent to paranasal sinuses is aggressively drilled, short of entering the sinus space. Inadvertent opening into paranasal sinuses or mastoid air cells must be recognized and appropriately sealed with muscle/fat graft or bone wax.

In 1983, Dolenc introduced an extensive extradural skull base technique to gain safe entry into the cavernous sinus. The critical steps of this technique, following a routine frontotemporal craniotomy and drilling of the lateral sphenoid wing, include complete bone removal around the superior orbital fissure (SOF), posterior orbitotomy, optic canal unroofing, extradural removal of the ACP, and removal of bone around the foramen rotundum and ovale. Meningiomas of the posterior orbital roof, cavernous sinus (CS), sphenoid wing or orbitosphenoid regions frequently cause hyperostosis of the orbital roof, and the greater and lesser sphenoid wing, including the ACP. For these tumors, the Dolenc approach, with modifications tailored to removal of only the involved bone, is an ideal technique.

In addition, the extensive sphenoid bone removal of the Dolenc approach, when coupled with the extradural exposure of the CS, facilitates removal of the involved dura, especially the portion of temporal dura covering the medial greater sphenoid wing, which simultaneously forms the outer lateral wall of CS. Following extradural bone removal as summarized above, the dural fold at the superolateral aspect of the SOF is sharply cut with microscissors tangential to the temporal dura. The temporal dura forming the outer lateral CS wall is then "peeled" off the underlying inner CS lateral wall. This process of separating the two-layered CS lateral wall is continued laterally and posteriorly until all three divisions of the trigeminal

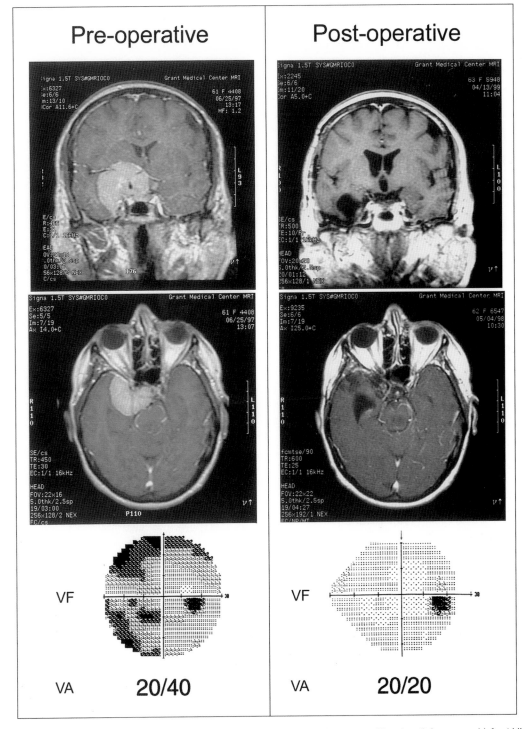

**Fig. 12.3.** Coronal and axial gadolinium-enhanced T1-weighted MR images of a 61-year-old patient (left upper and left middle) presenting with decreased visual acuity (20/40) and visual field (superior and inferior arcuate defects) (left lower). Following total resection (right upper and right middle), her vision returned to normal (right lower). VA, visual acuity; VF, visual field.

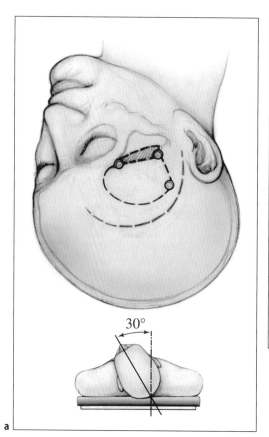

30°

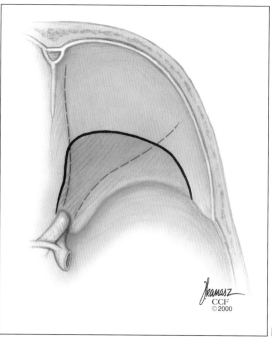

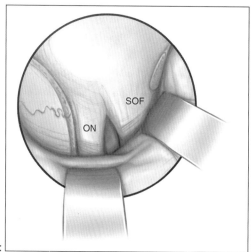

**Fig. 12.4. a** Operative position of the patient's head (Mayfield head-clamp not shown). The head of the bed is raised 20° and the patient's head is rotated 30° away from the side of surgery. A standard curvilinear frontotemporal skin incision is made behind the hairline (broken line). A frontotemporal craniotomy is turned (broken line connecting the three burr holes), following which the lateral sphenoid wing is drilled (shaded area). **b** The shaded area depicts the bone removed during the right-sided extradural skull base technique. The removed bone includes the lateral sphenoid wing, posterolateral orbital wall, posterior orbital roof, optic canal roof and ACP. The broken lines outline the orbit. **c** Extradural operative view of the exposed intracanalicular optic nerve and the opened SOF following complete removal of the ACP. ACP, anterior clinoid process; ON, optic nerve; SOF, superior orbital fissure.

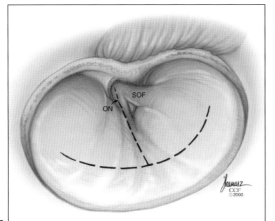

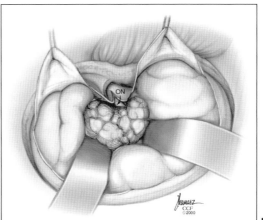

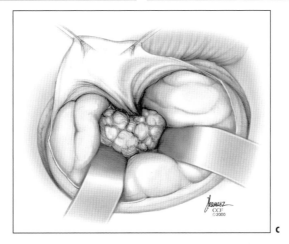

**Fig. 12.5. a** Extradural view after completion of the skull base technique, including: (1) frontotemporal craniotomy, (2) lateral sphenoid wing removal, (3) posterior orbitotomy, (4) SOF decompression, (5) optic canal unroofing, and (6) extradural anterior clinoidectomy. The dural incision (broken line) is made in two steps: First, a frontotemporal curvilinear opening is created, centered on the Sylvian fissure, followed by a bi-section of the dural flap toward the optic sheath and extending across the falciform ligament and to the anulus of Zinn. **b** The same clinoidal meningioma as depicted in c, following completion of the extradural skull base technique and extending the dural incision into the optic sheath. The optic nerve is readily identified in the exposed optic canal and completely decompressed at the onset of tumor removal. Tumor resection progresses by following the exposed optic nerve proximally. The combination of early optic nerve identification and decompression leads to prevention of intraoperative optic nerve injury. **c** The view of an exposed large clinoidal meningioma after the initial dural opening, using pterional craniotomy and standard frontotemporal dural opening only. Upon tumor exposure, it is noted to be covering the critical neurovascular structures (the optic and oculomotor nerves, ICA). The exact locations of the optic nerve and ICA are unknown to the surgeon, and the optic nerve remains in a compressed state. Tumor resection progresses slowly until the optic nerve and ICA are eventually identified. FL, frontal lobe; ON, optic nerve; SOF, superior orbital fissure; TL, temporal lobe.

nerve and the gasserian ganglion are exposed. In this manner, the lateral aspect of the CS is exposed entirely extradurally, freeing up the dura of medial temporal pole for removal as necessary, which would not have been possible to resect otherwise. This maneuver is particularly helpful in orbitosphenoid, CS and sphenoid wing meningiomas, which frequently involve the temporal polar dura (Figs. 12.6, 12.7).

## Post-operative Management

Follow-up evaluations consist of careful neurological examination and MRI scans with and without gadolinium. For patients with pre-operative diplopia and changes in vision, detailed neuro-ophthalmological evaluations are a critical part of follow-up management. Similarly, patients with posterior fossa meningiomas presenting with hearing loss, or those patients whose surgery involved dissection of the cranial nerve complex VII–VIII, should have thorough audiological evaluations as part of their post-operative management. Following resection of all meningiomas, a post-operative baseline MRI scan is obtained on day 1 or 2 after surgery. For benign tumors, following confirmation of total removal on post-operative MRI, further follow-up evaluation with imaging studies are performed every 1–3 years, depending on whether Simpson grade I or II removal

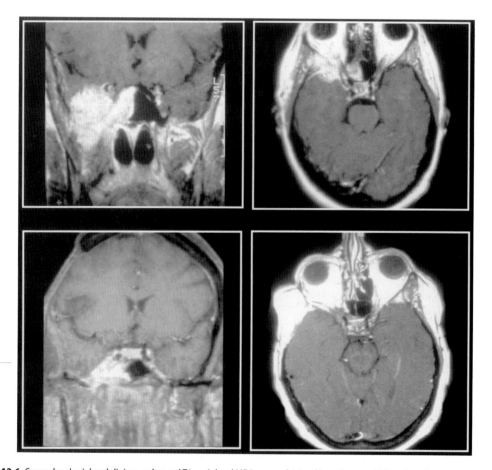

**Fig. 12.6.** Coronal and axial gadolinium-enhanced T1-weighted MR images obtained in a 47-year-old female patient presenting with a 3-year history of right-sided V2 numbness and mild proptosis (left upper and right upper). This large orbitosphenoid meningioma also extends into the infratemporal fossa and the nasal sinuses. Aggressive subtotal resection was achieved, with the residual tumor in the nasal sinuses only (left lower and right lower).

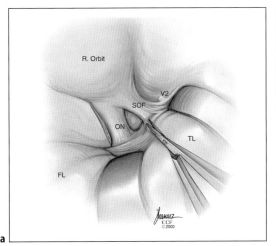

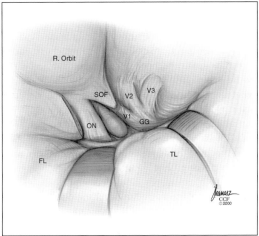

**Fig. 12.7. a** Following completion of the extradural skull base technique described in Figures 12.4 and 12.5, the process that allows for removal of the sphenoid bone involved by the tumor; the temporal dura forming the outer portion of the two-layered CS wall is "peeled off" the inner CS wall. This is best started by sharply and tangentially cutting the dural fold at the superiolateral aspect of the completely exposed SOF. **b** This "peeling" process is continued posteriorly and laterally until all three divisions of the trigeminal nerve and the gasserian ganglion are exposed. In this manner, the lateral aspect of the CS is exposed entirely extradurally, freeing up the anterior and medial temporal dura, commonly involved by CS or sphenoid wing/orbitosphenoid meningiomas, for aggressive removal along with the rest of the tumor. GG, gasserian ganglion; R, right.

was achieved. Following a subtotal removal, subsequent follow-up with MRI is done every year, with plans of adjuvant radiation if and when there is clinical or radiographic progression of the residual tumor. If the tumor is noted to be clinically and radiographically stable for a few years after initial surgery, the frequency of follow-up may be decreased to every 2–3 years. For atypical meningiomas, after initial post-operative MRI following either subtotal or total removal, subsequent evaluations with MRI are performed every 6 months for the first 2 years. As with benign tumors, radiation is considered in the presence of documented clinical or radiographic progression of the residual tumor. With malignant meningiomas, adjuvant radiation is administered shortly after surgery regardless of the extent of resection. However, if there is any reversible post-operative neurological deficit from brain swelling or cranial nerve manipulation, the timing of radiation therapy should be delayed to allow for adequate recovery. Depending on the extent of resection, follow-up MRI scans are performed every 3–6 months.

# Therapeutic Radiation

## Role of Radiation Therapy: an Overview

Radiation therapy (RT) represents an important treatment option for patients with benign and malignant brain tumors. Recent advances in computer and imaging technology as well as radiation delivery have greatly improved the radiation oncologist's ability to deliver high doses of radiation to the tumor bed while sparing the surrounding normal tissues. This should decrease complications and perhaps increase control of local disease. Despite these advances, however, the use of radiation therapy in the management of meningiomas remains controversial, partly because these tumors grow slowly and in an unpredictable pattern. Moreover, no randomized clinical trials have been performed to test the optimal timing and effectiveness of radiotherapy in the management of patients with meningiomas. In this section, the currently available radiation-therapy techniques and their results are presented.

## Conventional Radiation

Before the introduction of sophisticated planning computers and the integration of radiographic images to optimize radiation delivery, conventional radiation therapy was used to treat patients. With conventional therapy, radiation was delivered not only to the tumor bed but also to a margin (2 cm) to ensure adequate tumor coverage. This approach potentially delivered high doses of radiation to normal brain tissues. Early studies suggested that meningiomas were relatively insensitive to conventional radiation. More modern reports, however, found that RT resulted in excellent local control. Recently, Nutting et al. [30] reported a 5-year progression-free survival rate of 92%, and a 10-year progression-free survival rate of 83%, in 82 patients with benign meningiomas who were treated by surgery followed by external-beam RT.

Despite these impressive results, some have questioned the safety of conventional RT out of a concern over its potential long-term effects, including the induction of malignancies. Thus, researchers have been investigating ways to improve local control and minimize toxicities. This has led to the development of conformal radiation techniques, which enable radiation oncologists to increase the dose and minimize damage to the normal surrounding tissues and structures.

## Three-dimensional Conformal Radiotherapy (3D-CRT)

With this type of treatment, three-dimensional computer planning systems are used to deliver radiation that conforms to the shape of the tumor. During the initial planning phase (simulation), a thermoplastic mask is used to immobilize the patient to ensure reproducible, accurate set-ups. CT or MRI is used to localize the tumor. These images are then transferred to a high-speed computer. This allows the physician to contour the normal structures and tumor. A dosimetrist or physicist will then plan the field orientation and optimize the dose distribution. The beams may be shaped using custom-made blocks or collimators. A beam's eye view can be created to determine the orientation of the radiation beams, which helps to tailor the radiation dose around the tumor. Dose–volume histograms can be used to calculate a defined tumor volume that will receive a given percentage of the dose, which allows for the comparison of plans. The 3D-CRT has two main limitations: the accuracy of the results depends heavily on the planner's skills, and multiple iterations are required to develop an optimal plan.

## Intensity-modulated Radiation Therapy

Intensity-modulated radiation therapy (IMRT) extends the benefits of 3D-CRT by enabling radiation oncologists to deliver non-uniform beams of radiation. This allows for more conformal delivery of radiation to the tumor and possible dose escalation. The technique uses a computer optimization process that is based on prescribed doses to the target and constraints on normal, sensitive structures. Radiation delivery is further optimized by the use of a multileaf collimator (MLC) or complex compensators, which automatically shape the radiation beam. These two concepts – inverse treatment planning with computer optimization and computer-controlled intensity modulation of the radiation beam – form the basis of IMRT.

One of the more commonly used collimators for IMRT is the multivane intensity-modulating collimator (MIMiC), which attaches to the accessory tray of the linear accelerator (Peacock system, NOMOS Corp., Sewickley, PA). The MIMiC contains 40 small vanes, each of which can alter the intensity of the radiation beam during treatment. The system delivers the radiation dose using arc therapy and segmented fields. The beam can also be modified by using a dynamic MLC that passes across the treatment field or by superimposing a number of static fields. The patient's head can be affixed to the immobilization device either invasively or non-invasively.

Some radiation centers, including the authors' at the Cleveland Clinic, are using IMRT to treat meningiomas in the hopes of achieving excellent local control and minimizing acute and long-term side-effects. No large clinical experiences that have used IMRT to treat meningioma have been reported thus far.

## Brachytherapy

Brachytherapy is the implantation of radioactive isotopes into a tumor. This method delivers a high dose of radiation to the tumor while sparing most of the surrounding normal tissue. It may be a good choice for patients with poor health, advanced age, or unresectable or recurrent tumors. The most commonly used brachytherapy method for treating meningiomas is permanent implantation of I-125 seeds. These seeds deliver high levels of radiation for a period of months, which is a potential advantage for treating slow-growing tumors like meningiomas. The seeds can be placed stereotactically or directly sewed or glued into the tumor cavity.

The clinical results of brachytherapy for meningiomas are limited. Patil et al. reported on 26 patients with meningiomas undergoing I-125 seed implant [31]. All 26 patients experienced tumor regression. The authors have treated 14 patients with intracranial meningiomas at the Cleveland Clinic using stereotactic wand guidance. One to five I-125 seeds were placed in each tumor to provide a minimum peripheral dose of 10,000 centigray (cGy) total decay. Overall, the procedure has been well tolerated with encouraging initial results. However, the interest in using brachytherapy as a treatment for meningiomas has waned given the development of radiosurgical and conformal radiation techniques.

## Stereotactic Radiosurgery

In 1951, Dr Lars Leksell coined the term "stereotactic radiosurgery" (SRS), which is the delivery of a single, high dose of radiation via stereotactically directed beams into a small target. Presently, three main types of SRS techniques are used: heavy charged particles (proton beam), gamma irradiation from cobalt-60 sources (gamma knife), and high-energy photons from linear accelerators (LINACs). With all of these methods, a stereotactic headframe is used for patient positioning and target determination.

In the past 10 years, SRS has become an increasingly popular option in managing meningioma patients with tumors that are less than 3 cm in diameter. This technique is more advantageous than surgery for a number of reasons. It is minimally invasive, does not require general anesthesia, and can be performed as an outpatient procedure. In addition, it carries a minimal risk of bleeding and infection, and recovery time is minimal. Stereotactic radiosurgery also costs less than conventional surgery.

The gamma knife (Elekta Instruments, Atlanta, GA) is a dedicated machine that performs SRS. The machine uses 201 cobalt-60 sources arranged in a hemispheric dome around the patient's head. Since 1968, more than 100,000 patients with various tumors, vascular malformations and functional disorders have been treated with this device. The goal is to encompass the target area using multiple isocenters or shots to maximize conformality and to minimize the radiation dose to normal surrounding structures. The initial results from gamma knife radiosurgery have been encouraging. Kondziolka et al. reviewed the long-term results of 99 consecutive patients (89% had skull base tumors) who underwent gamma knife radiosurgery for meningiomas between 1987 and 1992 [32]. The patients were assessed using follow-up scans, patient survey, and physician-based evaluations. Using an average tumor dose of 16 Gy (range 9–25 Gy), the authors achieved clinical tumor control in 92 of the patients (93%). Sixty-one (63%) of the tumors decreased in size. Two factors seemed to predict local tumor progression: history of prior resection ($P = 0.02$) and history of multiple meningiomas ($P<0.00001$). The mean actuarial rate of post-radiosurgery complications was 4.85% at 31–120 months. Overall, 96% of the surveyed patients were satisfied with their outcome. Morita et al. [33] reviewed the results of a prospective study of 88 skull base meningiomas treated by gamma knife radiosurgery. With a median follow-up time of 35 months, the progression-free survival rate was 95% [33]. Follow-up scans showed that 68% of the tumors had decreased in size.

Modified and dedicated LINAC-based systems are also commonly used for SRS. To achieve multiple, convergent beams of radiation, the couch and gantry of the LINAC are rotated around the isocenter or target. This achieves the sharp, dose–gradient characteristic of SRS. The results of LINAC radiosurgery seem comparable to those of gamma knife SRS. Shafron [34] reported on 70 patients with 76 meningiomas. After a median follow-up of 23 months, no lesion had enlarged, and 21 out of 48 (44%) had decreased in size after at least 1 year of follow-up. Hakim et al. [35] reported on 106 benign meningiomas that were treated with LINAC radiosurgery. The 5-year actuarial tumor control rate was 89.3%.

## Fractionated Radiosurgery (Stereotactic Radiotherapy)

Based on the encouraging results of SRS and the concern about potential normal tissue toxicity from SRS, researchers developed a technique called "fractionated stereotactic radiosurgery" (FSR) or "stereotactic radiotherapy" (SRT). It combines the high-precision technology of SRS with the potential radiobiological benefits of fractionation. Examples of SRT systems include the Gill–Thomas–Cosman frame with a dental plate and strapping system and the bite plate with infrared light-emitting diodes.

Unlike the other methods, which require the use of a minimally invasive head frame, patients can be positioned with a frame that is non-invasive and re-locatable. The initial results of studies that have used SRT to treat meningiomas have been encouraging.

## Timing of Radiation Therapy

Although studies have shown that radiation therapy reduces the likelihood for tumor recurrence following subtotal resection and produces results similar to those of complete resection, the timing of radiation therapy is controversial. Given the potential side-effects of radiation and long natural history of this disease, some believe it is reasonable to use radiation therapy only when tumors recur [21]. Others believe that immediate treatment is warranted because any delay may shorten survival, decrease the interval between recurrences, increase the risk of malignant transformation, and decrease the likelihood of salvage with radiation as a result of increasing tumor burden.

For malignant histology, many oncologists recommend immediate radiation treatment (6000 cGy) following surgery, regardless of the extent of resection, owing to the very high rates of local recurrence [21]. For patients with atypical histology, the role of radiation therapy is not as clear, although patients who undergo gross total resection may not require adjuvant radiation. Patients with benign meningiomas who undergo complete resection do not benefit from radiation.

The Gamma Knife Meningioma Study Group evaluated 203 patients with histologically benign parasagittal meningiomas [36]. Based on their results, the authors recommended that patients should receive radiosurgery soon after surgical resection if the procedure leaves behind a residual tumor nodule or neoplastic dural remnant. No prospective, randomized trial has evaluated the timing (immediate vs delayed) of radiation therapy for meningiomas.

In conclusion, radiation therapy seems to play an important role in the overall management of patients with meningiomas. Its use as an adjunctive or primary therapy has thus far been valuable in the multi-modality approach for these patients. Innovative approaches with stereotactic radiosurgery, intensity-modulated radiation therapy, fractionated radiosurgery, and brachytherapy represent promising options. However, because some of these treatments do not have mature results, long-term follow-up is needed before we can make any definitive statements about their effectiveness.

# Tumor Biology

## Mechanisms of Tumorigenesis

Similar to tumorigenesis in other tissues, development of meningiomas is likely to result from complex interactions between genes and environment. The etiological role of environmental factors in meningioma development has been suggested for ionizing radiation, diet, smoking, head trauma, and occupational exposures to carcinogenic substances. Of these factors, the evidence is convincing only for an association between ionizing radiation and meningiomas. Elevated risk of meningioma development was shown in studies involving patients who received a low-dose radiation therapy for childhood tinea capitis. Meningiomas were also found to occur years after any type of therapeutic cranial irradiation. Moreover, an increased incidence of meningiomas has been recently reported in survivors of atomic bomb explosions. Radiation-induced meningiomas are often aggressive or malignant. They are also likely to be multiple, and they have a high recurrence rate following treatment. Furthermore, it is suggested that they display a distinct pattern of molecular genetic aberrations compared with sporadic meningiomas.

## Inherited Susceptibility Factors

In general, germline mutations and metabolic mutations (polymorphisms) are the two groups of genetic alterations that are associated with increased constitutional cancer risk. Both of these groups of inherited susceptibility factors have been implicated in meningioma development. The first group consists of genes that exhibit high penetrance but are present in a low frequency in human populations. The familial occurrence of meningiomas, usually multiple, occurs often in association with NF-2. Overall, more than 50% of NF-2 patients develop meningiomas. The phylogenetically conserved gene that is the target for NF-2 resides on chromosome 22q12 and was cloned in its entirety in 1993. Studies of both meningiomas from NF-2 patients and sporadically occurring meningiomas firmly place the NF-2 tumor suppressor gene in a causal role for tumorigenesis of meningiomas. It was recently shown that NF-2-associated and sporadic meningiomas share a common spectrum and frequency of allelic losses and similar proliferative activity. The NF-2 gene encodes for a protein of 595 amino acids termed "schwannomin" or "merlin". Schwannomin/merlin is a member of the band 4.1 superfamily of proteins that are thought to play crucial roles in linking cell membrane proteins with cytoskeleton, a previously unknown site of activation of tumor suppressor genes in humans.

Werner's syndrome (WS) is one of several rare genetic disorders characterized by genetic instability and premature onset of age-related diseases, such as atherosclerosis and an unusual spectrum of tumors that includes soft-tissue sarcomas, thyroid cancers and meningiomas. The gene mutated in WS patients – WRN gene – encodes for a DNA helicase, an enzyme that helps DNA unwind [37]. The WRN gene appears to function as a key element in resolving aberrant DNA structures that arise from DNA metabolic processes, such as replication, recombination and/or DNA repair, to preserve the genetic integrity of cells. The role of WRN gene product in tumorigenesis of WS-related and sporadic meningiomas, as well as in radiation-induced meningiomas, is unknown.

The second group of inherited susceptibility factors for meningioma consists of genes that exhibit low penetrance but appear in human populations with a high frequency. Glutathione S-transferase and cytochrome P450 are examples of genetic polymorphisms that affect the ability of the body to detoxify carcinogens, including those that can induce meningiomas in laboratory animals. Both GST-T1 null and P450 CYP2D6 poor metabolizer alleles are associated with a significantly elevated risk for meningioma development. Clearly, GST and P450 genes, as well as other polymorphic genes that are involved in the metabolism of carcinogenic compounds found in diet, cigarette smoke and some industrial chemicals, may be promising candidates to explain the gene–environment interactions in meningioma development.

## Somatic Alterations in Meningiomas

Cytogenetic studies and analyses of loss of heterozygosity of certain DNA markers in meningiomas suggested the existence of genes that play a role in meningioma development. In spite of the fact that meningiomas are cytogenetically among the best characterized solid tumors in humans, the responsible genes residing in the frequently affected chromosomes remain unidentified. Alterations of the chromosome 22 occur in about 60% of meningiomas, while other cytogenetic alterations such as loss of genetic material on chromosomes 1p, 14q, 10 and 18q, as well as gains on 20q, 12q, 15q and 1q, are less frequent. Some of these changes were associated with progression of meningiomas to more aggressive forms. To date, only the importance of a chromosome 22 deletion in meningioma tumorigenesis has been clearly demonstrated with the cloning of the NF-2 gene.

## Tumor Suppressor Genes

### NF-2 Tumor Suppressor

Mutational analyses of the NF-2 gene and studies of the NF-2 protein show that the NF-2 protein is often dramatically reduced or absent in about 50% of sporadic meningiomas, including those tumors that do not harbor mutations in the NF-2 gene. Interestingly, alterations in NF-2 gene and protein expression were rarely found in the meningothelial meningioma variant, suggesting the existence of other meningioma susceptibility gene(s).

In spite of intense study of NF-2 gene functions, the molecular mechanisms that enable the NF-2 protein to function as a tumor suppressor are largely unknown. As a member of the band-4.1 superfamily of proteins, the NF-2 protein is considered important in the regulation of actin cytoskeleton and in interactions between cytoplasmic proteins and membranes. A possible physiological role of the NF-2 protein was suggested by its antiproliferative effect on some cell types, including meningioma cells. The NF-2 protein has also been shown to modulate cellular adhesion [38]. Further clues about NF-2 protein functions come from identification of cellular proteins that physically interact with the NF-2 protein. The list of NF-2 protein-interacting molecules includes:

II-spectrin, an actin-binding protein, extracellular matrix receptor β1-integrin, and regulatory cofactor for an $Na^+/H^+$ exchanger. It is, therefore, possible that mutated/inactivated NF-2 protein contributes to meningioma tumorigenesis by impairing signal transduction from the extracellular matrix and/or ion channels to the cytoskeleton, and thus deleteriously alters molecular pathways that control cell differentiation, growth and survival. In addition, naturally occurring mutant forms of NF-2 protein, but not the full-length NF-2 protein that exhibits growth-suppressive activity, physically interact with a novel coiled-coil protein of unknown function, termed "SCHIP-1" [39]. Clearly, the NF-2 protein is a tumor suppressor that is regulated in a complex manner to control diverse biological functions.

## Other Tumor Suppressor Genes

Besides the loss of NF-2 tumor suppressor expression in about 50% of sporadic meningiomas, the expression of another member of the band-4.1 family of proteins was found to be lost in about 60% of these tumors [40]. This novel tumor suppressor gene, DAL-1 (differentially expressed in adenocarcinoma of the lung) from chromosome 18p11.3, appears to be important in the early stages of meningioma tumorigenesis. Recently, a gene from human chromosome 22 that belongs to the glycosyl-transferase gene family has been isolated. Abnormal function of that gene may be involved in meningioma tumorigenesis by altering the composition of gangliosides and other glycosylated molecules.

Because of a higher incidence of meningiomas in patients with a history of breast cancer, breast cancer genes BRCA1 and BRCA2 were examined for loss of heterozygosity in meningiomas. However, alterations of these tumor suppressor genes were not detected in meningiomas [41]. Similarly, another tumor suppressor gene, PTEN, was initially suspected as a meningioma tumor suppressor gene because of the gene's location on chromosome 10q, the region with allelic loss commonly associated with malignant progression of meningiomas. The PTEN gene was recently found to be unaltered in meningiomas, and it was therefore ruled out as a meningioma tumor suppressor gene.

Because the loss of p53 tumor suppressor functions is the most common genetic alteration in human cancer, several studies carried out mutational analysis of p53 gene and p53 protein expression levels in meningioma. While the frequency of p53 alterations in meningiomas varies among studies [42], the common finding is that accumulation of p53 protein is associated with meningiomas with a high proliferative potential, i.e. the anaplastic and recurrent tumors [42]. Mutational analysis of tumors with high level of p53 protein expression suggests that overexpressed p53 protein is often not a mutant, but rather a wild-type p53 protein. It was suggested, therefore, that the accumulation of p53 protein and mutations in p53 gene could be used as a potential marker to detect the progression of meningiomas.

Loss of heterozygosity at chromosome 1p, particularly in the 1p36 and 1p34-p32 regions, is frequently detected in meningiomas. Interestingly, the loss of chromosome 1p was shown to be associated with NF-2 gene alterations and more frequent tumor recurrence following surgery. Because of the large size of chromosome 1p, loss of many genes could account for the more aggressive behavior of meningiomas with monosomy of chromosome 1p. Because the tumor suppressor gene p18 resides on chromosome 1p32, its locus was analyzed for loss of heterozygosity in meningioma and excluded as a candidate meningioma gene [43]. Interestingly, the loss of tissue non-specific alkaline phosphatase protein encoded by gene that maps to 1p36.1-p34 was demonstrated in areas of meningioma with monosomy 1p, suggesting its possible role as a candidate tumor suppressor gene in meningiomas [44]. Further genetic research is likely to result in the discovery of novel meningioma-related tumor suppressor gene(s) residing on chromosome 1p and other chromosomes implicated in meningioma tumorigenesis.

## Growth Factors and Ras Signal Transduction Pathway

Besides loss of tumor suppressor functions, an enhanced signal transduction through the polypeptide growth factors and protein tyrosine kinase (PTK) receptors is the best-characterized group of molecular alterations that are associated with meningioma tumorigenesis. Growth factors and their receptors, which transduce their signals through Ras GTPase proteins, are overexpressed on the same population of tumor cells compared with normal, precursor leptomeningeal cells. The Ras proto-oncogene family encodes four closely related plasma membrane proteins of 21 kDa that are essential for entry into the mitotic cell cycle, for maintenance of proliferation, and for regulation of differentiation, adhesion molecule expression and cytoskeletal actin organization. Therefore, overexpression of growth factors and their receptors enhances signal transduction through the Ras pathway with a consequent aberration of cellular functions that are considered critically important in meningioma tumorigenesis.

The list of aberrantly overexpressed molecules is long and includes epidermal, platelet-derived, fibroblastic, insulin-like and vascular endothelial growth factors (EGF, PDGF, FGF, IGF, VEGF, respectively) and their PTK receptors. At present, it is not known which growth factors and/or receptors are the most critical in meningioma tumorigenesis. Nevertheless, the expression of VEGF by tumor cells appears to be prognostically relevant. Elevated expression of VEGF is found in most meningiomas, and it correlates with the development of meningioma blood supply from cerebral arteries and

emergence of peritumoral brain edema. Further-more, high levels of VEGF expression were recently identified as the most powerful predictor of meningioma recurrence.

The clinical importance of frequent expression of the hepatocyte growth factor (HGF) and c-met, a proto-oncogene that encodes receptor for HGF by meningioma cells, is not known, but HGF and c-met may represent an important link with the NF-2 tumor suppressor pathway. It was recently shown that the HGF-regulated tyrosine kinase substrate physically interacts in vivo and in vitro with NF-2 tumor suppressor protein [45]. At present, it is not clear exactly how the HGF and NF-2 molecular pathways cross-talk. Another line of evidence suggests that the NF-2 protein antiproliferative action may occur downstream of Ras proteins. Overexpression of the NF-2 protein is able to reverse some aspects of the Ras-protein-induced malignant phenotype, such as anchorage-independent growth in a soft agar, and to restore contact inhibition of cell growth.

## Sex Hormones

One of the most consistent findings in epidemiological studies of meningiomas is that these tumors are about twice as common in women as in men. The proposed role of sex hormones in meningioma tumorigenesis is further supported by an observation that breast cancer and meningiomas appear to occur together more frequently than would be expected by chance, and by detection of estrogen and progesterone receptors in meningiomas. While it is well recognized that human meningiomas express progesterone receptors, there is still uncertainty about the presence of estrogen receptors in these tumors. However, the use of polymerase chain reaction method, which is more sensitive than the immunohistochemical or ligand binding assays, reveals that both receptors may be present in most meningiomas. At present, it is not clear whether these receptors are functional in meningioma and whether the therapeutic use of progesterone and/or estrogen inhibitors is beneficial. Nevertheless, the presence/absence of progesterone receptors in meningiomas may have prognostic and therapeutic implications. For example, proliferating meningioma cells do not express progesterone receptors, and tumors with a high proliferative

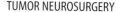

index are more likely to express no or low levels of progesterone receptors. In addition, meningiomas that are progesterone-receptor-negative appear to be more likely to recur. Further investigations are required to delineate the definitive significance of sex hormones in meningiomas.

# Future Therapy

A more detailed understanding of molecular mechanisms involved in meningioma tumorigenesis has opened the door for new anticancer treatment approaches that are based on the concept of target-specific therapies. Molecular-based treatment strategies targeting the precise molecular abnormalities that create and drive the neoplastic phenotype offer a great hope as future meningioma treatments. These approaches include gene therapy to restore the functions of inactivated NF-2 gene and other meningioma-associated tumor suppressors, and the use of gene therapy or several promising small molecule agents that inhibit signal transduction molecules responsible for overactivation of the growth factor/Ras signaling pathway.

Besides trying to replace a defective tumor suppressor gene with a functional allele, or to deliver genes that can help kill tumor cells, gene therapy technology encompasses many additional applications, such as adoptive immunotherapy, anti-angiogenesis, and anti-telomerase approaches to cancer treatment. For example, virus-mediated delivery was successfully used to introduce functional NF-2 tumor suppressor gene into NF-2-gene-deficient meningioma cell lines. It is likely that such an approach can be used to deliver other meningioma-associated tumor suppressor genes, such as DAL-1 and p53, to target early and late stages of meningioma progression, respectively.

The elevated expression of a large number of polypeptide growth factors and their tyrosine kinase receptors is a hallmark of meningioma tumorigenesis. Many polypeptide growth factors implicated in meningioma tumorigenesis transduce their proliferative signal through Ras proteins. As expected, inhibition of Ras proteins by the adenovirus-mediated transfer of the dominant negative Ras mutant potently suppressed proliferation of exponentially growing and growth-arrested meningioma cells stimu-lated with serum. As shown in several models, another anti-cancer gene therapy approach to specifically target Ras proteins is to use anti-sense oligonucleotide inhibitors or antisense ribozymes, catalytic RNA molecules [46,47]. Another attractive molecular target of the growth factor activated Ras pathway is the Raf-1 protein. The application of the antisense oligonucleotide directed against the human Raf-1 kinase (ISIS 3521) has now reached the phase II stage of anti-cancer therapy development. If the evidence for anti-tumor effect is provided, this therapeutic approach may be applied to meningioma treatment in the future.

Anti-angiogenic gene therapy approaches are particularly attractive for meningioma treatment because of the well-documented role of VEGF in meningioma tumorigenesis and tumor recurrence. Targeting of telomerase represents an exciting new approach to cancer therapy. Because telomerase activation occurs frequently in atypical and anaplastic meningiomas, and anti-telomerase gene therapy approaches have been successfully used in animal and tissue culture models for treatment of malignant gliomas and other malignancies, there is no reason to question the applicability of this gene therapy approach to the treatment of meningiomas. The major limiting factor of successful clinical use of gene therapy for treatment of cancer, including meningiomas, is the lack of selectivity and low efficiency of the currently available vector delivery systems. Improved vectors and anti-sense oligonucleotides, and new formulations for enhanced delivery, are likely to circumvent degradation and delivery difficulties and thus improve the clinical application of gene therapy technology.

At present, however, treatment of meningiomas by small molecule compounds that target molecular abnormalities can be a more promising approach to treat meningiomas in humans. For example, recently developed selective kinase inhibitors of PDGF, EGF and VEGF receptors may one day serve as novel therapeutic agents for the treatment of meningiomas [48]. Unfortunately, it is not clear which PTK receptors are the most critical in meningioma tumorigenesis, and therefore, simultaneous specific targeting of several PTK receptors, or use of broad-spectrum PTK inhibitors, is likely to be required to achieve therapeutic response in humans.

A better approach, however, may be to target Ras proteins or molecules downstream of Ras proteins through which meningioma-associated growth factors transduce their signals. These include small molecule inhibitors of the enzyme farnesyl-protein transferase (FPTase) and mevalonate pathway inhibitors that suppress those enzymes that are involved in production of farnesyl diphosphate, the substrate for FPTase. Because farnesylation is critical for converting a cytoplasmic and biologically inactive precursor Ras protein into a functional membrane-associated protein, several pharmaceutical companies are currently assessing anticancer activities of FPTase inhibitors in clinical trials.

Considering the nature of molecular alterations in meningiomas, one can hypothesize that inhibition of proteins that function downstream of the growth factor/Ras pathway by small molecule compounds can also be therapeutically useful. For example, a novel inhibitor drug, PD 184352, was recently discovered to directly and specifically inhibit the Mek-1 kinase, a protein that acts downstream of Ras proteins to activate extracellular signal-regulated kinases Erk-1 and Erk-2. This Mek-1 inhibitor significantly suppressed the growth of human colon and ovarian xenograft tumors in mice without unacceptable side-effects [49].

It is well established that activation of the growth factor/Ras pathway causes increased turnover of the arachidonic acid metabolism, including production of prostaglandins and leukotrienes, by regulating the activity of cytosolic phospholipase A2, cyclooxygenases (COX-1 and COX-2) and 5-lipoxygenase (5-LO), respectively. Dramatically elevated concentrations of arachidonic acid, prostaglandins and leukotrienes have been reported to occur in meningiomas compared with normal brain tissue, and are believed to be important mediators of peritumoral brain edema. One can therefore speculate that inhibitors of these lipid enzymes, such as COX-2-specific and 5-LO inhibitors, may be of use to prevent or treat meningiomas and peritumoral edema. At least six cancer trials with a COX-2-specific inhibitor, celecoxib, are currently underway [50]. Boswellic acids, naturally occurring compounds isolated from the gum-resin exudate from the stem of the tree Boswellia serrata (frankincense), are potent inhibitors of 5-LO. At low micromolar, physiologically achievable concentrations, boswellic acids are cytotoxic for meningioma and glioma cells [51]. A phase I/II clinical trial to establish the effects of boswellic acids on peritumoral edema in glioblastoma patients is currently in progress (at www.medizin.uni-tuebingen.de/~webnonk/clinical.html ).

Clearly, an improved understanding of the biological functions of known genes that play a critical role in meningioma development, as well as identification of novel molecular abnormalities, will provide potential targets for new therapeutic approaches that are both more effective and better tolerated than the traditional therapies.

## Key Points

- *Surgical approaches may vary in meningioma surgery depending upon the tumor location and size.*
- *The amount of residual tumor after surgery is a major determinant of the rate of recurrence.*
- *Radiation therapy often plays an important role in the overall management of patients with meningiomas.*
- *Radiosurgery is playing an increasingly important role in skull base meningiomas.*
- *The treatment of meningiomas will continue to advance through continued research at the subcellular level coupled with advances in molecular therapy.*

## References

1. Rachlin JR, Rosenblum ML. Etiology and biology of meningiomas. In: Al-Mefty O, editor. Meningiomas. New York: Raven Press, 1991; 27–35.
2. DeMonte F, Al Mefty O. Meningiomas. In: Kaye AH, Laws ER Jr, editors. Brain Tumors. New York: Churchill Livingstone, 1995; 675–704.
3. Kurland LT, Schoenberg BS, Annegers JF et al. The incidence of primary intracranial neoplasms in Rochester, Minnesota. Ann N Y Acad Sci 1982;381:6–16.
4. Nakasu S, Hirano A, Shimura T et al. Incidental meningiomas in autopsy study. Surg Neurol 1987;27:319–22.
5. Fan KJ, Pezeshkpour GH. Ethnic distribution of primary central nervous system tumors in Washington DC, 1971–1985. J Natl Med Assoc 1992;84:858–63.
6. Haddad G, AL-Mefty O. Meningiomas: an overview. In: Wilkins RH, Rengachary SS, editors. Neurosurgery. New York: McGraw-Hill, 1996; 833–41.

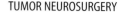
7. Drake JM, Hoffman HJ. Meningiomas in children. In: Al-Mefty O, editor. Meningiomas. New York: Raven Press, 1991; 145–52.

8. Ersahin A, Ozdamar N, Demirtas E, Karabiyikoglu M. Meningioma of the cavernous sinus in a child. Childs Nerv Syst 1999;15(1):8–10.

9. Giangaspero F, Guiducci A, Lenz FA, Mastronardi L, Burger PC. Meningioma with meningoangiomatosis: a condition mimicking invasive meningiomas in children and young adults: report of two cases and review of the literature. Am J Surg Pathol 1999;23:872–5.

10. Inskip PD, Mellelkjaer L, Gridley G, Olsen JH. Incidence of intracranial tumors following hospitalization for head injuries (Denmark). Cancer Causes Control 1998;9(1):109–16.

11. Parent AD. Multiple meningiomas. In: Al-Mefty O, editor. Meningiomas. New York: Raven Press, 1991;161–8.

12. Levy WJ Jr, Bay J, Dohn D. Spinal cord meningiomas. J Neurosurg 1982;57:804–12.

13. Fox J. Meningiomas and associated lesions. In: Al-Mefty O, editor. Meningiomas. New York: Raven Press, 1991;129–36.

14. Iida A, Kurose K, Isobe R, Akiyama F, Sakamoto G, Yoshimoto M et al. Mapping of a new target region of allelic loss to a 2-cM interval at 22q13.1 in primary breast cancer. Genes Chromosomes Cancer 1998;21(2):108–12.

15. Kuratsu JI, Kochi M, Ushio Y. Incidence and clinical features of asymptomatic meningiomas. J Neurosurg 2000;92:766–70.

16. Jaaskelainen J, Haltia M, Laasonen E, Wahlstrom T, Valtonen S. The growth rate of intracranial meningiomas in its relation to histology. An analysis of 43 patients. Surg Neurol 1985;24:165–72.

17. Cho K, Hoshiro T, Nagashima T, Murovic J, Wilson C. Predication of tumor doubling time in recurrent meningiomas. J Neurosurg 1986;65:790–4.

18. Shino A, Nakasu S, Matsuda M, Handa J, Morikawa S, Inubushi T. Noninvasive evaluation of the malignant potential of intracranial meningiomas performed using proton magnetic resonance spectroscopy. J Neurosurg 1999;91:928–34.

19. Simpson D. The recurrence of intracranial meningiomas after surgical treatment. Neurol Nerosurg Psychiat 1957;20:22–39.

20. Melamed S, Sahar A, Beller AJ. The recurrence of intracranial meningiomas. Neurochirurgie 1979;22:47–51.

21. Chan R, Thompson G. Morbidity, mortality, and quality of life following surgery for intracranial meningiomas. A retrospective study in 257 cases. J Neurosurg 1984;60:52–60.

22. Mirimanoff RO, Dosoretz DE, Linggood RM, Ojemann RG, Martuza RL. Meningioma: analysis of recurrence and progression following neurosurgical resection. J Neurosurg 1985;62:18–24.

23. Kallio M, Sankila R, Hakulinen T, Jaaskelainen J. Factors affecting operative and excess long-term mortality in 935 patients with intracranial meningiomas. Neurosurgery 1992;31:2–12.

24. Jaaskelainen J, Haltia M, Servo A. Atypical and anaplastic menigiomas: radiology surgery, radiotherapy, and outcome. Surg Neurol 1986;25:233–42.

25. Kakinuma K, Tanaka R, Onda K, Takahashi H. Proliferative potential of recurrent intracranial meningiomas as evaluated by labeling indices of BUdR and KI-67, and tumor doubling time. Acta Neurochir (Wien) 1998;140:26–31.

26. May P, Broome J, Lawry J, Buxton R, Battersby R. A flow cytometric study of paraffin-embedded archival material. J Neurosurg 1989;71:347–51.

27. Mantle R, Lach B, Delgado M, Baeesa S, Belanger G. Predicting the probability of meningioma recurrence based on the quality of peritumoral brain edema on computerized tomography scanning. J Neurosurg 1999;91:375–83.

28. Nakasu S, Nakasu Y, Nakajima M, Matsuda M, Handa J. Preoperative identification of meningiomas that are highly likely to recur. J Neurosurg 1999;90:455–62.

29. Lee JH, Evans JJ, Kosmorsky G. Surgical management of clinoidal meningiomas. Neurosurgery 2001;48:1012–21.

30. Nutting C, Brada M, Brazil L et al. Radiotherapy in the treatment of benign meningiomas of the skull base. J Neurosurg 1999;90:823–7.

31. Patil AA, Kumar P, Leibrock LG. Response to extra-axial tumors to stereotactically implanted high-activity I-125 seeds. Stereotactic Funct Neurosurg 1995;64:139–52..

32. Kondziolka D, Levy EI, Niranjan A, Flickinger JC, Lunsford LD. Long-term outcomes after meningioma radiosurgery: physician and patient perspectives. J Neurosurg 1999;91:44–50.

33. Morita A, Coffey RJ, Foote RL, Schiff D, Gorman D. Risk of injury to cranial nerves after gamma knife radiosurgery for skull base meningiomas: experience in 88 patients. J Neurosurg 1999;90:42–9.

34. Shafron DH, Friedman WA, Buatti JM, Bova FJ, Mendenhall WM. Linac radiosurgery for benign meningiomas. Int J Radiat Oncol Biol Phys 1999;43:321–7.

35. Hakim R, Alexander E 3rd, Loeffler JS et al. Results of linear accelerator-basedradiosurgery for intracranial meningiomas. Neurosurgery 1998;42:446–53.

36. Kondziolka D, Flickinger JC, Perez B. Judicious resection and/or radiosurgery for parasagittal meningiomas: outcomes from a multicenter review. Gamma Knife Meningioma Study Group. Neurosurgery 1998;43:405–13.

37. Shen J-L, Loeb LA. The Werner syndrome gene: the molecular basis of RecQ helicase-deficiency diseases. Trends Genet 2000;16:213–20.

38. Huynh DP, Pulst SM. Neurofibromatosis 2 antisense oligodeoxynucleotides induce reversible inhibition of schwannomin synthesis and cell adhesion in STS26T and T98G cells. Oncogene 1996;13:73–84.

39. Goutebroze L, Brault E, Muchardt C, Camonis J, Thomas G. Cloning and characterization of SCHIP-1, a novel protein interacting specifically with spliced isoforms and naturally occurring mutant NF2 proteins. Mol Cell Biol 2000;20:1699–1712.

40. Gutmann DH, Donahoe J, Perry A, Lemke N, Gorse K, Kittiniyom K et al. Loss of DAL-1, a protein 4.1-related tumor suppressor, is an important early event in the pathogenesis of meningiomas. Hum Mol Genet 2000;9:1495–1500.

41. Kirsch M, Zhu JJ, Black PM. Analysis of the BRCA1 and BRCA2 genes in sporadic meningiomas. Genes Chromosomes Cancer 1997;20:53–9.

42. Cho H, Ha SY, Park SH, Park K, Chae YS. Role of p53 gene mutation in tumor aggressiveness of intracranial meningiomas. J Korean Med Sci 1999;14:199–205.

43. Santarius T, Kirsch M, Nikas DC, Imitoal J, Black PM. Molecular analysis of alteration of the p18INK4c gene in human meningiomas. Neuropathol Appl Neurobiol 2000;26:67–75.

44. Mueller P, Henn W, Niedermayer I, Ketter R, Feiden W, Steudel WI et al. Deletion of chromosome 1p and loss of expression of alkaline phosphatase indicate progression of meningiomas. Clin Cancer Res 1999;5:3569–77.

45. Scoles DR, Huynh DP, Chen MS, Burke SP, Gutmann DH, Pulst S-M. The neurofibromatosis 2 tumor suppressor protein interacts with hepatocyte growth-factor regulated tyrosine kinase substrate. Hum Mol Genet 2000;9:1567–74.

46. Cooper C, Jones HG, Weller RO et al. Production of prostaglandins and thromboxane by isolated cells from intracranial tumors. J Neurol Neurosurg Psychiatry 1984;47:579–84.

47. Scanlon KJ, Kashani-Sabet M. Ribozymes as therapeutic agents: are we getting closer? J Natl Cancer Inst 1998;90:558–9.

48. Levitzki A. Protein tyrosine kinase inhibitors as novel therapeutic agents. Pharmacol Ther 1999;82:231–9.

49. Sebolt-Leopold JS, Dudley DT, Herrera R et al. Blockade of the MAP kinase pathway suppresses growth of colon tumors in vivo. Nat Med 1999;5:810–16.

50. Smigel K. Arthritis drug approved for polyp prevention blazes trail for other prevention trials. J Natl Cancer Inst 2000;92:297–9.

51. Park YS, Lee JH, Harwalkar JA, Bondar J, Safayhi H, Golubic M. Acetyl-11B-Boswellic Acid (AKBA) is cytotoxic for meningioma cells and inhibits phosphorylation of the extracellular-signal regulated kinase 1 and 2. In: Honn KV, Nigam S, Marnett IJ, Dennis E, editors. Proceedings of the 6th International Conference on Eicosanoids and Other Bioactive Lipids in Cancer, Inflammation and Related Diseases. New York: Plenum Publishing, 2000.

# 13

# Intraventricular and Pineal Region Tumors

Sandeep Kunwar, G. Evren Keles, Mitchell S. Berger

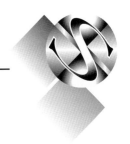

## Summary

Intraventricular and pineal region tumors represent 2% of all primary central nervous system tumors but have many unique features. Because many patients present with symptomatic hydrocephalus, urgent treatment of the tumor or hydrocephalus is often needed. Both benign and malignant tumors can arise in these regions, and often radiographic imaging is non-diagnostic. Surgery remains the main therapeutic approach for these tumors but is complicated by the central location of these lesions. A successful resection of intraventricular and pineal region tumors is based on a thorough knowledge of the relevant cerebral anatomy and the deep vascular system, avoidance of functionally eloquent areas and use of limited retraction.

## Intraventricular Tumors

Brain tumors located in the ventricles constitute 1.4% of all primary central nervous system tumors, and 5.4% of all central nervous tumors in the pediatric age group [1]. The most common primary neoplasms of the third ventricle are neuroepithelial tumors [2]. These tumors include juvenile pilocytic astrocytoma, astrocytoma, subependymal giant cell astrocytoma, ependymoma and glioblastoma multiforme. Although juvenile pilocytic astrocytomas most often originate from the floor of the third ventricle, they may arise from the posterior pituitary or optic system and extend into the ventricle. Low-grade astrocytomas, as well as anaplastic astrocytoma and glioblastoma multiforme, typically originate from the thalamic region. Ependymomas, and less frequently subependymomas, originate from the ventricular wall. These lesions are more common in the lateral ventricles. Subependymal giant cell astrocytoma, which may be associated with tuberous sclerosis, often originates at the foramen of Monro and is more frequently seen in the lateral ventricle. Colloid cysts are the most common lesions located in the third ventricle [3]. Although rare, epidermoid and dermoid tumors may occur in the third ventricle, and usually are solid rather than cystic at this location. Meningiomas originating from the velum interpositum and choroid plexus papillomas are also seen in the third ventricle. Craniopharyngioma and suprasellar germinomas can invade the floor of the third ventricle. Another main group of tumors that may grow into the third ventricle originate from the pineal gland and will be discussed in detail later in this chapter. In addition to these primary neoplasms, metastatic tumors may occur in the third ventricle and invade its floor or lateral walls.

Regarding lateral ventricle tumors, in a study excluding tumors that originated in the brain parenchyma with secondary extension into the ventricles, the authors found that the most common histologic diagnosis in adults was astrocytoma, followed by meningioma [2]. In the pediatric age group, the most common diagnosis was subependymal giant cell astrocytoma. In another series [4], the most frequent tumor types were subependymal giant cell astrocytoma, choroid plexus tumors, ependymoma and astrocytoma. The most common location for lateral ventricular tumors was the trigone (38%), followed by the cella media (33%) and the frontal horn (27%) [2].

Intraventricular meningioma, although rare, is a well circumscribed tumor, most often located in the trigone, and constitutes approximately 0.5–2% of all intracranial meningiomas [3] (Figure 13.1). Approximately 80% occur in the lateral ventricles, more commonly in the left trigone, but can occur in the third ventricle, and less frequently in the fourth ventricle. Most patients present in the fourth to the sixth decades, and these tumors are more common in women. The intraventricular location of these slow-growing tumors provides a compensatory mechanism in the form of reserve space, which contributes to the delay in clinical demonstration of symptoms and signs. They may either arise from the choroid plexus and grow within the ventricle, or arise from the tela choroidea and grow partly within the ventricle and partly into the surrounding brain tissue. Imaging characteristics are similar to those of other meningiomas, being sharply defined and globular.

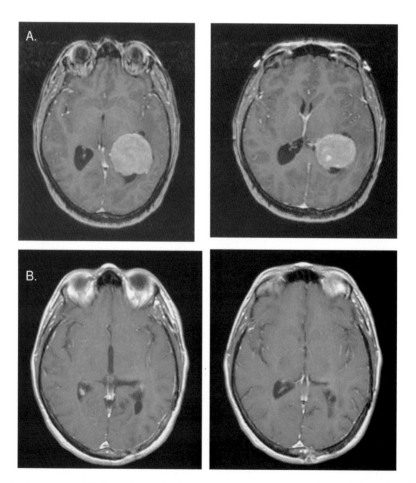

**Fig. 13.1. a** Despite the large size of the tumor, the patient had minimum symptoms and presented with headaches. **b** Postoperative images after resection via the superior parietal lobule. Because of the location within the dominant hemisphere, a posterior middle temporal gyrus approach would carry risk of speech impairment.

Intracranial ependymomas represent about 2% of brain tumors in adults, and 5.2–6.9% of all tumors in the pediatric population [1]. Approximately one-third of childhood ependymomas arise from the supratentorial ventricular system, and supratentorial lesions are more common in children over the age of 3 years. Adult patients tend to be relatively young, with most series reporting median ages under 45 years [5–7]. Although controversial, age, tumor location, tumor grade and extent of surgical resection have been suggested to be of prognostic significance. Subependymomas are benign, usually asymptomatic, nodules on the ventricular wall and are most commonly detected as an incidental autopsy finding.

Subependymal giant cell astrocytomas are seen in 6–19% of patients with tuberous sclerosis, and may also occur in the absence of this autosomal dominant phakomatosis [8,9]. Despite the benign nature of these tumors, they mostly arise near the foramen of Monro and may grow large enough to obstruct the foramen and cause obstructive hydrocephalus. Intratumoral hemorrhage and malignant differentiation have also been reported.

Choroid plexus tumors are more common in the lateral ventricles when compared with the third ventricle. In contrast to adults, in whom the majority of choroid plexus tumors are located in the fourth ventricle and the cerebellopontine angle, approximately 75% of choroid plexus tumors in children are found in the lateral ventricles, mostly located in the atrium. In a recent meta-analysis including 566 well documented choroid plexus tumors, histology was the most important prognostic factor, as 5- and 10-year projected survival rates were 81 and 77% for choroid plexus papillomas (n = 353) compared to 41 and 35% in choroid plexus carcinomas, respectively (P < 0.0005) [10]. Surgery was also a statistically significant prognostic factor for both choroid plexus papillomas and choroid plexus carcinomas.

## Relevant Anatomy

As a variety of eloquent structures surround the third and lateral ventricles, a thorough knowledge of the related anatomy, including neural and vascular structures, is essential in evaluating neuroimaging studies and in planning surgery.

The roof of the third ventricle is formed by the tela choroidea and the forniceal body. The anterior wall is formed by the lamina terminalis, forniceal columns, optic recess and the foramen of Monro. Medial surface of the thalamus forms the posterosuperior aspect of the lateral wall of the third ventricle. Separated by the hypothalamic sulcus, the hypothalamus constitutes the antero-inferior aspect of the lateral wall. The third ventricle floor consists of the optic chiasm, the tuber cinerum and infundibulum, mammillary bodies, posterior perforated substance and the superior aspect of the tegmentum. Pericallosal arteries, medial posterior choroidal arteries, internal cerebral veins and the branches of the circle of Willis inferiorly are vascular structures of critical importance in this region.

The lateral ventricles extend from the foramen of Monro anteriorly into the frontal lobe as the frontal horn. The walls of each frontal horn are formed by the genu of the corpus callosum anteriorly; by the septum pellucidum, the foramen of Monro and the forniceal column medially; and by the head of the caudate nucleus laterally. The floor is formed by the rostrum of the corpus callosum. The choroid plexus passes through the foramen of Monro and curves posteriorly to line the roof of the third ventricle. The anteromedially located septal vein joins the posterolaterally located thalamostriate vein at the foramen of Monro to form the inferior cerebral vein. The body of each lateral ventricle extends from the posterior aspect of the foramen of Monro to the junction of the corpus callosum with the fornix. The body is surrounded by the body of the caudate nucleus laterally and by the corpus callosum superiorly. The striothalamic sulcus divides the thalamus from the caudate nucleus and houses the thalamostriate vein and the stria terminalis. Tumors located in the body of the lateral ventricles derive most of their blood supply from the posterior lateral choroidal arteries. Caudal to the thalamus, the lateral ventricle curves laterally and anteriorly forming the temporal horn. Posteriorly from the junction of the body and the temporal horn extends the occipital horn. The triangular expansion of the ventricle between the occipital and temporal horns is the atrium, i.e. the trigone. The visual projection fibers are located laterally to the atrium. Tumors located in the atrium are supplied from the anterior choroidal and posterior lateral choroidal arteries.

## Pre-operative Evaluation

Intraventricular tumors are often slow-growing and benign. These lesions frequently grow large before clinical manifestations and, ultimately, produce symptoms secondary to hydro-cephalus, either by obstruction of the normal pathways of cerebrospinal fluid flow or by its overproduction. Most patients present with headaches [2]. Colloid cysts, which typically occur anteriorly and superiorly within the third ventricle, have a tendency to intermittently obstruct the foramen of Monro, resulting in acute lateral ventricular hydrocephalus with symptoms of intracranial hypertension. Visual loss, impotence and diabetes insipidus may be caused by tumors invading the floor of the third ventricle. Asymmetric bitemporal hemianopia, starting with inferior temporal field loss, may occur due to dilatation of the third ventricle with pressure on the optic chiasm from above. The extension of the tumor may cause a variety of visual field defects, including homonymous hemianopia, binasal field defects, arcuate defects and central scotoma [11].

The standard preoperative imaging study is MRI. An MR scan provides information regarding the size of the tumor, its degree of invasion, its relationship with the surrounding anatomical structures and the extent of hydrocephalus. Information regarding the relationship of the tumor with surrounding venous structures is also critical in planning surgery. The exact location of the tumor, e.g. posterior third ventricle versus pineal or quadrigeminal, is of crucial importance in planning the surgical approach.

Neuroendocrinologic evaluation may be necessary, depending on the degree of hypothalamic involvement. Germ cell markers that will be detailed later in this chapter should be obtained if the tumor is suspected of being of germ cell origin. Visual field testing is obtained if the visual pathways are affected, and for patients undergoing a posterior approach to a tumor of the occipital horn or atrium.

Any lesion that appears to be highly vascular on MRI may be studied angiographically. Although not routine, angiography is important for large tumors and when the deep venous system should be visualized. Angiography will also provide information regarding the status of the bridging veins between the cerebral hemisphere and the sagittal sinus, useful for surgical planning. Less detailed information regarding the status of vascular structures may be obtained with MR angiography/venography in a non-invasive manner.

In addition to neoplasms covered in this chapter, differential diagnosis should include histiocytosis, sarcoidosis, neurocysticercosis, fungal and indolent bacterial infections and, although very rare, abscesses.

## Outcome

Although the main therapeutic approach is surgical resection, the decision to operate on an intraventricular tumor should be based on several factors, including the patient's age, neurological and medical status and expected survival, as well as tumor-related factors such as documented progression and resectability. The surgical approach to be selected must take into account the vital anatomical structures encountered in reaching them and the potential neurologic sequelae. The use of preoperative angiography and embolization, together with intraoperative neuronavigational guidance, may significantly facilitate the operation. A successful resection of intraventricular tumors is based on a thorough knowledge of the relevant anatomy, avoidance of functionally eloquent areas, use of limited retraction and early control of the main blood supply. For patients with no significant surgical morbidity, survival is directly linked to the histopathological characteristics of the tumor. Unlike a patient with a totally resected meningioma, survival for a patient with a totally resected glioblastoma multiforme is not favorable.

# Pineal Region Tumors

Tumors of the pineal region can be divided into germ cell tumors, pineal cell tumors and other tumors (including astrocytoma, ependymoma and meningioma) (Figure 13.2). The true incidence of pineal region tumors from historical data is difficult to extrapolate because of the variety of histopathology and often confusing nomenclature associated with them. In the most comprehensive series analyzing "pineolomas" in 4,865 cases of brain tumors, these tumors make up 0.6% of all adult brain tumors and 1–3% of pediatric brain tumors [1,12]. Several

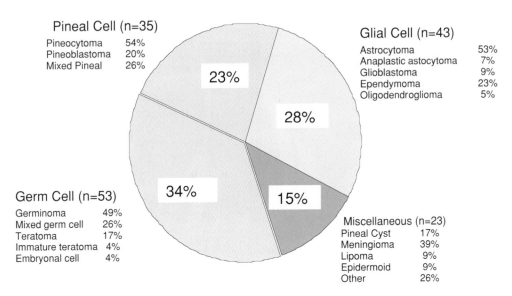

**Pineal Cell (n=35)**

| Pineocytoma | 54% |
|---|---|
| Pineoblastoma | 20% |
| Mixed Pineal | 26% |

**Glial Cell (n=43)**

| Astrocytoma | 53% |
|---|---|
| Anaplastic astocytoma | 7% |
| Glioblastoma | 9% |
| Ependymoma | 23% |
| Oligodendroglioma | 5% |

**Germ Cell (n=53)**

| Germinoma | 49% |
|---|---|
| Mixed germ cell | 26% |
| Teratoma | 17% |
| Immature teratoma | 4% |
| Embryonal cell | 4% |

**Miscellaneous (n=23)**

| Pineal Cyst | 17% |
|---|---|
| Meningioma | 39% |
| Lipoma | 9% |
| Epidermoid | 9% |
| Other | 26% |

**Fig. 13.2.** Pathological summary of 154 patients surgically treated for pineal region tumors reviewed by Bruce et al. (1995).

studies have suggested a greater incidence in Japan, ranging from 4 to 6% [13,14]. However, a prospective study of actual population-based incidence between the number of pineal region tumors seen in Niigata, Japan and Western Australia failed to show a statistically significant difference (0.07 vs 0.06 per 100,000 person-years, respectively) [15].

## Epidemiology

The most common location of extragonadal germ cell tumors occurs in two midline sites: the mediastinum (thymus) and the diencephalopineal (pineal and infundibulum) region. The origin of these non-neuroectodermal tumors remains unknown but may be related to the persistence of primordial germ cells which disseminate widely throughout many tissues and organs in the early embryo. These extra-gonadal germ cells typically have an ephemeral existence and undergo an apoptotic death. It is possible that some of these cells may survive and, over time, transform into a neoplasm. This is in contrast to the theory that the presence of these cells is related to a migrational defect. The pineal gland is the most common site of intracranial germ cell tumors (37–45%), followed by the suprasellar region (27–35%), with 10% of tumors involving both regions at presentation

[16,17] (Figure 13.3). Intracranial germ cell tumors occur most frequently between ages 10 and 21 years (70%) and 95% occur before age 33 [16]. These tumors have a marked predominance in males. Jennings et al. (1985) showed that males are 2.2 times more likely to be affected, while Bruce et al. (1995) showed a stronger male preponderance of 8.5:1. Interestingly, there is an equal sex distribution, or perhaps a bias towards females, among suprasellar germ cell tumors [12,16].

Intracranial germ cell tumors represent a heterogeneous group of tumors, divided into germinomas and non-germinomatous germ cell tumors (NGGCT). NGGCT include teratomas, embryonal cell tumors, choriocarcinomas and endodermal sinus tumors (yolk sac carcinoma). Germinomas are the most common intracranial germ cell tumor, comprising between 40 and 65% of all germ cell tumors [16,18]. Teratomas (18–20%), endodermal sinus tumors (5–7%), embryonal cell tumors (3–5%), and choriocarcinomas (3–4%) are less frequent [16,18]. Furthermore, large series with extensive tissue sampling have shown mixed germ cell histology in up to 25% of germ cell tumors [17]. Thus, it is imperative to establish an adequate histological diagnosis prior to proceeding with radiation or chemotherapy because the management and prognosis of patients with germ cell tumors vary

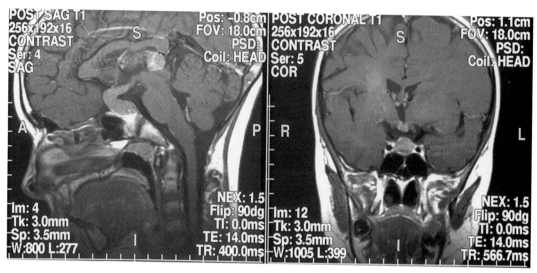

**Fig. 13.3.** Eight-year-old child with a pineal and suprasellar germinoma. Involvement of the suprasellar and pineal region is most consistent with a germ cell tumor.

greatly on histology. Germinomas, for example, can be cured by radiotherapy alone or in combination with chemotherapy in the majority of cases. NGGCT, however, do not have as good prognosis but, with aggressive surgical resection, high-dose chemotherapy and radiotherapy, long-term control can be achieved. Mature teratomas, which are the least common, are slow-growing and can be cured with surgery alone [16,18].

Parenchymal pineal tumors are neoplasms arising from pinealocytes and account for 0.4–1.0% of the 17,000 primary brain tumors diagnosed each year [19]. These tumors have been categorized as pineocytoma (low-grade), pineoblastoma (high-grade) and mixed [17,19]. Approximately 30–57% of pineal parenchymal tumors are pineocytomas, 23–50% are pineoblastomas and 20% are mixed tumors [17]. The mean age of presentation for all pineal cell tumors was 22 years, ranging from 11 months to 77 years. Pineoblastoma, the more malignant variety, has been found to occur in younger populations with a mean age of 18 years [17,19]. There is no gender preference for these tumors, although a slight male predominance has been suggested in the Japanese literature [14]. Pineoblastoma is associated with bilateral retinoblastomas (trilateral retinoblastoma) and, in such, arise from germ line mutations in the

retinoblastoma (Rb) gene. Pineoblastomas have similar histological and clinical behavior as PNETs [17,20] (Figure 13.4).

Other tumors that involve the pineal region include glial cell tumors (astrocytoma, ependymoma, oligodendroglioma), choroid plexus tumors, pineal cysts, meningiomas and metastases, which are rare in this region.

## Pathological Appearance

Macroscopically, germinomas are usually soft, grayish pink and friable; some may have a granular consistency. Focal hemorrhages and small cysts may be present. Smaller tumors can appear encapsulated, confined to the pineal region, whereas larger tumors tend to be poorly defined and infiltrate the adjacent structures, including the quadrigeminal plate, the posterior commissure, thalamus and the roof of the third ventricle [17]. Suprasellar germinomas tend to infiltrate the lamina terminalis, the optic chiasm, the septum pellucidum and the hypothalamus. Sometimes, these tumors can appear highly infiltrative without a definite mass, and may mimic an infiltrating glioma. Occasionally, suprasellar growth may extend into the sella turcica and compress the anterior lobe anteriorly or cause compression of the optic chiasm.

Embryonal carcinomas and endodermal sinus tumors have variable gross appearances

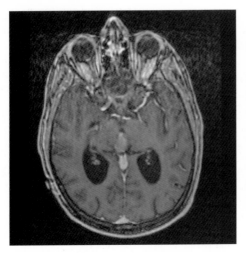 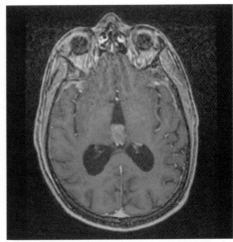

**Fig. 13.4.** Pineal region tumor presenting with progressive hydrocephalus from aqueductal obstruction. Pathology showed pineoblastoma.

depending on the degree of mixed cell types. Choriocarcinoma is often well demarcated and may contain regions of hemorrhage and necrosis. Teratomas are usually well defined, with an irregular or lobulated outer surface. These tumors may contain cartilage, bone and hair (rarely, teeth) [17]. Typically, the tumor has multiple cysts containing whitish fluid from the desquamation of the dermoid cell lining. Immature teratomas contain hemorrhage and central necrosis and have more invasive features.

Microscopically, germinoma is composed of two clearly distinguishable cell types: large germ cells and small lymphocytes [17]. The germ cells are large, polygonal or spheroidal cells with well defined cell boundaries and an eosinophilic, sometimes vacuolated, cytoplasm with large central spherical nuclei and pale nucleoplasm containing a central nucleolus. Mitotic figures and microscopic mineralization can be present. The second cell type consists of infiltrating lymphocytes clustered around tumor blood vessels. This is thought to represent a granulomatous reaction, although the significance of the immunological reaction is unknown, particularly since this cellular reaction may be completely absent in some cases. The immunological reaction has been found to be primarily a T-cell infiltrate. Occasionally, the local T-cell response predominates the histology, with the germinoma cells being few and difficult to

identify. In these cases, confusion with primary cerebral lymphoma may occur. Occasionally, multinucleated syncytiotrophoblast giant cells can be seen, which stain for human chorionic gonadotropin (bHCG). Immunohistochemical stains are useful, since germinomas will stain positive for placental alkaline phosphatase and may show variable staining for cytokeratins, the epithelial membrane antigen or vimentin [17].

Embryonal carcinoma is the least differentiated, having a monotonous pattern with aggregates of primitive epithelial cells in sheets and ribbons [17]. These tumors have the potential to differentiate toward embryonal structures, forming yolk sac or trophoblastic structures. Thus, embryonal carcinoma may give rise to mixed tumors and pure CNS embryonal carcinomas are exceedingly rare. Endodermal sinus tumor is histologically quite close to embryonal carcinomas. The key distinction is the predominance of retiform arrangements, papillary structures, PAS-positive alpha-fetoprotein (AFP)-containing hyaline globules and Schiller–Duvall bodies. Endodermal sinus tumor forms papillary projections constructed of low cuboidal epithelium.

Choriocarcinoma features two predominant cell types: cytotrophoblast and multinucleated syncytiotrophoblast. The cytotrophoblast is recognized by its epithelioid appearance, with clear cytoplasm and a single nucleus. The syncytiotrophoblasts have a very basophilic, vacuolated cytoplasm and multiple hyperchromatic nuclei which stain positive for HCG. Hemorrhage and necrosis are common.

Teratoma is composed of well differentiated tissues from all three germ cell layers (endoderm, mesoderm and endoderm). Mature teratoma may contain solid or cystic foci of squamous epithelium, cartilage or glandular or tubular structures, lined by tall columnar mucus-secreting cells. Teratoma will often contain neuroepithelial tissue showing varying degrees of glial and neuronal differentiation. It is important to differentiate any primitive features, typically in only one of the three germinal layers, which define an immature teratoma. Immature teratomas contain poorly differentiated non-neuroepithelial cells in high density, often staining positive for CEA, cytokeratins or epithelial membrane antigen (EMA) [17].

Pineoblastoma macroscopically is a soft tumor that is pinkish-gray in color and may contain hemorrhagic, necrotic or cystic components. It can be relatively well circumscribed or ill defined and invasive into local surrounding structures, often destroying the pineal gland with growth. By contrast, pineocytoma is well defined and has a pale gray color and lobulated surface. Necrosis, hemorrhage and invasion into adjacent structures are rare findings in pineocytomas. Calcification may be grossly obvious on inspection or on imaging.

Microscopically, pineoblastoma cells are highly cellular, with small, round nuclei resembling cerebellar medulloblastomas. Mitotic figures may be numerous and the tumor cell cytoplasm is scanty. The cells are usually in amorphous sheets, but ill defined Homer-Wright rosettes may be present. Occasionally, perivascular orientation of the cells may be seen. Pineoblastomas also have a propensity to seed the subarachnoid space. Pineocytoma, on the other hand, can be cellular but less so than pineoblastoma. There is a strong resemblance to normal pineocytes, with tumor cells arranged in sheets or diffuse lobules. Giant cells may be present, but mitotic figures are uncommon. Pineocytoma cells may differentiate into mature astrocytes or neurons, or both [17]. Mixed tumors may contain features of both pineocytoma and pineoblastoma, although no consensus exists on where the transition from well differentiated pineoctyoma to undifferentiated pineoblastoma occurs. Some mixed tumors have been designated when divergent differentiation exists along neuronal, glial or both lines; however, more recent designation of mixed tumors relates to the presence of pineoblastoma and pineocytoma elements [19].

The pathological appearances of other tumors (astrocytoma, ependymoma and meningioma) in the pineal region are not site-specific and are histologically similar when found within other areas of the brain.

## Relevant Anatomy

The pineal gland has a central location in the brain, such that the distance between it and the surface of any portion of the scalp is almost the same, regardless of which surgical approach is taken to this region. The anatomy of the parenchymal tissue and, more importantly, the vascular structures are critically important in considering the most appropriate approach to these tumors. Pineal tumors occupy the posterior aspect of the third ventricle and the quadrigeminal cistern. They may involve the quadrigeminal plate inferiorly, the posterior commissure and thalamus anterolaterally and the roof of the third ventricle and splenium superiorly. The arterial supply to the pineal gland is from the medial posterior choroidal artery. The draining veins from the pineal body and habenular trigone are the superior and inferior pineal veins that flow into the vein of Galen or the internal cerebral veins. The veins for the superior and inferior colliculi, the superior and inferior quadrigeminal or tectal veins also flow into the vein of Galen or the superior vermian vein. The basal veins of Rosenthal are lateral to the pineal gland and drain into the vein of Galen or the internal cerebral veins. Immediately superior to the pineal gland are the internal cerebral veins, converging and draining into the vein of Galen, sitting superior and posterior to the gland. The superior vermian vein and precentral cerebellar vein lie posterior and inferior to the pineal gland and drain into the vein of Galen as well. From a supratentorial approach, the posterior pericallosal vein and internal occipital vein can also be visualized draining into the vein of Galen.

## Pre-operative Evaluation

Patients with primary pineal region tumors present with signs and symptoms of hydrocephalus secondary to compression or involvement of the tectum, occluding the Sylvian aqueduct, including headaches, diplopia, lethargy and ataxia. Compression of the tectum may also cause Parinaud's syndrome, resulting in vertical gaze paresis, impaired pupillary light reflex and convergence nystagmus. The clinical presentation for germ cell tumors is dependent upon the sites of involvement. Suprasellar involvement, particularly with germinomas, may be associated with a long prodrome (month to several years) of signs and symptoms of hypopituitarism. Diabetes insipidus is most common because of the involvement of the infundibulum, but growth failure and hypothyroidism or precocious puberty can also be seen. Children with diabetes insipidus or hypopituitarism may harbor germ cell tumors and should be followed expectantly with MRI scans at regular intervals. Visual field or acuity impairments may occur related to compression of the optic chiasm or direct involvement of the optic nerve. Germinomas can spread directly along the floor and walls of the third ventricle or via CSF pathways. NGGCT have a higher incidence of metastatic dissemination than germinomas, with estimates ranging from 5 to 57%. Etraneural metastasis has been reported in up to 3% of all germ cell tumors, with lung and bone being the most common sites [16].

MRI is the radiographic imaging of choice in evaluating patients with pineal region tumors. CT, however, can be helpful in looking for calcification of the pineal region, which can be seen in the normal gland, germinomas, pineocytomas and teratomas, or for assessing hemorrhage and degree of ventriculomegaly. On MRI scans, germinomas are often isointense to gray matter, and slightly hyperintense on T2-weighted images. These tumors have homogeneous and dramatic contrast enhancement. Cystic areas can occasionally be seen. It is important to assess the suprasellar region and lateral and third ventricles for tumor involvement. There are no typical radiographic features of NGGCT, but they are often heterogeneous on MRI scans and tend to have infiltrating borders with variable degrees of enhancement. Teratomas, in particular, have marked heterogeneity, loculations and irregular enhancement related to lipid, soft tissue and cystic components as well as calcification. Malignant teratomas have similar features but demonstrate invasion into the surrounding structures [21]. Pineoblastomas are often heterogeneous on T1-weighted sequences and tend to be hyperintense on T2-weighted sequences. There is usually strong enhancement with some heterogeneous areas within the tumor (Figure 13.4). These tumors are aggressive and frequently disseminate in the neuraxis. There may be regions of necrosis or hemorrhage contributing to the heterogeneity. Pineocytomas are typically iso or hypointense on T1-weighted imaging with homogeneous and intense enhancement. However, pineocytomas can have variable appearance and can be associated with a hypointense cyst on T1-weighted images, similar to pineal cysts. MRI also provides critical anatomic information when considering surgical approach, extension of the tumor, the degree of brainstem involvement and the relationship of the deep venous system to the tumor.

All patients with pineal region tumors should undergo a high-resolution MRI scan with gadolinium of the head and screening MRI of the spinal axis (post-contrast sagittal view). Patients also require CSF and serum measurements of AFP, human chorionic gonadotropin (HCG) and CEA levels. CSF should also be sent for cytology. Evaluation of pituitary function should be performed if endocrine abnormalities are suspected and formal visual field examination in patients with evidence of suprasellar involvement.

## Management and Outcome

Surgery has assumed an important role in the management of pineal region tumors. Radiographic features are not diagnostic and therapy and outcome are dependent on tumor type. Management of hydrocephalus requires urgent attention, since patients can develop acute obstruction and a herniation syndrome. Nearly all patients with pineal region tumors present with symptomatic hydrocephalus. The standard of care has been placement of a ventriculoperitoneal shunt (VPS), at which time CSF can be collected. More recently, endoscopic management of obstructive hydrocephalus with a ventriculostomy, CSF sampling and biopsy of the tumor has gained popularity. Disadvantages of a permanent VPS for the initial management of hydrocephalus in these patients include shunt malfunction, infection and, rarely, peritoneal seeding of tumors. In many cases, if the tumor can be removed, the patient may not need the shunt at all. Endoscopic third ventriculostomy allows for successful treatment of the obstructive hydrocephalus, collection of CSF for markers and cytology and allows for multiple biopsies under direct endoscopic vision as a one-step procedure [22]. We have utilized this approach in the initial management of all patients with pineal region tumors presenting with hydrocephalus. If the biopsy is adequate and demonstrates a germinoma or primary malignant glioma without significant mass effect, the patient is managed with radiation and chemotherapy. For NGGCT, pineal cell tumors and large glial tumors, the patient can then undergo a more elective craniotomy appropriate for the location and size of tumor. Stereotactic biopsy of tumors of this region has also gained popularity but still carries a risk of damage to the complex venous anatomy. A concern with either endoscopic or stereotactic biopsy is sampling error. Germinomas can contain nests of malignant germ cell tumor that would significantly alter therapy and outcome. Likewise, a glial tumor may contain mixed cell types or focal areas of a higher-grade neoplasm, although this is less of a problem since radiographic appearance can help in choosing the most appropriate region to biopsy.

There are many surgical approaches to the pineal region (Figure 13.5). Three surgical approaches are most commonly used: infratentorial supracerebellar, suboccipital transtentorial and paramedian transcallosal. The surgeon's degree of comfort and experience with the procedure and the size and extension of the tumor should determine the most appropriate approach chosen in order to minimize complications.

Surgical results depend more on the tumor's invasiveness and relationship with surrounding structures than on which approach is utilized. The deep location of these tumors makes surgery risky, with possible damage to the tectum, thalamus or deep venous system. The supratentorial approaches are best suited for

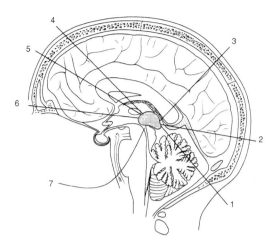

**Fig. 13.5.** Approaches to the pineal region and tumors of the posterior third ventricle. 1. Infratentorial, supracerebellar. 2. Suboccipital, transtentorial. 3. Posterior interhemispheric, transcallosal. 4. Anterior transcallosal, subchoroidal/transvelum interpositum. 5. Transcortical or interhemispheric transforaminal. 6. Translamina terminalis. 7. Posterior transventricular.

large tumors that have a significant lateral or supratentorial component. Supratentorial approaches have the disadvantage of requiring retraction of the occipital lobe, resulting in a hemianopsia and an obstructed view of the tumor by the deep venous system. In most cases, we prefer the infratentorial, supracerebellar approach because it allows the most direct access to these midline tumors. Typically, the deep venous anatomy is displaced superiorly, facilitating tumor resection. In the past, the sitting approach was utilized, which allows gravity to help in retracting the cerebellar hemispheres and facilitating dissection [18]. However, because of the risks of air embolism and cortical collapse, we prefer a modified "Concorde" position in which the surgeon operates over the patient's left shoulder. There is a growing appreciation of the value of aggressive tumor removal for improving the prognosis of patients; however, this is dependent on tumor type. With benign tumors, complete resection is usually curative [18]. With malignant tumors, radical debulking is thought to improve the outcome and response to adjuvant therapy [12,13,18].

All patients with malignant germ cell or pineal cell tumors require radiation therapy.

The concomitant use of chemotherapy, the extent of tumor involvement and the presence of dissemination have impacted on the field of radiation therapy. For certain tumors, such as ependymoma and malignant astrocytoma, focal radiotherapy is indicated. For pineoblastomas and some germ cell tumors, craniospinal radiotherapy is more appropriate. Radiotherapy has been the primary curative treatment for germinomas arising in the pineal and suprasellar regions. Long-term control rates of 65–90% are well documented for germinomas [23,24]. The control of NGGCT and pineoblastomas with radiotherapy alone is poor, necessitating multimodality therapy. Radiosurgery has been used in boosting the primary site of tumor or in the primary management of low-grade pineal tumors (pineocytomas) [25].

Chemotherapy is being evaluated with increasing enthusiasm for germinoma and certain NGGCT. For germinomas, attempts have been made to reduce or defer radiotherapy after a trial of adjuvant chemotherapy. Recurrence rates as high as 49% for germinomas treated with chemotherapy alone support the continued need for radiotherapy in these tumors [26]. Multimodal therapy for patients with NGGCT with radiotherapy and chemotherapy (bleomycin, vinblastine, carboplatin and etoposide) have shown a 4-year progression-free survival of 67% [27]. Multimodality therapy is also utilized for patients with pineoblastoma, similar to medulloblastomas. In the Childrens Cancer Group protocol, there was a 3-year progression free survival rate of 61% with combined surgery, radiotherapy and chemotherapy [28]. In adults, a review of 11 patients treated at our facility with multimodality therapy showed a median survival of 30 months for patients with positive staging, with all five patients with negative staging having progression-free survival at 26 months [20].

Treatment for patients with primary glial tumors of the pineal region are similar to tumors in other locations and are not specific to this region. However, these patients need to be monitored closely for evidence of CSF dissemination.

# Key Points

- *Intraventricular and pineal region tumors often present with hydrocephalus.*
- *Diagnosis is usually based on characteristic imaging features. Serum or CSF markers can add additional diagnostic information in some tumors.*
- *Surgical approaches to anterior intraventricular tumors are accomplished using open surgery or endoscopic techniques.*
- *Pineal region tumors comprise a number of histologic subtypes, some of which are exquisitely sensitive to radiotherapy.*
- *Posterior surgical approaches to pineal tumors are effective in safely resecting these tumors and establishing the diagnosis. Additional chemotherapy and/or radiotherapy is indicated for some tumors.*

# References

1. CBTRUS Statistical Report. Primary brain tumors in the United States, 1995–1999. Hinsdale, Illinois: Central Brain Tumor Registry of the United States, 2002.
2. Pendl G, Ozturk E, Haselsberger K. Surgery of tumours of the lateral ventricle. Acta Neurochir (Wien) 1992;116:128–36.
3. Morrison G, Sobel DF, Kelley WM, Norman D. Intraventricular mass lesions. Radiology 1984;153:435–42.
4. Zuccaro G, Sosa F, Cuccia V, Lubieniecky F, Monges J. Lateral ventricle tumors in children: a series of 54 cases. Childs Nerv Syst 1999;15:774–85.
5. Shaw EG, Evans RG, Scheithauer BW, Ilstrup DM, Earle JD. Postoperative radiotherapy of intracranial ependymoma in pediatric and adult patients. Int J Radiat Oncol Biol Phys 1987;13:1457–62.
6. Donahue B, Steinfeld A. Intracranial ependymoma in the adult patient: successful treatment with surgery and radiotherapy. J Neurooncol 1998;37:131–3.
7. Schwartz TH, Kim S, Glick RS, Bagiella E, Balmaceda C, Fetell MR, Stein BM, Sisti MB, Bruce JN. Supratentorial ependymomas in adult patients. Neurosurgery 1999;44:721–31.
8. Shepherd CW, Scheithauer BW, Gomez MR, Altermatt HJ, Katzmann JA. Subependymal giant cell astrocytoma: a clinical, pathological, and flow cytometric study. Neurosurgery 1991;28:864–8.
9. Kingsley DP, Kendall BE, Fitz CR. Tuberous sclerosis: a clinicoradiological evaluation of 110 cases with particular reference to atypical presentation. Neuroradiology 1986;28:38–46.
10. Wolff JE, Sajedi M, Brant R, Coppes MJ, Egeler RM. Choroid plexus tumours. Br J Cancer 2002;87:1086–91.
11. Gradin WC, Taylon C, Fruin AH. Choroid plexus papilloma of the third ventricle: case report and review of the literature. Neurosurgery 1983;12:217–20.

12. Hoffman HJ, Yoshida M, Becker LE, Hendrick EB, Humphreys RP. Pineal region tumors in childhood: experience at the Hospital for Sick Children. Pediatr Neurosurg 1983;21:91–103, 1994;discussion 104.
13. Sano K. Pineal region tumors: problems in pathology and treatment. Clin Neurosurg 1983;30:59–91.
14. Koide O, Watanabe Y, Sato K. Pathological survey of intracranial germinoma and pinealoma in Japan. Cancer 1980;45:2119–30.
15. Ojeda VJ, Ohama E, English DR. Pineal neoplasms and third-ventricular teratomas in Niigata (Japan) and Western Australia: a comparative study of their incidence and clinicopathological features. Med J Aust 1987;146:357–9.
16. Jennings MT, Gelman R, Hochberg F. Intracranial germ-cell tumors: natural history and pathogenesis. J Neurosurg 1985;63:155–67.
17. Russell D S, RLJ. Tumors of specialized tissues of central neuroepithelial origin. In: Russell D S, RLJ, editor Pathology of tumors of the nervous system. Baltimore: Williams & Wilkins, 1989;351–420.
18. Bruce JN, Stein BM. Surgical management of pineal region tumors. Acta Neurochir (Wien) 1995;134:130–5.
19. Schild SE, Scheithauer BW, Schomberg PJ, Hook CC, Kelly PJ, Frick L, Robinow JS, Buskirk SJ. Pineal parenchymal tumors: clinical, pathologic, and therapeutic aspects. Cancer 1993;72:870–80.
20. Chang SM, Lillis-Hearne PK, Larson DA, Wara WM, Bollen AW, Prados MD. Pineoblastoma in adults. Neurosurgery 1995;37:383–90, discussion 390–1.
21. Tien RD, Barkovich AJ, Edwards MS. MR imaging of pineal tumors. AJR Am J Roentgenol 1990;155:143–51.
22. Pople IK, Athanasiou TC, Sandeman DR, Coakham HB. The role of endoscopic biopsy and third ventriculostomy in the management of pineal region tumours. Br J Neurosurg 2001;15:305–11.
23. Jenkin D, Berry M, Chan H, Greenberg M, Hendrick B, Hoffman H, Humphreys R, Sonley M, Weitzman S. Pineal region germinomas in childhood treatment considerations. Int J Radiat Oncol Biol Phys 1990;18:541–5.
24. Linstadt D, Wara WM, Edwards MS, Hudgins RJ, Sheline GE. Radiotherapy of primary intracranial germinomas: the case against routine craniospinal irradiation. Int J Radiat Oncol Biol Phys 1988;15:291–7.
25. Kondziolka D, Hadjipanayis CG, Flickinger JC, Lunsford LD. The role of radiosurgery for the treatment of pineal parenchymal tumors. Neurosurgery 2002;51:880–9.
26. Balmaceda C, Heller G, Rosenblum M, Diez B, Villablanca JG, Kellie S, Maher P, Vlamis V, Walker RW, Leibel S, Finlay JL. Chemotherapy without irradiation: a novel approach for newly diagnosed CNS germ cell tumors: results of an international cooperative trial. The First International Central Nervous System Germ Cell Tumor Study. J Clin Oncol 1996;14:2908–15.
27. Robertson PL, DaRosso RC, Allen JC. Improved prognosis of intracranial non-germinoma germ cell tumors with multimodality therapy. J Neurooncol 1997;32:71–80.
28. Jakacki RI, Zeltzer PM, Boyett JM, Albright AL, Allen JC, Geyer JR, Rorke LB, Stanley P, Stevens KR, Wisoff J, et al. Survival and prognostic factors following radiation and/or chemotherapy for primitive neuroectodermal tumors of the pineal region in infants and children: a report of the Childrens Cancer Group. J Clin Oncol 1995;13:1377–83.

**14**

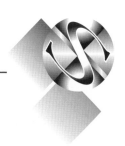

# Cerebello-pontine Angle Tumors

Peter C. Whitfield and David G. Hardy

## Summary

This chapter describes the clinical and radiological features of cerebellopontine angle (CPA) tumors. A detailed account of the management of these lesions is provided, with particular reference to the details of microsurgical treatments. The complications of CPA surgery are protean and may significantly impair the quality of a patient's life. A multidisciplinary approach to the management of these problems is advocated.

## Introduction

CPA tumors comprise about 8–10% of all intracranial neoplasms. About 80–85% of CPA tumors are acoustic neuromas, with meningiomas and a wide variety of other lesions accounting for the remainder [1]. This chapter describes the anatomy, pathology and management of these lesions.

## Anatomy

The CPA is the wedge-shaped space formed anteriorly by the dural-coated face of the petrous temporal bone, and posteriorly by the ventral surfaces of the pons and cerebellum. It contains the superior CSF cistern, which is traversed by the trigeminal, abducens, facial and vestibulocochlear nerves, the anterior inferior cerebellar artery (AICA) and the superior petrosal vein with its tributaries. The CPA has important relationships with surrounding structures. The cisterna ambiens, containing the trochlear nerve and the superior cerebellar artery, is located superiorly. Inferiorly lies the cerebellomedullary (inferior cerebellopontine) cistern containing the glossopharyngeal, vagal, accessory and hypoglossal nerves, along with the vertebral artery, origin of the PICA and the inferior petrosal vein. Medially lies the prepontine cistern which invests the basilar artery and the origin of the abducens nerve.

The cerebellar hemisphere wraps itself around the postero-lateral aspect of the pons forming the V-shaped cerebellopontine fissure. The middle cerebellar peduncle, flocculus and foramen of Luschka lie in the floor of the apex of the cerebellopontine fissure. The latter, with its tuft of protruding choroid plexus, is an important landmark for the emergence of the VII and VIII cranial nerves in CPA surgery.

### Cranial Nerves

The trigeminal nerve, comprising a small motor root and a larger sensory root, arises from the lateral aspect of the rostral pons. It courses, in an anterior, lateral and slightly superior direction, towards the porus trigeminus at the entrance to Meckel's cave. The IX, X and XI nerves arise in the longitudinal sulcus lateral to the olive. They course through the inferior cerebellopontine cistern to the jugular foramen. The facial nerve arises 2 or 3 mm superior to the rostral rootlets of the glossopharyngeal nerve, from the lateral aspect of the pontomedullary sulcus. The VIII nerve leaves the pontomedullary sulcus about 1 mm lateral to the facial nerve. The nervus intermedius is usually closely applied to the VIII nerve at this point. The VII and VIII nerves then become apposed as they course toward the porus acousticus (internal auditory meatus). The presence of transverse and vertical (Bill's bar) crests of bone within the internal auditory canal enable the surgeon to identify with certainty the location of the facial nerve and the subdivisions of the vestibulo-cochlear nerve. The superior and inferior vestibular nerves occupy the postero-superior and postero-inferior quadrants of the canal, respectively. The antero–superior quadrant is occupied by the facial nerve and nervus intermedius, whilst the cochlear nerve lies antero–inferiorly. Since most acoustic neuromas arise from one of the vestibular nerves, the cochlear and facial nerves are usually displaced anteriorly.

## Clinical Presentation

Lesions within the CPA may present with symptoms and signs of:

- cranial nerve dysfunction: unilateral hearing loss; tinnitus; dysequilibrium and vertigo; diplopia due to an abducens palsy; facial paraesthesia, anaesthesia, or pain. Facial weakness or spasms are unusual at presentation. Large lesions may lead to dysphonia, dysarthria and dysphagia due to involvement of the IX and X cranial nerves.
- cerebellar and/or brainstem compression: impaired co-ordination, upper motor neurone signs in the limbs.
- raised intracranial pressure secondary to associated hydrocephalus, or occasionally to the mass of the lesion itself.
- pain localized to the ear/mastoid regions, or sometimes non-localizing headache.

With the widespread availability of MRI, an increasing number of patients present relatively early. Unilateral hearing loss frequently presents as impaired speech discrimination noted during the use of a telephone by patients with small acoustic neuromas. However, hearing loss may be sudden and profound in 12–15% of patients with CPA tumors, suggesting a vascular basis for the symptom in some cases [2].

## Clinicopathological Correlates

Table 14.1 details the relative incidence of the different tumor types found in the CPA.

**Table 14.1.** Relative incidence of cerebellopontine angle masses. This table represents 438 patients with CPA lesions operated on in Cambridge, UK between 1981 and 1994 [1].

| Pathology | | Patients (n) | Percentage of CPA lesions |
|---|---|---|---|
| Acoustic schwannoma | | 369 | 84 |
| Meningioma | | 31 | 7.1 |
| Other schwannoma | V | 2 | |
| | VII | 6 | 3.2 |
| | VIII, IX, X | 6 | |
| Primary epidermoid (cholesteatoma) | | 10 | 2.3 |
| Glomus jugulare (Fisch Type D) | | 5 | 1.1 |
| Metastasis | | 1 | 0.2 |
| Cerebellar astrocytoma | | 1 | 0.2 |
| Lymphoma | | 1 | 0.2 |
| Dermoid cyst of the fourth ventricle | | 1 | 0.2 |

## Acoustic Neuromas

Acoustic neuromas arise from Schwann cells at the Schwann cell–glial junction, which is usually found in the internal auditory canal. Around 40% of patients with sporadic acoustic neuromas show loss of heterozygosity in the region of the tumor suppressor NF-2 gene on chromosome 22, suggesting that an underlying genetic predisposition exists in many patients [3]. Indeed the presence of bilateral acoustic neuromas is diagnostic for neurofibromatosis-2, further implicating dysfunction of this gene in the pathogenesis of these tumors.

Acoustic neuromas arise almost exclusively from the vestibular branches of the VIII nerve complex; hence, they are more correctly referred to as vestibular schwannomas. They expand the porus acousticus forming a cone-shaped mass with a canalicular and CPA component in 61% of patients. In 21% of cases, the canalicular component becomes sausage-shaped and "mushrooms" out of the porus into the CPA, leading to a dumbbell appearance. In the remainder (18%), the tumors appear to be largely confined to the CPA with no significant intracanalicular component [4]. The laterally arising tumors tend to present earlier with audiovestibular symptoms. Those arising within the CPA are more likely to present with signs of trigeminal compression, cerebellar dysfunction and raised intracranial pressure. A recent analysis of 473 patients with acoustic neuromas treated in Cambridge shows that 89.3% presented with typical audiovestibular symptoms. Of the 10.7% with an atypical presenting symptom, facial numbness (6.4%), headache (2.1%), otalgia (1%), visual changes (0.6%), taste disturbance (0.2%) and facial weakness (0.2%) were all recorded. A high degree of clinical acumen is required to avoid inadvertent delays in the diagnosis of the lesion in this group of patients.

Macroscopically, the superior cerebellopontine cistern is invaginated by the tumor, forming a double arachnoid plane around the lesion. Whilst many tumors are homogeneous in texture, macrocyst formation occurs.

Histological examination reveals regions characterized by spindle-shaped cells with hyperchromatic, elongated nuclei (Antoni A type) and other regions where vacuolated cells with pleomorphic nuclei are embedded in a loose eosinophilic matrix in which microcystic change may be prominent (Antoni B). Malignant change in acoustic neuromas is exceptional, with few cases reported in the world literature.

## Meningiomas

Meningiomas of the petrous face comprise around 7% of all CPA lesions. They present in patients aged 30–70 years and are five times more common in women. Most patients have symptoms of vestibulocochlear nerve dysfunction. About 80% complain of hearing loss, with a dead ear being evident in 19%. Tinnitus (60%), impaired balance (26%), trigeminal signs (45%) and facial weakness (10%) may also occur. Imaging investigations show that the mean tumor size is 3.5 cm at the time of diagnosis [1]. Risk factors probably include previous radiotherapy, e.g. for childhood leukaemia. Inactivation of the NF-2 tumor suppressor gene appears to be important in the pathogenesis of sporadic meningioma in up to 60% of cases.

Meningiomas of the CPA can arise in close proximity to the porus acousticus, or from a separate origin on the face of the petrous bone. Meningiomas of the CPA possess similar pathological features to those found at other, more common intracranial sites. The World Health Organisation classifies meningothelial cell tumors into many subtypes. Anaplastic and atypical meningiomas have a higher propensity for local recurrence, and complete local resection, along with dural attachments and any abnormal bone, are mandatory to minimize the risk of tumor recurrence.

## Epidermoid Tumor (Cholesteatomas)

Primary epidermoid tumors, or cholesteatomas, are non-neoplastic, cystic lesions lined with a simple stratified squamous epithelium. They are considered to be congenital, arising from misplaced epidermal cell rests [5]. Cholesteatomas of the CPA must be differentiated from the acquired lesions that occur secondary to middle-ear suppurative disease. The latter are usually restricted to the tympano–mastoid region, but erosion of the petrous bone may occur, with the appearance of a petrous apex cholesteatoma. These acquired lesions are about 1.5 times more frequent in our experience. CPA cholesteatomas present in adults of either sex with a mean age of 43 years. They contain lamellae of desquamated keratin, cell debris and a variable number of cholesterol crystals. Macroscopically, the lesions resemble clusters of pearls. They grow slowly, by a process of desquamation, and infiltrate the cisternal spaces. Cranial nerve palsies dominate the clinical presentation [1].

## Glomus Tumors

Glomus tumors result from neoplastic transformation in paraganglionic "jugular bodies". Since spread of these tumors follows the path of least resistance, large tumors may present within the CPA [6]. The presenting symptoms include hearing loss, pulsatile tinnitus, dysequilibrium, dysphonia, dysphagia and aural bleeding.

## Other CPA Lesions

Schwannomas may occur on any of the lower cranial nerves. The facial and trigeminal nerves are more frequently affected than the bulbar nerves [1]. These lesions may occur entirely within the CPA but, in the case of trigeminal schwannomas, dumbbell extension through Meckel's cave into the middle cranial fossa is usual.

Cerebellopontine angle arachnoid cysts are rare and often present with headache and ataxia, rather than cranial nerve compression syndromes. If symptoms are few, observation is advocated. However, symptomatic lesions require treatment. This is most safely met through a wide fenestration procedure rather than excision or shunting [7].

Basilar artery ectasia and posterior circulation aneurysms can present as a mass in the CPA. With modern imaging techniques and careful history taking these lesions should be recognised at a stage that enables appropriate neurovascular management to be directed at them.

The foramen of Luschka provides a communication between the fourth ventricle and the CPA. In view of this, lesions of the ventricular system, such as ependymomas, choroid plexus tumors and dermoid tumors, may protrude into

the CPA. Presentation may be related to cranial nerve compression, mass effect or hydrocephalus. Other rare tumors of the CPA include chordomas, haemangioblastomas, metastases and lipomas. Whilst MRI findings may provide diagnostic information, an accurate pre-operative diagnosis is often not possible.

# Management of CPA Tumors

Since 80–85% of CPA lesions are acoustic neuromas, much of this discussion concerns the management of these lesions.

## Investigations

### MRI Scanning

Contrast-enhanced MRI is the investigation of choice in patients with symptoms and/or signs of CPA disease. Thin sections in axial and coronal planes can detect acoustic neuromas as small as 2 mm in diameter. CT scans provide complementary information on bone anatomy, but the beam-hardening artefact caused by the petrous bone reduces the resolution of the technique within the CPA. Typical MRI appearances of CPA lesions are shown in Fig. 14.1. Acoustic neuromas and meningiomas may both appear isointense on T2-weighted images and enhance with paramagnetic contrast. Cystic appearances can be present in either lesion. However, meningiomas appear broad-based and form an obtuse angle with the petrous dura. A tail of dural enhancement is frequently present and is a pathognomic sign. Acoustic neuromas characteristically expand the porus acousticus but, if hyperostosis is associated with a meningioma, the porus may be narrowed.

### Otoneurological Findings

Otoneurological investigations are indicated when a patient presents with symptoms suggestive of vestibulocochlear nerve dysfunction. Using pure tone audiometry, four patterns of sensorineural hearing loss are recognized in patients with acoustic neuromas. High-frequency loss is seen in 65% of patients. In 22% of patients, hearing loss is depressed equally

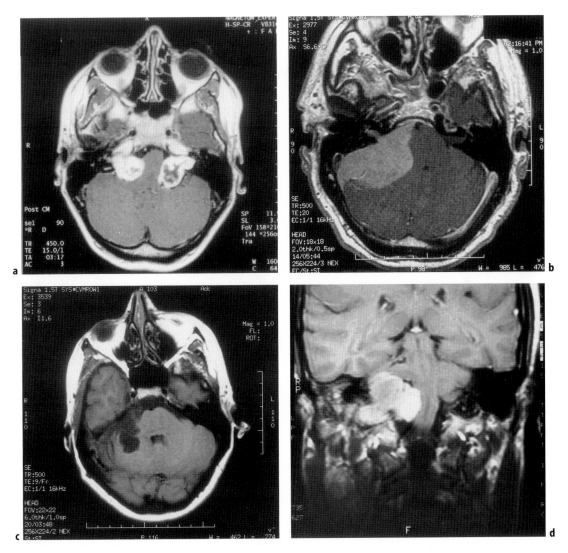

**Fig. 14.1.** Radiological appearances of CPA lesions. **a** T1-weighted axial image with contrast. Bilateral acoustic neuromas in a patient with NF-2. **b** T1-weighted axial image with contrast showing a CPA meningioma. Notice the normal appearance of the internal auditory meatus and the broad origin of the tumor. The T2-weighted image showed increased signal in the compressed cerebellar hemisphere. **c** T1-weighted axial image showing a CPA cholesteatoma. This lesion did not enhance following contrast injection. **d** T1-weighted coronal image with contrast showing a large CPA glomus jugulare tumor.

across all frequencies. In 7%, low tone loss is evident whilst, in 6%, a trough-shaped loss is seen, with relative preservation of hearing at high and low frequencies [8].

Speech discrimination tests determine the ability of the patient to identify a taped series of words presented at 40 dB above the speech threshold. The quality of hearing can be classified according to the speech discrimination

score combined with the pure tone audiogram loss [9]. Hearing is described as excellent if there is a pure tone loss of 0–30 dB with 70–100% speech discrimination. Other grades (serviceable, non-serviceable, poor and absent) represent increasingly poor auditory function. Poor speech discrimination that is out of proportion to the degree of pure-tone loss is a feature of acoustic neuromas. This is attributed to the finding that up to 75% of cochlear fibers may be damaged before the pure-tone deficit is evident. The ability to discriminate speech is of importance when considering the appropriate management strategies, such as hearing preservation surgery, for an individual patient.

Although widely used, the specificity and sensitivity of caloric tests, brainstem auditory evoked responses and acoustic decay reflexes are inferior to MRI as screening tests in patients with symptoms and/or signs of CPA pathology. A recent retrospective analysis has shown that pure tone audiometry was normal in 25% of patients with CPA meningiomas, further supporting the use of MRI as the investigation of choice in patients with symptoms indicative of CPA disease, including patients presenting with unilateral audiovestibular symptoms.

## Treatment Strategies in Patients with Acoustic Neuromas

When considering the management of a patient with an acoustic neuroma, several factors preside. The size of the tumor is of paramount importance. In the Cambridge series of 473 patients presenting between 1983 and 1995, 47% of tumors were large (more than 2.5 cm), 32% medium (1.5–2.5 cm) and 21% small (less than 1.5 cm). Large tumors may cause the life-threatening complications of symptomatic hydrocephalus, and direct mass effect. We advocate initial insertion of a ventriculoperitoneal shunt, or, in suitable cases, a third ventriculostomy, to alleviate hydrocephalus. If mass symptoms are evident, early surgery to remove the tumor should be considered. The initial presentation of these tumors in this way is now rare.

At presentation, most acoustic neuromas present with audiovestibular symptoms and do not constitute a threat to life at that time. A complete understanding of the natural history, surgical morbidity and success of radiosurgery is of importance in deciding the appropriate management of patients with these tumors.

### Natural History

Intracanalicular acoustic neuromas frequently present early with audiovestibular symptoms, and may be very small at presentation. Imaging studies show that the rate of growth of these tumors varies both between individual tumors

and within a specific lesion. Whilst a growth rate of around 2 mm per year is usual, tumors can grow by as much as 17 mm per annum [10]. This information, combined with the fact that quality of life is reduced after surgery for very large tumors, make a strong case for treatment in the young patient with a small acoustic neuroma. A "wait and see" policy condemns the patient to indefinite follow-up, an uncertain future and substantial costs for regular MR scans. However, in the elderly patient with comorbidity, a conservative approach with careful clinical and radiological follow-up is a reasonable alternative strategy. Although assessment of growth and volumetric estimation of tumor size are complex, repeat imaging for comparative studies usually provides sufficient information for clinical decision making. In such patients, we recommend a repeat MRI scan 6 months after diagnosis, annually for 4 years and then bi-annually, provided tumor growth is not progressive.

## Surgery for Acoustic Neuromas

Much has been written about the relative merits of the translabyrinthine, retrosigmoid and middle fossa approaches in the treatment of acoustic neuromas. A synopsis of the historical milestones in acoustic neuroma surgery is shown in Table 14.2.

### Intraoperative Monitoring

Intraoperative facial nerve monitoring is useful and widely practiced. A pre-requisite for electromyographic monitoring is that the patient is

**Table 14.2.** Historical milestones in acoustic neuroma surgery.

| Year | Event |
|------|-------|
| 1891 | McBurney attempts removal of an acoustic neuroma |
| 1894 | Charles Ballance successfully removes an acoustic neuroma |
| 1903 | Krause describes the sub-occipital approach |
| 1904 | Panse describes the translabyrinthine approach |
| 1917 | Cushing's acoustic neuroma monograph is published |
| 1931 | Cairns successfully preserves the facial nerve |
| 1964 | House describes microsurgical translabyrinthine approach |
| 1979 | Mortality is reduced to 2.6% in a series of 500 patients |

not paralyzed with neuromuscular agents when assessing facial nerve responses. A bipolar stimulating electrode provides a spatially precise means of stimulating the facial nerve, enabling EMG potentials to be recorded using needle electrodes in facial muscles (e.g. orbicularis oculi and oris). The signals are amplified and made audible to the surgeon. Although a randomized study of this technique has not been performed, few surgeons now operate without such monitoring. For large CPA lesions and other skull base tumors, the technique can be adapted to monitor the motor components of other cranial nerves. The trigeminal nerve can be assessed by inserting electrodes into the masseter and/or temporalis muscles. The lower motor cranial nerves can be monitored by inserting electrodes into the soft palate (IX), taping electrodes to the endotracheal tube to assess laryngeal muscle function (X), or inserting electrodes in the sternocleidomastoid and trapezius muscles (XI) or the tongue (XII). Other monitoring systems have been developed based upon mechanotransducers, the stimulus for development being the artifact caused in EMG recording by electrocoagulation. However, newer generation multichannel EMG monitoring devices are likely to become the monitoring tools of choice.

A variety of techniques may be used to monitor intraoperative cochlear nerve function. These include brainstem auditory evoked responses (BAERs) and auditory compound action potentials (CAPs) [11]. BAERs are recorded from vertex and upper cervical electrodes. Sound stimuli at 20 pulses per second at 65 dB above normal threshold are used via earphones. A continuous waveform can be displayed to show the effects of surgery upon cochlear nerve function. The principal drawback of this technique is the time delay between anatomical or physiological disruption of the cochlear nerve and a change in the BAER. This limits the clinical utility of the method. To overcome this problem, direct recording of CAPs from either the cochlear nerve or the cochlear nucleus have been used. Whilst this form of monitoring may reduce intraoperative trauma to the cochlear nerve, an effect upon the outcome of hearing preservation surgery has not been demonstrated.

## Translabyrinthine Approach

This approach provides the shortest, most direct route to the CPA. Cerebellar retraction is minimized and the lateral end of the facial nerve is clearly visualized. William House popularized this approach, and we advocate its use in patients with hearing loss and in virtually all patients with large neuromas.

The patient is placed supine with the head turned 70° away from the side of the lesion. The head is flexed, but the chin must remain clear of the contralateral clavicle. The head is tilted so the malar is uppermost. A sandbag is placed beneath the ipsilateral shoulder. The thigh is also prepared to enable fascia lata and fat to be harvested in preparation for wound closure. We use a "hockey stick" incision, curving from just above the posterior-superior aspect of the auricle, descending to a point 1 cm behind and below the mastoid tip. Careful attention is given to opening the scalp in two layers. The periosteum is then reflected anteriorly, exposing the posterior aspect of the external auditory canal and the spine of Henle. Care must be taken not to perforate the skin of the canal during placement of the self-retaining retractor. The temporal bone is then drilled in a systematic fashion to provide a corridor of access to the CPA.

Drilling of the temporal bone is performed in four phases:

- Extended mastoidectomy with exposure of the facial nerve.
- Removal of the semicircular canals.
- Exposure of the bony internal auditory canal. To improve access the jugular bulb can be uncovered and retracted inferiorly.
- Removal of bone around the lateral 270° of the canal.

The dura is then opened longitudinally in the inferior half of the internal auditory canal. The canalicular portion of the tumor is readily evident and the facial nerve identified. The posterior fossa dura is then opened in continuity with the already exposed internal auditory canal, increasing access into the CPA.

The tumor usually displaces the facial nerve anteriorly. This relationship needs to be clarified during resection of the tumor. The superior and inferior poles of the tumor are sequentially inspected, enabling the lateral aspect of the brainstem to be identified. Care must be taken to preserve all blood vessels passing over the surface of the tumor. Many of the arteries looping over the tumor will supply the brainstem. The trigeminal nerve and superior petrosal vein can usually be identified superiorly. Lintine strips are eased into the plane around the tumor capsule to protect the brainstem. Inferiorly, the lower cranial nerves and posterior inferior cerebellar artery are protected from the tumor. Care must be taken in larger tumors not to over-retract either the neuraxis or the tumor. In such tumors, early attention to CSF drainage helps, but exposure of the tumor margins must be performed in an incremental fashion. The surface of the tumor is diathermied to reduce vascularity during this phase of exposure. The canalicular and anterior aspects of the tumor are left undisturbed at this point.

The tumor surface is then incised and the tumor debulked from within using an ultrasonic aspirator. Care is taken not to perforate the tumor during this maneuver. After debulking the tumor, further exposure of the capsule can be made taking care to protect the brainstem structures. Sequential exposure and debulking can then be performed. The brainstem end of the facial nerve requires exposure. Essential landmarks are the choroid plexus of the Foramen of Luschka, the line of the glossopharyngeal nerve and the pontomedullary sulcus. Once the facial nerve has been identified the cochlear and vestibular nerves are sacrificed at the brainstem end. The tumor is then rolled laterally towards the internal auditory canal. The position of the facial nerve is carefully observed. The tumor is then dissected from the facial nerve using microscissors under a modestly irrigated operating field. The tumor may be adherent to the dural margins of the porus acousticus. The ring of dura enveloping the tumor needs to be opened at both shoulders of the tumor. The facial nerve is often very thin and splayed at this point. At times, the facial nerve can be followed from lateral to medial, gently retracting the tumor into the CPA whilst dissecting the tumor from the nerve. Eventually, the tumor will be removed. After ensuring resection is complete, hemostasis is secured, using irrigation and application of a monolayer of oxidized cellulose patches to the brainstem.

The principal objective during closure of the wound is to ensure that CSF leakage cannot occur. The eustachian tube and middle ear are sealed with small pieces of fat and fibrin glue (Tisseel, Immuno IG, Vienna, Austria). A patch of fascia lata (2 × 2.5 cm), secured with fibrin glue, is then placed over the drilled surface of the petrous bone to cover the middle ear. Three finger-sized strips of fat are then placed just into the CPA and anchored superficially with fibrin glue. The mastoid air cells are sealed with bone wax. The pericranium is then closed. The galea, reinforced with a fascia lata patch, is sutured. Finally, the scalp is closed in two layers.

To minimize the risk of CSF leak, we recommend daily lumbar punctures, reducing the CSF pressure to +5 cm on the first three postoperative days. These are performed in preference to leaving a lumbar drain in situ to encourage early ambulation. The post-operative hospital stay is variable, but is around 5 or 6 days in healthy ambulant patients.

## Retrosigmoid Approach

Historically, this approach was favored for the removal of acoustic neuromas. However, cerebellar retraction, which in large lesions may be considerable, and difficult access to the lateral internal auditory canal have reduced the utility of the approach in favor of the translabyrinthine exposure in the majority of patients. Furthermore, headache appears to be more persistent than after a translabyrinthine approach. We use the retrosigmoid approach in an attempt to preserve hearing in patients with socially useful hearing (Gardner–Robertson Grade I). We also use this approach in patients with Grade II hearing accompanied by contralateral hearing loss.

The patient is positioned supine with the head turned 80° to the contralateral side, with the neck flexed and the ear uppermost. Brain relaxation is achieved by inducing an osmotic diuresis during exposure. A curvilinear incision commencing posterior to the auricle and descending 2 cm behind and below the mastoid process is used. The sub-occipital muscles and fascia are divided in the line of the incision in separate layers. Care is taken to avoid cutting the occipital artery. The periosteum is then retracted to expose the mastoid tip and the superior nuchal line. A sub-occipital, retrosigmoid craniectomy is performed, exposing the transverse and sigmoid sinuses. The latter is followed inferiorly for about 4 cm. The foramen magnum is not opened. The dura is then opened in a cruciate fashion. A self-retaining retractor is introduced to retract the cerebellum posteriorly. Early drainage of CSF facilitates the exposure, minimizing neuraxis retraction. This is performed by identifying the lower cranial nerves and opening the inferior cerebellopontine cistern. These cranial nerves are then protected with a cottonoid pattie. The tumor is then examined and the arachnoidal plane around the superior and posterior poles opened. If the tumor is small, the proximal VII and VIII nerve complex will be seen at this early stage. Care must be taken to ensure that the facial nerve passes anterior to the tumor rather than taking an aberrant course over the posterior or superior aspects of the tumor. With larger tumors internal debulking, preferentially performed with the cavitating ultrasonic surgical aspirator, will be required prior to identification of the neural structures. Careful dissection of the tumor is then performed, with the objective of preserving the facial and auditory nerves. The vestibular nerves are divided.

Rather than follow the tumor mass along the internal auditory canal, the safest approach is to drill off the posterior wall of the internal auditory canal. The petrous dura is incised and retracted, enabling the posterior lip of the porus and the opening for the endolymphatic sac to be identified. Radical removal of the porus acousticus can inadvertently fenestrate the inner ear, destroying auditory function. After opening the internal auditory canal, the dura is incised, exposing the intracanalicular tumor and the distal nerves. The facial and cochlear nerves are preserved, whilst the vestibular nerves are divided. The tumor is then dissected towards the porus acousticus. With meticulous attention, this most adherent part of the tumor can be removed. Hemostasis is secured, and the drilled petrous bone is sealed with bone wax and covered with a piece of fascia lata (2 × 2 cm) secured with fibrin glue. The dura is closed in a watertight fashion with fascia lata to bridge any defects. Fat patches are placed over the dura. The pericranium, muscles, fascia, subcutaneous fat and skin are closed in separate layers.

## Middle Fossa Approach

This approach is utilized for intracanalicular tumors in which an attempt at hearing preservation is desirable. The drawbacks of the approach are temporal lobe retraction, which can result in seizures and focal neurological signs, limited access if the tumor has extended beyond the porus into the CPA and the difficulty in identifying landmarks on the petrous ridge.

The patient is positioned supine with the head turned to the contralateral side, with the ear uppermost. Brain relaxation using osmotic diuretics and/or lumbar CSF drainage is mandatory. A pre-auricular incision is used and a middle fossa free flap craniotomy performed. This must be made as low as possible to minimize the amount of bone that needs to be removed with ronguers. The petrous bone is then exposed extradurally. The arcuate eminence and greater petrosal nerve are useful landmarks to localize the internal auditory canal. Once located, the internal auditory canal must be opened widely. The dural sleeve is opened along the long axis of the canal. The position of the facial nerve is confirmed. The tumor is then excised, with careful dissection from the nerves and vessels in the canal. The cochlear nerve is usually only revealed once the tumor has been resected. A small plug of fat is placed in the tumor bed. The dura is repaired and the craniotomy closed in standard fashion.

# Results of Acoustic Neuroma Surgery

The objective of acoustic neuroma surgery is the total removal of the neoplasm with minimal morbidity and mortality. Objective recording of cranial nerve function, CSF leak rates, meningitis incidence and quality-of-life assessments can assess morbidity. Extent of tumor removal can be determined intraoperatively, and recurrence can be monitored with MRI scans.

In the modern era, total tumor removal should be achieved. This was the case in 99.6% of patients with unilateral tumors in Cambridge. Recurrence of acoustic neuromas is exceptional, and has only been seen in two patients in our center between 1982 and 1998. In one of these cases (a patient with NF-2), the tumor was histologically malignant. We perform MRI scans 2 and 5 years post-operatively to ensure recurrence has not occurred.

The mortality of surgery for acoustic neuromas has reduced dramatically over the course of this century. Whilst Cushing's overall operative mortality was 11.4% [12], mortality figures of around 20% were reported in other historical series. However, microsurgical advances have reduced death rates, initially to 5%, then to around 2–3%. In the total Cambridge series of 660 acoustic neuroma operations, we have encountered eight deaths (1.2%). The causes of death include hematomas in the CPA or cerebellum, brainstem infarction and post-operative meningitis, in addition to concomitant medical complications.

## Facial Nerve Outcome

Facial nerve function can be assessed using the House–Brackmann scale [13]. This grades facial weakness as normal (Grade I) through mild (II), moderate (III), moderately severe (IV), severe (V) and total paralysis (VI). This method of assessment has a high degree of interobserver reliability and has become widely adopted.

In the Cambridge series (1982–1998), the facial nerve was anatomically intact following tumor resection in 94% of cases. Loss of the facial nerve in patients with small tumors was exceptional. In the 372 patients with long-term facial nerve follow-up, 76% of patients undergoing translabyrinthine surgery achieved a Grade I–III result. Retrosigmoid resection results were slightly better, with 79% achieving a Grade I–III result at 12 months. Table 14.3 shows results for facial nerve function related to tumor size. When the series is analyzed in 5-year time-blocks the Grade I–III facial nerve results improved from 56% (1982–1987), through 81% (1988–1992) to 85% (1993–1997). This indicates that the experience of the surgical team is critical in facial nerve preservation surgery [14].

Multivariate analysis has shown that the most important independent risk factors for poor facial nerve outcome (House–Brackmann Grade IV–VI) are increasing patient age, tumor size greater than 2.4 cm, the translabyrinthine approach and lack of intraoperative facial nerve monitoring [15]. The explanations behind these findings are largely speculative. With increasing age, the vascularity of the facial nerve may become compromized. Risk factors implicating the translabyrinthine route may include thermal injury generated during drilling of the temporal bone, and post-operative facial nerve oedema.

### Management of Facial Nerve Palsy

Although Ballance successfully performed the first removal of an acoustic neuroma nearly 100 years ago, the patient required subsequent enucleation of the eye due to trigeminal and facial nerve complications. Exposure keratitis can occur in patients with severe facial palsy due to decreased lacrimation and reduced closure, particularly if associated with trigeminal sensory loss and a poor Bell's phenomenon. Decreased lacrimation can be treated with methyl cellulose eye drops and liquid paraffin eye ointment. The eye should be protected, particularly at night. If eye closure is deficient 1 week post-operatively, botulinum toxin injection or a lateral tarsorrhaphy should be performed. If a facial nerve palsy persists, static (e.g. gold weight in eye lid, fascial slings) or dynamic procedures (e.g. muscle transfers) can be used to protect the eye and improve the cosmetic appearance. If the nerve remained in continuity at operation, spontaneous regeneration offers a better prospect of a good result compared with a reanimation procedure [16].

**Table 14.3.** Post-operative facial nerve function at 1 year after surgery for small, medium and large acoustic neuromas: Cambridge results.

| House Grade | Percentage of patients in each group | | |
|---|---|---|---|
| | Small (<1.5 cm) | Medium (1.5–3 cm) | Large (>3 cm) |
| I | 58 | 42.5 | 18 |
| II | 16.5 | 19.5 | 19 |
| III | 15 | 22 | 26 |
| IV | 1.5 | 4.5 | 22 |
| V | 4.5 | 4.5 | 5 |
| VI | 4.5 | 7 | 21 |

The latter should therefore be delayed 1 year from the time of surgery unless the facial nerve has been severed. Post-operative electroneuronography 1 week post-operatively has been shown to be of prognostic value. Incomplete degeneration is associated with a Grade I or II outcome whereas complete degeneration forecasts a protracted, incomplete recovery [17].

If the facial nerve is divided at operation a primary repair is the procedure of choice. This may be feasible due to stretching of the nerve by the tumor and by mobilization of the nerve within the petrous bone. A posterior auricular or sural nerve cable graft is useful if a primary repair is technically not possible. Where a reanimation procedure is subsequently performed, a variety of options exist. Several groups currently favor hypoglossal–facial nerve anastomosis. The principal drawback of this operation, namely hemiatrophy of the tongue, is small compared with other potential donor nerves such as the glossopharyngeal, spinal accessory and phrenic. A hypoglossal–facial anastomosis can either be performed by complete division of the hypoglossal nerve, or by fashioning a bifurcation in the nerve at the level of the descendens hypoglossi, leaving some innervation to the tongue intact. In a meta-analysis, good results were reported in 65% of more than 500 cases. After nerve transfer procedures, motor activity takes 6 months to commence and may improve over a few years. The patient needs to learn that manipulating the tongue results in facial movements.

Involuntary and emotional movements of the face do not occur as a result of hypoglossal–facial anastomosis. Such movements require innervation from the facial nerve nucleus in the brainstem. A cross-facial nerve transfer consists of a peripheral nerve interposition graft (usually sural nerve) between a distal facial branch on the normal side to a complementary branch on the affected side. This procedure can improve expressive movements of selected facial muscle groups.

Nerve transfer procedures require relatively lengthy surgery with uncertain, often disappointing, results that take months or even years to achieve a desirable result. A careful selection process is pertinent in performing these procedures. We reserve reanimation surgery for young, well motivated patients with a robust psychological approach to their disease. Static and dynamic cosmetic procedures are more suitable for the majority of patients with severe permanent facial nerve palsy.

## Hearing Preservation

What constitutes useful hearing is debatable. Whilst many consider Gardner–Robertson Grade II hearing useful, the distortion and imbalance may be annoying and distracting to many patients. However, if the contralateral ear is damaged, Grade II hearing preservation is highly desirable. Generally, we consider hearing preservation surgery in patients with 70% speech discrimination and a pure tone audiogram within 30 dB of the non-affected side (Grade I). We consider severe pre-operative tinnitus a relative contraindication to hearing preservation surgery. In selected patients the results of attempts at hearing preservation are variable. A recent analysis of 50 hearing preservation operations performed in Cambridge via the retrosigmoid approach has shown that only 4.8% of patients had normal post-operative hearing and 8% had serviceable hearing. A further 18% had some hearing at post-operative assessment [18]. Hearing was preserved in 24% of patients treated at the Mayo Clinic via the retrosigmoid approach [19]. In contrast, of 25 patients with serviceable hearing (Grade I or II) operated upon via the middle fossa approach, 18 (72%) retained hearing post-operatively; however, in only seven (28%) was the post-operative hearing of Grade I quality [20]. The success of hearing preservation is dependent upon tumor size, with dismal results in patients with large tumors.

## Nervus Intermedius Function

Although pre-operative symptoms related to dysfunction of this nerve are uncommon, post-operative symptoms are frequent. The nervus intermedius carries secretomotor fibers to the submandibular, sublingual and minor salivary glands, the nasal and palatine mucus glands and the lacrimal gland. It also carries taste from the anterior two-thirds of the tongue and hard palate, and some somatic afferent fibers from the external auditory meatus. Damage to the nervus intermedius is common in CPA surgery. Reinnervation or transephaptic transmission probably accounts for the onset of lacrimation during eating ("crocodile tears") which is present in 44% of patients post-operatively. A reduction in tear production is present in 72% of patients, whilst 48% admit to changes in taste sensation post-operatively [21]. To reduce the distress caused by these symptoms all patients should be adequately counselled pre-operatively.

## CSF Leakage and Meningitis

Excluding facial nerve damage, CSF leakage is the most common complication after translabyrinthine or retrosigmoid acoustic neuroma surgery. Most authors report a rate of 10–15%, although meticulous refinement of closure techniques can reduce the incidence to 5% or less [22]. The principal complication of post-operative CSF leakage is meningitis, which occurs in around 2–5% in the major series. This may present some weeks after discharge from hospital, and diligence is required not to overlook the diagnosis. In the Cambridge series, CSF leakage occurred in 5% of patients, although a subset of 188 consecutive patients were operated upon with a leak rate of only 1.6%. CSF leakage usually settles with a period of lumbar CSF drainage. However, 2% of the whole series required re-exploration and wound re-closure.

## Quality of Life

Whilst the past four decades have seen a reduction in the mortality rates from 16 to 2–3% and an increase in normal facial nerve function from 3 to 50–60%, a significant hidden morbidity exists in patients undergoing acoustic neuroma surgery. This has been measured in 227 patients using an acoustic neuroma specific questionnaire coupled with the European Organisation for Research into the Treatment of Cancer (EORTC) core questionnaire. This showed that life quality was reduced to 85% (normal = 100%) in patients with acoustic neuromas. In patients with tumors of more than 1.5 cm in diameter, life quality was significantly reduced further to 77%. However, the post-operative life quality did not differ between patients with tumors 1.5–2.5 cm in diameter compared with tumors of more than 2.5 cm. This information carries the implication that surgery in patients with small tumors is justified to prevent the tumor reaching a larger size where quality of life after surgery is reduced further. Despite the findings of this sensitive quality-of-life analysis,

only 3% of patients were dependent upon others for important daily activities, with 79% of patients returning to their normal lifestyle. This apparent discrepancy illustrates the difficulties involved in measuring quality of life.

## Stereotactic Radiosurgery in the Treatment of Acoustic Neuromas

Stereotactic radiosurgery is increasingly being used in the treatment of small and medium acoustic neuromas. The rapid return to normal activity and avoidance of an open procedure are attractive alternatives to microsurgery. The treatment aims to prevent further tumor growth, maintain neurological function and minimize the risk of new neurological deficits. Worldwide experience with the technique is increasing and long-term results require careful scrutiny. Treatment protocols are evolving as experience with the technique increases [23]. Careful planning using stereotactic MRI enables precise isodose curves with steep radiation fall-off outside the tumor margin to be used in the treatment of small and medium acoustic neuromas. Doses of between 12 and 16 Gy at the treatment margin and 16–24 Gy at the tumor core are being used. If hearing preservation is sought, doses are at the lower limits of these ranges.

Of 162 consecutive patients followed up for a minimum of 5 years in Pittsburgh, tumor size diminished in 62%, remained static in 33% and showed slow growth in 6%. Normal facial and trigeminal nerve function was evident in 79 and 73%, respectively, at follow-up [24]. Preservation of useful hearing was reported in 50% of the 18 patients with useful pre-treatment hearing treated in Sheffield [25]. In the small number of patients we have operated upon following failed radiosurgery, dissection of the tumor from the facial nerve is more difficult due to increased adherence, particularly at the porus acousticus.

To date, no randomized trial has been performed to compare the treatment options in patients with acoustic neuromas. The indications for radiosurgery are relative and are evolving. Patients with co-existing medical ailments, recurrent tumors, which are very rare in our experience, and neurofibromatosis-2 are all suitable. Patients in whom microsurgery is an option need to be counselled, bearing in mind the resources and outcome information currently available.

## Bilateral Acoustic Neuromas

Bilateral acoustic neuromas are diagnostic of neurofibromatosis-2. This disease is caused by mutations in the NF-2 tumor suppressor gene on chromosome 22, and follows an autosomal dominant pattern of inheritance. Treating these patients is always difficult. Bilateral facial palsies, deafness and the prospect of other CNS tumors developing point to a miserable existence. Management options include observation or subcapsular removal to minimize risk to the audiovestibular nerves and stereotactic radiosurgery. Both require careful consideration. Other options include early treatment of the smaller neuroma to maximise the chance of hearing preservation or treatment of the larger tumor first, with the aim of delaying surgery on the contralateral side if it remains the only source of useful hearing after the first procedure. The treatments in each of these unfortunate patients require individualization and supportive aftercare. The development of brainstem implant technology to augment auditory function may prove useful in these cases in the future.

# Management of Other CPA Tumors

Pre-operative imaging can provide information that is of diagnostic value in many patients with CPA tumors. Most CPA masses require surgical removal, although, increasingly, stereotactic radiosurgery provides an alternative treatment, and may become more important as long-term cohort studies are reported. The surgical approach to CPA is dependent upon the exact location of the tumor, and the presence of associated pre-operative cranial nerve lesions.

## Meningiomas

The treatment of choice for meningiomas is complete surgical excision of the tumor, its dural attachments and any abnormal bone. For CPA meningiomas, this may be accomplished by any of the standard approaches described for acoustic neuroma excision, depending upon the hearing status and the precise location of the tumor. Complete macroscopic surgical excision is usually achieved in this group of patients. This objective is only accomplished in about 70% of patients with "non-acoustic neuroma like" meningiomas – a group that includes clival and petrous apex tumors. In the Cambridge series of 31 patients (1981–1994) with CPA meningiomas, the retrosigmoid approach was used in 16 cases. Grade I hearing was present in nine of these patients and Grade II in two patients pre-operatively. Grade I hearing was preserved in six patients (67%) and Grade II in two patients. Other groups have reported similar results. Furthermore, a case has been reported of a patient in whom meningioma excision resulted in a dramatic improvement in hearing. Serious consideration should be given to the retrosigmoid approach rather than the translabyrinthine approach in patients in whom the pre-operative imaging suggests a meningioma. In the Cambridge series normal facial nerve function was present in 65% post-operatively, with 84% having a House Grade I–III result. Other cranial nerve palsies observed in small numbers of post-operative patients involved the IV, V, VI, IX, X and XI cranial nerves [1].

Alternative treatments for meningiomas are not evidence based. Whilst stereotactic radiosurgery may be applicable in some selected patients, the relatively large tumor size at presentation (3.5 cm mean) mitigates against this approach in the majority of patients.

## Other Schwannomas

Facial nerve neuromas are usually indistinguishable from acoustic lesions until the tumor is encountered at surgery [1]. Surgery is therefore performed either by the translabyrinthine or retrosigmoid approach according to the patient's pre-operative hearing. Neuromas of the trigeminal nerve often present with a dumbbell mass present in both the posterior and middle cranial fossae. We usually remove such lesions via a pre-sigmoid combined posterior fossa/middle fossa approach. The otic capsule is left intact during drilling of the temporal bone. The petrous face dura is opened to gain access to the posterior fossa. If the tumor is large, the dura in the retrosigmoid region should be exposed and opened. If necessary, the sigmoid sinus is divided to improve access. If this is contemplated, pre-operative venous angiography is advised. A low, middle fossa craniotomy is performed to enable the middle fossa component of the tumor to be adequately exposed. The tentorium cerebelli is divided to greatly enhance simultaneous access into the middle and posterior fossae. The line of division should be parallel to the petrous apex, but just posterior to where the trochlear nerve pierces the dura at the medial edge of the tentorium.

Neuromas of the vagus, glossopharyngeal and spinal accessory nerve are exceedingly rare. Total resection was achieved in all five patients reported in the Cambridge series. All patients had at least one cranial nerve palsy, but only one required phonosurgery (teflon injection to vocal cord), and all swallow satisfactorily.

## Primary Cholesteatomas of the CPA

Cholesteatomas usually present with features of audiovestibular nerve dysfunction. The surgical approach is determined by the clinical presentation. If hearing is preserved, a retrosigmoid approach is favored (6/10 in the Cambridge series), whereas a transpetrous approach is used if useful hearing has been lost pre-operatively [1]. Despite this, the chance of preserving hearing is low, with only one of the six patients operated on via the retrosigmoid approach retaining hearing. If the lesion extends far medially, the cochlea may require removal to provide sufficient access. Cholesteatomas usually envelop a multitude of cranial nerves and vascular structures. Whilst the soft contents of the lesion can readily be removed, the capsule, which is usually adherent to vascular and neural structures, needs to be excised to avoid recurrence. Although the mortality from surgery to remove these lesions is low, neurological morbidity in the form of post-operative cranial nerve lesions is frequent. This is most commonly the facial nerve, and is most frequently confined to a House–Brackmann Grade II weakness, but complete lesions can occur. Lower cranial nerve lesions were also present in around 30–40% of cases in the Cambridge series [1].

## Glomus Tumors

Historical studies have shown only 29% surviving 10 years in patients with glomus jugulare tumors managed with a variety of modalities ranging from no treatment to craniotomy with radiotherapy. Surgical excision offers a potential cure in the treatment of these patients. We advocate a combined trans and infratemporal approach to Type C (tympanomastoid with infralabyrinthine or petrous apex destruction) and D (intradural extension) tumors as described by Fisch. Pre-operative angiography with tumor embolization, where possible, is mandatory. Preliminary control of the internal carotid artery, the sigmoid sinus and the cavernous sinus is necessary to avoid a vascular catastrophe. Blind sac closure of the external auditory canal is performed, followed by a radical mastoidectomy. This exposes the middle and posterior fossa dura and the venous sinuses. The facial nerve distal to the geniculate ganglion is fully skeletonized and transposed anteriorly when necessary. A wide dural opening, sometimes in combination with transection of the sigmoid sinus and the tentorium cerebelli, is performed. The infralabyrinthine petrous bone needs to be removed to expose the petrous portion of the carotid artery and the jugular bulb. The intradural tumor is dissected using a technique of capsular diathermy and sharp dissection. The lower cranial nerves are frequently inseparable from the tumor in the region of the posterior lacerate canal (jugular foramen). The jugular vein is divided and the attachment of the tumor to the carotid artery is removed. This portion of the dissection may be quite hemorrhagic because of the contribution of caroticotympanic vessels to the tumor circulation. Once the tumor has been removed, time needs to be spent effecting a watertight closure.

One or more of the lower cranial nerves were sacrificed in 40% of patients in the Cambridge series. However, patients showed a remarkable ability to accommodate to the neurological deficit [6]. Whilst dysphonia was initially a problem in 6/15 patients, Teflon injection or thyroplasty significantly alleviated symptoms such that it was a persisting problem in only one patient. Persistent dysphagia was a feature in only two patients. Both were treated with a feeding gastrostomy. The remarkable tolerance of these patients to cranial nerve sacrifice may be related to the presence of mild pre-operative cranial nerve deficits present in most patients. Pre-existing cranial nerve dysfunction appears to lead to an increased capacity for functional adaptation. Traditionally, facial nerve transposition has been considered to lead to a permanent House–Brackmann Grade III palsy in the post-operative phase. However, a permanent facial nerve palsy was evident in only 6/15 of our cases at long-term follow-up. A quality of life assessment showed that 70% of patients had an "excellent", 10% a "good" and 20% a "poor" outcome from surgery for large glomus tumors. Long-term follow-up has shown that a small number of patients may develop local tumor recurrence (3/15). We therefore advocate early post-operative MRI to assess residual disease and provide a baseline for future reference. If tumor recurrence occurs, further surgery and/or radiotherapy needs to be considered.

## Conclusion

Acoustic neuromas are relatively common neoplasms of the CPA. Surgical approaches are well described, and the treatment outcomes, namely complete tumor removal with minimum mortality and morbidity, well established. Other tumors of the CPA are very rare. These tumors may have very complex relationships with cranial nerves, blood vessels and the skull base. Whilst surgery remains the mainstay in the treatment of all of these lesions, technical difficulties abound. Extended routes of access are frequently used to achieve maximal excision with minimal morbidity. Considerable experience at treating CPA acoustic neuromas is therefore highly desirable before embarking upon surgery for CPA rarities. Due to the large number of problems that these patients may present, a multi-faceted-team approach is advocated at all stages of treatment. In view of the rarity of these tumors, we strongly advocate a tertiary referral system to allow patients to benefit from the pooling of both experience and resources.

## Key Points

- *MRI scans can usually provide the surgeon with an accurate pre-treatment diagnosis for lesions in the CPA.*

- *Microsurgical excision, stereotactic radiosurgery and a "watch, wait and re-scan" policy all have merits in different patients with CPA lesions.*
- *Attention to detail, coupled with operator experience, minimize surgical complications.*
- *A multi-faceted-team approach is required to manage post-operative cranial nerve palsies optimally.*

## Self-assessment Questions (based on genuine patients)

☐ Discuss the management of a 30-year-old lady presenting with tinnitus in whom an MRI scan revealed a 2-cm acoustic neuroma.

☐ A 13-year-old girl presented with dizzy turns and life-long facial asymmetry. An MRI scan of the brain demonstrated bilateral intracanalicular acoustic neuromas, a 2.5-cm trigeminal neuroma, a 1-cm intraventricular tumor and a 1-cm cervico-medullary meningioma. Discuss the management of the child and her family.

☐ Describe the anatomical basis for the features of a complete facial nerve palsy.

☐ Describe the management of a patient with a House Grade IV facial nerve palsy after acoustic neuroma excision.

## References

1. Grey PL, Moffat DA, Hardy DG. Surgical results in unusual cerebellopontine angle tumors. Clin Otolaryngol 1996;21:237–43.
2. Pensak ML, Glasscock ME, Josey AF, Jackson CG, Gulya AJ. Sudden hearing loss and cerebellopontine angle tumors. Laryngoscope 1985;95:1188–93.
3. Irving RM, Moffat DA, Hardy DG et al. A molecular, clinical, and immunohistochemical study of vestibular schwannoma. Otolaryngol Head Neck Surg 1997;116:426–30.
4. Moffat DA, Golledge J, Baguley DM, Hardy DG. Clinical correlates of acoustic neuroma morphology. J Laryngol Otol 1993;107:290–4.
5. Michaels L. Origin of congenital cholesteatoma from a normally occurring epidermoid rest in the developing middle ear. International Journal of Pediatric Otorhinolarngology 1988;15:51–65.
6. Whitfield PC, Grey P, Hardy DG, Moffat DA. The surgical management of patients with glomus tumors of the skull base. Br J Neurosurg 1996;10:343–50.

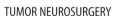
7. Jallo GI, Woo HH, Meshki C, Epstein FJ, Wisoff JH. Arachnoid cysts of the cerebellopontine angle: diagnosis and surgery. Neurosurgery 1997;40:31–8.

8. Maceri DR, Fox CM. Audiological assessment of the acoustic neuroma patient. Techniques in Neurosurgery 1997;3:89–94.

9. Gardner G, Robertson JH. Hearing preservation in unilateral acoustic neuroma surgery. Ann Otol Rhinol Laryngol 1988;97:55–66.

10. Bederson JB, von Ammon K, Wichmann WW, Yarsagil MG. Conservative treatment of patients with acoustic neuromas. Neurosurgery 1991;28:646–51.

11. Møller AR. Intraoperative monitoring in acoustic neuroma operations. Techniques in Neurosurgery 1997;3: 109–21.

12. Cushing H. Intracranial Tumors. Springfield, Illinois: Charles C. Thomas, 1932.

13. House JW, Brackmann DE. Facial nerve grading system. Otolaryngol Head Neck Surg 1985;93:146–7.

14. Moffat DA, Hardy DG, Grey PL, Baguley DM. The operative learning curve and its effect on facial nerve outcome in vestibular schwannoma surgery. Am J Otol 1996;17:643–7.

15. Grey PL, Moffat DA, Palmer CR, Hardy DG, Baguley DM. Factors which influence the facial nerve outcome in vestibular schwannoma surgery. Clin Otolaryngol 1996;21:409–13.

16. Erickson DL, Ausman JI, Chou SN. Prognosis of seventh nerve palsy following removal of large acoustic tumors. J Neurosurg 1977;47:31–?

17. Croxson GR, Moffat DA, Hardy DG, Baguley DM. Role of post-operative electroneuronography in predicting facial nerve recovery after acoustic neuroma removal: a pilot study. J Laryngol Otol 1989;103:60–2.

18. Moffat DA, da Cruz MJ, Baguley DM, Beynon GJ, Hardy DG. Hearing preservation in solitary vestibular schwannoma surgery using the retrosigmoid approach. Otolaryngol Head Neck Surg 1999 (In Press).

19. Ebersold MJ, Yamamoto Y, Harner SG, Beatty CW, Quast LM. The retrosigmoid approach for acoustic neuromas: the Mayo Clinic experience. Techniques in Neurosurgery 1997;3:122–30.

20. Haines SJ, Levine S. Middle fossa approach for acoustic neuroma. Techniques in Neurosurgery 1997;3:143–9.

21. Irving RM, Viani L, Hardy DG, Baguley DM, Moffat DA. Nervus intermedius function after vestibular schwannoma removal: clinical features and pathophysiological mechanisms. Laryngoscope 1995;105:809–13.

22. Hardy DG, MacFarlane R, Moffat DA. Wound closure after acoustic neuroma surgery. B J Neurosurg 1993; 7:171–4.

23. Kondziolka D, Lunsford LD, Flickinger JC. Stereotactic radiosurgery for acoustic tumors: Technique and results. Techniques in Neurosurgery 1997;3:154–61.

24. Kondziolka D, Lunsford LD, McLaughlin MR, Flickinger JC. Long-term outcomes after radiosurgery for acoustic neuromas. New Eng J Med 1998;339:1471–3.

25. Forster DMC, Kemeny AA, Pathak A, Walton L. Radiosurgery: a minimally interventional alternative to microsurgery in the management of acoustic neuroma. Br J Neurosurg 1996;10:169–74.

# 15

# Skull Base Tumors

R.S.C. Kerr and C.A. Milford

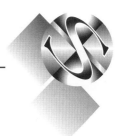

## Summary

Skull base tumors are rare, accounting for less than 1% of intracranial tumors. Management options include a conservative approach with serial scans, conventional surgery or radiotherapy/stereotactic radiosurgery. Surgery is difficult because of problems with access, involvement of basal blood vessels/cranial nerves and the potential for post-operative cerebrospinal fluid leakage.

This book contains other chapters that deal specifically with the management of:

- Sellar and parasellar tumors.
- Meningiomas.
- Cerebellopontine angle tumors.

Clearly, these tumors comprise a large number of the cases that a skull base team will see. Readers are therefore referred to other chapters for those specific lesions, and we will deal only with those tumors of the skull base not included in the above.

In the past, the skull base has been a surgical "no-man's land", and the discipline of skull base surgery owes its development to individuals in many disciplines who were prepared to tackle the almost impossible problems confronting them at the time. It began near the turn of the century, with resections of acoustic tumors and approaches to the pituitary. It was not until the pioneering work of Ketcham et al. [1], whose first report appeared in 1963, that co-ordinated efforts between surgical disciplines produced the first series of skull base procedures.

The modern skull base unit comprises a multidisciplinary team, which will include (as a minimum) a neuroradiologist, neurosurgeon, otolaryngologist, plastic and reconstructive surgeon, neuroanaesthetist and intensive care specialist. Nursing and ancillary staff with an interest in neurosurgical/neurological rehabilitation is also mandatory. No one surgeon can obtain, much less sustain, all the skills required to deal with all lesions in this area. Multidisciplinary management is the only approach that is likely to lead to improved outcomes for patients with these difficult problems – successful skull base surgery is a team effort!

The surgery involved in skull base tumors is often lengthy. The teamwork helps not only in bringing together expertise from different specialties but also provides an opportunity for intermittent relaxation during a prolonged surgical procedure.

Whatever the make up of the skull base team, the neurosurgeon often assumes a major responsibility for the patients in the post-operative period, as the majority of the major complications are related to the brain and its coverings.

# Presentation of Patients with Skull Base Lesions

Lesions at the skull base are often occult and not easily diagnosed early. Symptomatology varies greatly, depending on the size, site and nature of the tumor.

## Lesions of the Anterior Cranial Fossa

Localizing symptoms of lesions in the anterior fossa often include nasal or visual dysfunction. Symptoms may include nasal obstruction as well as pain, epistaxis and hyposmia/anosmia. Optic problems may include visual loss (acuity or visual field), diplopia and proptosis. For lesions involving the frontal lobes, alteration in personality, memory and concentration may also be apparent, especially with bi-frontal changes.

Examination should include endoscopy of the nose/nasopharynx, as well as a full neurological examination.

## Lesions of the Middle Cranial Fossa

These may be divided into sphenoid/parasellar mid-line lesions (including nasopharyngeal lesions), and pathologies affecting the true middle cranial fossae on either side of the mid-line structures. The sphenoid lesions may present with endocrine abnormalities through effects on the pituitary and/or cranial neuropathies of nerves II, III, IV, V and VI through effects on the cavernous sinus. Nasopharyngeal lesions may present with nasal symptoms or otologic problems related to secondary Eustachian tube dysfunction, as well as a trigeminal neuropathy. Finally, if more laterally placed, symptoms due to temporal lobe involvement may be apparent, including seizures and visual field defects.

## Lesions of the Posterior Fossa

Symptoms and signs of pathology in the posterior fossa are related primarily to dysfunction in cranial nerves V–XII, changes due to brain stem compression and cerebellar ataxia. Symptoms may include facial nerve weakness/spasm, hearing loss, tinnitus and imbalance, dysphonia and dysphagia. In association with larger tumors, patients may develop symptoms of raised intracranial pressure due to hydrocephalus.

In many instances, the pathological diagnosis of a skull base tumor has rested entirely on its imaging characteristics, unless it arises from a site accessible to biopsy, e.g. a paranasal sinus tumor with a nasal component. Increasingly, pathology involving the anterior and middle fossa is amenable to endoscopic biopsy via the nose/nasopharynx/paranasal sinuses. Reliance on imaging characteristics alone is therefore becoming less common. (In our unit, endoscopic biopsy via the paranasal sinuses has led to the pre-operative histologic diagnosis of trigeminal neuroma, lymphoma, meningioma, fibrous dysplasia, ossifying fibroma, plasmacytoma, chordoma and secondary renal carcinoma.)

# Imaging of the Skull Base

The skull base represents a bony partition between the intracranial cavity and the orbits, nose, paranasal sinuses, nasopharynx and ear. Imaging characteristics are important in establishing:

- The anatomic location and identity of the tumor.
- The extent of the tumor, especially in relation to the major vessels and cranial nerves, dura and intracranial structures.

MRI and CT are complementary in most areas of evaluation of skull base lesions.

CT is better at detecting calcification and at evaluating the effect of tumors on the bone of the skull base. It can be particularly helpful as part of the assessment of the paranasal sinuses and the temporal bone, and where the tumor is itself calcified. Its disadvantages consist mainly of the inadequately detailed display of intracranial structures.

MRI is superior in demonstrating the relationship of a skull base tumor to soft tissue structures, the carotid artery, sigmoid sinus/internal jugular vein, dura and brain. As far as the carotid artery is concerned, MRA is helpful for assessing patency and its relationship to the tumor. However, conventional angiography probably remains the "gold standard" if there is debate regarding its involvement and for demonstrating small vessel detail. It may also be required in:

- Embolization of the tumor pre-operatively. This is indicated in the case of juvenile angiofibroma, jugulotympanic paragangliomas, vagal paragangliomas and vascular meningiomas.

- Balloon test occlusion of the ICA. This is important if the carotid artery appears to be invaded by tumor, a temporary trial occlusion of the ICA can be used to identify those patients with no flow reserve who are at high risk of developing neurologic sequelae if the carotid is permanently occluded.

# General Principles of Skull Base Surgery

It is clearly important that any patient with a skull base tumor should be told the long-term outlook of the tumor itself, i.e. the natural history of the pathology. They also need to be informed of all the management options available and these would usually include:

- Conservative management – monitoring the tumor with serial imaging.

- Conventional surgery – again, patients need information regarding outcomes, surgical morbidity and mortality. The figures one quotes need to relate to your own experience, as well as figures taken from the literature.

- Radiotherapy/stereotactic radiosurgery.

There will be occasions when combinations of the above are appropriate, e.g. where partial removal and post-operative radiotherapy may be the most suitable option.

The choice of management option will rely on such factors as the age of the patient and their general medical status, the natural history of the tumor, the location and size of the tumor, the potential risks of the surgery/radiotherapy/

radiosurgery and, importantly, the skill and experience of the skull base team.

As far as the operation is concerned, the surgeon should be guided by one overriding principle: removal of adequate amounts of bone from the cranial base should provide sufficient access without the necessity to retract dura/brain. Remove bone before considering retracting brain, dura or the cranial nerves.

Even though many neoplasms involving the skull base are benign or locally confined malignant lesions, radical resection of extensive lesions remains difficult. The reasons for this include:

- The necessity to retract the brain to achieve tumor exposure (even when adequate bone removal has occurred), with the possibility of retraction-related cerebral injury.

- The involvement by tumor of basal blood vessels, injury to which may lead to stroke and/or death.

- The involvement of the cranial nerves, injury to which may result in significant functional deficits. In any surgical procedure which involves risk to the facial nerve, use of intraoperative electro-physiologic monitoring of the nerve is mandatory.

- The potential for CSF leakage through the skin, paranasal sinuses or nasopharynx, which may be followed by meningitis and death. In any case where the risk of post-operative CSF leak is high, use of a lumbar drain in the post-operative period should be considered.

In the past, the surgical treatment of skull base tumors has been associated with a high rate of local recurrence (related to the problems of gaining good surgical access and the involvement/close proximity of vital structures). Post-operative monitoring is therefore an extremely important part of their management and this will involve serial imaging. A 'base line' scan would usually be performed about 3 months following the surgery and then at regular intervals (often between 6 and 12 months). The choice of imaging may vary occasionally, although MRI will be the modality of choice in the majority of instances.

In some areas of the skull base, e.g. the nose/paranasal sinuses, imaging may be supplemented by endoscopic follow-up. Certainly, in extracranial skull base tumors in this area, endoscopic examination and biopsy will provide a more sensitive follow-up than any imaging modality currently available. The follow-up period varies according to the pathology, but often would be for a minimum of 5 years.

# Workload of the Oxford Skull Base Unit

Skull base tumors are rare, probably accounting for less than 1% of intracranial tumors [2], and it is difficult to obtain accurate figures regarding their incidence. Looking at our workload in Oxford does provide some insight into the incidence of these rare problems and their relative incidence in terms of benign and malignant tumors. During the 7-year period up to 2000, we have together seen 501 cases.

Their management involved the following:

- Surgery in 255 cases (51%).
- Conservative management with serial scans in 205 cases (41%).
- Radiotherapy/stereotactic radiosurgery in 41 cases (8%).

This workload represents approximately 71 new cases per year. As our unit serves a population of approximately 3 million, the 71 new cases per year represent an incidence of approximately 1:40,000 population per year. Our figures seem to compare to the few groups who have published details of workload. Sekhar and Janecka (1993) in Pittsburgh, USA, saw a total of 780 cases in a 7-year period, and these patients included 605 with neoplasms who underwent surgery, 487 (76%) with benign tumors and 118 (24%) with malignant tumors. This surgical workload represented approximately 69 surgical procedures per year. Donald (1998), in Sacramento, USA, saw a higher percentage of malignant lesions (37% malignant and 63% benign) and had a surgical workload of 27 cases per year.

# Pathology of Skull Base Tumors

Primary tumors of the skull base are rare. It is more common for involvement to occur consequent upon spread from either a primary intracranial or an extracranial neoplastic process. Whether arising primarily from the skull base or involving it secondarily, these tumors are uncommon.

Tumors may be classified as:

- Primary skull base lesions – those arising from the bone and/or cartilage.
- Intracranial – those that arise at the base of the brain, with a tendency to invade the basicranium. They may arise from the neural, vascular or meningeal tissues within the cranium.
- Extracranial – those originating from tissues just below the cranium and invading the skull base secondarily. They often involve the paranasal sinuses, the infratemporal fossa, or the parapharyngeal space.

## Primary Skull Base Lesions

### Benign Primary Skull Base Lesions

*Osteoma*

This is a slowly growing, benign tumor that may affect any area of the skull base, most commonly the frontal and ethmoid sinuses. Osteomata may require surgical treatment if they produce orbital or cosmetic problems. They are rarely associated with leakage of CSF or a pneumatocele through involvement of the anterior cranial fossa.

*Fibro-osseous Lesions/Fibrous Dysplasia*

The term "fibro-osseous lesion" has been used as a general description for a group of tumors and proliferative disorders that may involve any of the cranial fossae. They comprise a number of specific clinical entities, in which the clinical, radiological and histological features often overlap, resulting in confusion for both pathologists and clinicians concerned with diagnosis and management.

The common denominator is the replacement of normal bone architecture by tissue composed of collagen, fibroblasts and varying amounts of osteoid or bone. The two most common conditions falling within this group are ossifying fibroma and fibrous dysplasia.

- Ossifying fibroma is an encapsulated benign neoplasm consisting of fibrous tissue and containing varied amounts of metaplastic bone and mineralized masses. It mainly affects bones which are ossified in membrane, usually presenting as a painless mass. Radiological changes are of a discrete mass with a distinct boundary and thinning of the cortical bone, resulting in an eggshell appearance. In most instances, the mass is surrounded by smooth, well defined cortical bone, which differentiates it from fibrous dysplasia where "blending" into the surrounding bone is universal. Its behaviour is that of a benign neoplasm and hence it continues to grow after skeletal maturity is reached. It normally, therefore, warrants surgical treatment at some point.

- Fibrous dysplasia is a benign, localized bone disorder of unknown aetiology that results in extreme thickening of bone owing to the presence of intraosseous proliferating connective tissue. It may be monostotic (affecting one bone) or polyostotic (affecting several bones). It is a self-limiting process that starts in childhood but, due to a very slow growth rate, may not cause symptoms until adulthood. Growth can be expected to slow or stop after puberty in monostotic disease. The most characteristic radiologic feature is a diffusely blending margin in marked contrast to the sharply demarcated ossifying fibroma (although the features are non-specific, they depend upon the age of the lesion and degree of metaplastic bone formation).

Differential diagnosis of these conditions relies on the correlation of histopathologic and radiologic findings. Both are usually required to provide a definitive diagnosis.

The most common presentation would be with a slow-growing, asymmetrical, painless swelling (see Fig. 15.1). It manifests craniofacial involvement in about 10% of cases and gives

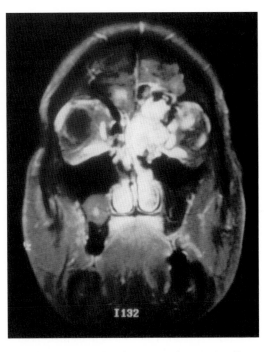

**Fig. 15.1.** Coronal MRI of patient with extensive fibrous dysplasia involving the anterior cranial fossa.

rise to cosmetic deformity, proptosis and, more seriously, compression of the optic nerve in the optic canal. Cosmetic concerns of the patient may give rise to pressure for consideration of surgical treatment but, on the whole, the management would be conservative in view of the slow natural history. However, signs of optic nerve compression are an absolute indication for surgery, as is the development of other intracranial complications, e.g. cerebrospinal fluid rhinorrhea.

## Malignant Primary Skull Base Lesions

### Chondrosarcoma

These are malignant tumors of cartilage that may arise in bone or soft tissues. They comprise 6% of skull base neoplasms [5]. Approximately 75% of all cranial chondrosarcomas occur at the base of the skull, and most of these are found in the middle cranial fossa.

These tumors affect both sexes equally and occur over a broad age range, with a peak distribution at between 30 and 50 years of age. Symptoms vary according to the site of origin but the most common include headaches, visual disturbance, cranial neuropathies, hearing loss and disturbances of gait. Imaging shows mottled calcification within the soft tissue mass on CT scanning.

Chondrosarcoma tends to act less aggressively than other sarcomas but nevertheless pursues a slow and intractably progressive course, which ultimately kills the patient in many cases. The history therefore tends to be long and is punctuated by multiple local recurrences. Distant metastases are relatively rare, occurring in only about 8% of cases [6].

Surgery is the primary treatment modality. Conventional radiotherapy has been used as an adjunct. More recently, some workers have advocated proton beam radiation therapy as the adjuvant radiation modality of choice. This form of irradiation is of interest to the radiation oncologist because of its improved dose localization capabilities in comparison to high-energy X-rays (photons). It is suggested [7] that proton radiation therapy after maximal surgical resection represents the best management policy currently available for patients with chondrosarcomas (and chordomas) of the skull base.

### Chordoma

These are slow-growing, locally aggressive malignant neoplasms, derived from vestigial remnants of the notochord found along the axial skeleton. They account for less than 1% of all intracranial neoplasms [8]. They can be divided into three main groups, depending upon the site of origin: cranial (35%), sacrococcygeal (50%) or vertebral (15%). Cranial lesions tend to affect a younger age group (range 20–40 years) compared to the sacrococcygeal group (40–60 years). Men are more commonly affected than women (3:1).

The location of a chordoma within the clivus determines the nature and path of its growth, the associated anatomic structures involved, the clinical symptomatology, and the approach for surgical management. However, whatever their position within the clivus and their symptoms, presentation is usually late after intracranial extension has occurred.

Lesions arising near the inferior tip of the clivus, the basion, usually produce lower brain stem compression as they expand and present clinically with hypoglossal nerve lesions. Tumors arising from the body of the clivus are the most common. They may expand ventrally and produce a nasopharyngeal mass with obstruction, or they may expand dorsally and stretch the sixth cranial nerve as it runs along and penetrates the clival dura, leading to diplopia. Tumors arising at the rostral end of the clivus involve the sella turcica and may present with hypopituitarism. With suprasellar extension, a chiasmal syndrome with bitemporal hemianopia may result. Lateral extension of rostral clival chordomas may produce a parasellar mass or extend into the cavernous sinus, affecting cranial nerves III–VI. Postero-lateral extension of mid-clival chordomas can produce otologic symptoms of deafness, vertigo and tinnitus, with risk of facial weakness through involvement of the petrous temporal bone.

The position of the tumor rarely allows complete surgical resection and thus recurrence rate after surgery remains high. In view of the high local recurrence rate, conventional radiotherapy has been used, with varying success. As mentioned above, it is suggested that proton radiation therapy after maximal surgical resection seems to represent the best management policy currently available for patients with chordomas of the skull base.

# Intracranial Skull Base Tumors

## Benign Intracranial Skull Base Tumors

### Schwannoma (Neurilemmoma)

Clearly, the VIII cranial nerve is the most common site for this tumor. However, other cranial nerves may be affected.

### Trigeminal Schwannoma

These tumors account for 2% of intracranial schwannomata. They may originate in any section of the fifth cranial nerve, from the root to the distal extracranial branches; as a result, a variety of symptoms and signs may develop, depending on the direction and extent of tumor growth. Fifty percent of all intracranial trigeminal schwannomata arise from the trigeminal ganglion and remain predominantly localized to the middle fossa. Patients typically present with pain/paraesthesia in a trigeminal distribution, which may spread from one to all three divisions, often followed by progressive sensory loss and, less commonly, by wasting of the muscles of mastication (most easily seen in temporalis).

Approximately 20% arise from the trigeminal root and remain primarily infratentorial within the posterior fossa. They present with ataxia, hearing loss, tinnitus and facial nerve dysfunction, together with trigeminal symptoms. Approximately 25% grow above and below the tentorium ("hourglass tumors") and produce a combination of clinical findings reflecting involvement of both the middle and posterior fossae. Finally, there are a small group of patients where the tumor arises from the distal intracranial branches of the V nerve and extend extracranially, e.g. producing a mass in the pterygopalatine/infratemporal fossa.

On CT, these tumors are usually isodense or slightly hyperdense in comparison to surrounding brain and enhance homogeneously after administration of intravenous contrast. On MRI, they are generally well circumscribed, show decreased signal intensity on T1-weighted images, increased signal on T2-weighted images and show homogeneous enhancement after administration of gadolinium.

Trigeminal schwannomas displace rather than invade adjacent structures and tumor removal can therefore often be accomplished without significant neurological injury (other than anaesthesia in the distribution of the affected branch of the nerve), provided an appropriate operative approach is chosen.

## Facial Nerve Schwannoma

Primary tumors of the facial nerve are rare. When they do occur, they can be found along the entire course of the nerve, but most frequently either within the temporal bone or extracranially. As they originate from the Schwann cells of the nerve sheath, their finding within the internal auditory canal or intracranially must be explained on the basis of embryonic rests of ganglionic cells from the geniculate ganglion.

Clinical presentation varies, depending on the site of tumor origin. Schwannomas found along the extracranial course of the nerve present primarily as a parotid mass, with facial nerve weakness being an unusual presenting complaint. If the tumor originates within the temporal bone (and that may be anywhere from the geniculate ganglion to the stylomastoid foramen), it usually produces otologic symptoms and is commonly associated with facial weakness (presumably related to compression

within a tight bony canal). Intracranially, these tumors will give rise to the symptoms associated with most other lesions of the cerebellopontine angle.

Both CT and MRI may be helpful in localizing the lesion. They may detect widening of the fallopian canal or bone erosion/soft tissue mass in relation to the intratemporal course of the facial nerve.

The aims of management include:

- Establishing a diagnosis.
- Attempting to preserve continuity of the facial nerve.
- Completing tumor resection.
- Facial nerve reconstruction/facial paralysis rehabilitation.

Because the cell of origin lies within the nerve sheath, it is theoretically possible to consider tumor removal without a nerve transection. In practice, it rarely proves possible and, hence, surgery results in complete facial nerve palsy in the vast majority of cases. There is therefore often a case for a period of conservative management whilst the facial nerve function remains normal or near normal, unless it gives rise to some more serious problems. When surgery is eventually undertaken, complete tumor removal should be confirmed by frozen section examination of the proximal and distal nerve margin. Reconstruction will usually involve an interposition nerve graft (the greater auricular nerve is a convenient local source of a cable graft). The quality of recovery following such a procedure would be between Grades III and V (House–Brackman) at best.

## Jugular Foramen Schwannoma

As with trigeminal and facial schwannomas, these are rare. The patient usually presents with a unilateral lesion of cranial nerves IX, X or XI or a combination of the three nerves. When the majority of the tumor is below the skull base, there is rarely a neuropathy and presentation, in our experience, is with the non-specific features of a parapharyngeal mass.

Diagnosis is made from CT and/or MRI. The CT scan demonstrates a smooth-edged enlargement of the jugular foramen, with extension inferiorly into the neck, posteriorly into the posterior fossa or directly into the skull base. MRI may be useful regarding soft tissue relations, particularly in the neck. Carotid angiography may be indicated for assessing cerebral cross-circulation if there is any question that surgery might compromise the internal carotid artery.

Management lies between a conservative approach with the use of serial imaging or surgery. Recommendations for treatment relies on the age of the patient and their general medical health, the size of the tumor, whether it is creating any mass effect in the posterior fossa and the presence or absence of cranial neuropathies. Certainly, older patients do not tolerate the rapid change in lower cranial nerve function that surgery may produce, and are therefore at risk of developing serious pulmonary complications from laryngeal aspiration. In this age group, patients are more likely to adapt to these lower cranial neuropathies if they occur slowly as the disease progresses; a conservative policy may therefore be the most appropriate.

## Malignant Intracranial Skull Base Tumors

### Olfactory Neuroblastoma (Esthesioneuroblastoma)

An uncommon neuroectodermal tumor that arises from the olfactory nasal epithelium, high up in the nasal roof within the olfactory cleft (the space between the superior nasal septum and the middle and superior turbinates on the lateral wall of the nose), attached to the cribriform plate. It affects both sexes equally and occurs in all age groups. Presentation is often non-specific, with nasal obstruction, epistaxis and, less commonly, anosmia and visual problems.

Although the diagnosis relies on biopsy and histology, imaging allows assessment of the extent of the tumor. Woodhead and Lloyd (1988) reviewed imaging in a series of 24 patients and concluded that there were no specific features to identify this tumor. However, a tumor within the ethmoid and upper nasal airway, expanding into the orbit and eroding the roof of the fronto–ethmoid complex or cribriform plate unilaterally in a young patient, is likely to be an olfactory neuroblastoma (see Fig. 15.2).

The natural history of this malignancy is both variable and unpredictable. Metastasis to cervical lymph nodes occurs in 10–30% of patients during the course of the disease and systemic metastasis (lung and bone) in 8–46% of cases [10–13]. Although often slow-growing, it must be considered as a highly malignant neoplasm, requiring radical initial treatment.

Treatment normally involves a combination of radical surgery and radiotherapy. Survival rates of 60% at 3 years and 40% at 5 years are

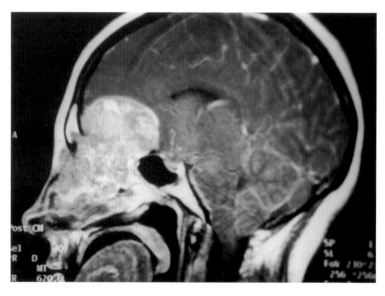

**Fig. 15.2.** Sagittal MRI of patient with large olfactory neuroblastoma.

quoted [14] for those patients having surgically accessible lesions treated with combinations of excisional surgery and radiotherapy.

# Extracranial Skull Base Tumors

## Benign Extracranial Skull Base Tumors

### Juvenile Angiofibroma

Highly vascular and locally invasive, juvenile angiofibromas occur almost exclusively in adolescent males. Although morphologically benign, these tumors can exhibit aggressive local growth, extending along planes of least resistance or pre-formed pathways and, when large, can invade directly by bone erosion.

Juvenile angiofibromas represent less than 0.05% of all head and neck tumors, with a median age at presentation of around 13 years. It is thought the hormonal changes at puberty are the primary influence on the growth of this tumor. The site of origin is unclear but is likely to be from the sphenopalatine foramen. The tumor spreads laterally into the pterygopalatine fossa, thereby gaining access into the infratemporal fossa as well as the nasal cavity/paranasal sinuses and nasopharynx posteriorly, and the orbit superiorly. Intracranial spread into the anterior cranial fossa may occur, but more likely is invasion into the middle cranial fossa (although it usually remains extradural). Early symptoms of nasal obstruction and intermittent epistaxis are found in over 80% of patients. Nasendoscopy invariably confirms the presence of a mass obstructing the posterior nares. At diagnosis, approximately two thirds of patients have localized disease, and 20% have intracranial involvement [15]. Erosion of the medial pterygoid plate associated with enlargement of the sphenopalatine foramen is a constant feature on CT scan. Involvement of the sphenoid sinus, infratemporal fossa, orbit or middle cranial fossa may be demonstrated but is more easily demonstrated on MRI. The distinction between the mass and fluid in an obstructed sinus and the vascularity of the lesion (signal voids from the vessels within the tumor) can also be made on MRI.

There is little factual evidence to support a common belief that, with increasing age, angiofibromas will show spontaneous involution. It must be assumed that all untreated angiofibromas possess potential for aggressive growth.

Management usually involves surgery (rarely radiotherapy may be indicated in extremely extensive tumors where surgery may carry a high risk of operative mortality). In view of its vascularity, the majority of surgeons would seek the help of the interventional neuroradiologist, with pre-operative angiography and embolization. About 10% of cases recur after surgical resection (probably a reflection upon the difficulty of gaining good surgical access to this area).

### Glomus Tumors (Paraganglioma) of the Temporal Bone

Paragangliomas are a group of histologically similar benign neoplasms that arise from neuroectodermally derived paraganglionic cells associated with autonomic ganglia. Two sites of these extra-adrenal paraganglia include:

- Intravagal – these are at the level of the jugular or nodose ganglion. Tumors arising here give rise to glomus vagale tumors.
- Jugulotympanic – these occur along Jacobson's nerve (tympanic branch of IX) and Arnold's nerve (tympanic branch of X), but the majority are found in the adventitia of the jugular bulb in the jugular fossa. Tumors arising from these sites give rise to glomus tympanicum (arising within the tympanic, or middle ear, cavity) and glomus jugulare tumors (arising from the jugular bulb).

Glomus vagale tumors usually present as a parapharyngeal mass, with no obvious neurologic problems. Their involvement of the jugular foramen and possible spread along the internal carotid artery towards the cavernous sinus can make their management difficult.

Jugulotympanic paragangliomas usually present with a unilateral hearing loss and pulsatile tinnitus. More rarely, they present with neuropathy involving the lower cranial (IX,X, XI,XII) or facial nerves. On examination, a vascular mass is seen behind the tympanic membrane or, in larger tumors, the mass may have eroded though the drum and floor of the bony ear canal to present within the ear canal itself.

Multiple or synchronous tumors occur in 3–10% of patients [16], and there is a familial incidence with an autosomal dominant mode of transmission (these patients have a higher incidence of synchronous paragangliomas).

These tumors demonstrate a slow and insidious pattern of growth. They tend to migrate through the temporal bone by vascular channels, naturally occurring fissures and foramina and, most importantly, along air cell tracts. Intracranial extension into the posterior and middle fossae does occur and increases potential morbidity and mortality. Rarely, these tumors may metastasize, usually to cervical lymph nodes.

The clinical picture of jugulotympanic paragangliomas is characteristic, but the clinical findings non-diagnostic. The mainstay of tumor diagnosis is radiological and the main diagnostic objectives are:

- Determine the site and extent of the tumor.
- Determine the presence of synchronous lesions.
- Determine the degree of major vascular involvement.
- Identify any intracranial extension.
- Determine central nervous system collateral circulation.

High-resolution CT scanning or MRI may assess the site and extent of tumor. MRI is superior in assessing intracranial extension and is useful for identifying synchronous tumors. Bilateral carotid angiography is used to determine involvement of the internal carotid artery (ICA) in larger tumors and the degree of collateral blood flow. It will also identify an aberrant ICA/intrapetrous carotid artery aneurysm (both are included in the differential diagnosis of a vascular lesion behind the tympanic membrane), as well as the rare case of anomalous venous drainage, where all intracranial venous return occurs via a single sigmoid sinus/internal jugular vein on the involved side (a contraindication to surgery). If performed pre-operatively, it also allows embolization of the lesion.

The management options for these tumors once again include:

- Conservative management.
- Surgery.
- Radiotherapy (or possibly stereotactic radiosurgery in some cases). This may have a place as a primary form of treat-

ment in some cases, and may be the treatment modality of choice in recurrent/residual disease. The aim of treatment is to prevent further growth rather than to eradicate the disease.

The intricate temporal bone anatomy, the extent of tumor invasion and tumor vascularity combine to make these tumors difficult to manage by any mode of therapy. The critical question to be asked is whether the disease is likely to cause the patient serious problems in the natural course of his/her remaining years. At one end of the spectrum, a large tumor in a young, fit patient almost certainly warrants surgical treatment, whereas a small tumor in an elderly patient probably needs nothing more than careful review. Unfortunately, there is a "gray area" between these two ends of the spectrum although, currently, many would consider surgery as the first-line treatment. The judicious use of surgery is imperative, since an iatrogenic deficit involving the last four cranial nerves may pose life-threatening complications to an older patient with poor respiratory reserve.

Contraindications to surgical treatment include:

- Carotid involvement in the presence of poor collateral circulation.
- Contralateral vagus lesion – surgery that compromises the only functional vagus is a relative contraindication.
- Unresectable tumor – a neurosurgically unresectable intracranial extension is a relative contraindication.
- Anomalous venous drainage – where all intracranial venous return occurs via a single sigmoid sinus on the involved side. In this situation, it may be better to await complete occlusion of the jugular bulb (which allows progressive opening of collateral venous channels) before operating.

## Malignant Extracranial Skull Base Tumors

### Carcinoma of the Paranasal Sinuses

Virtually all types of malignancy may present in this area but the most frequent are forms of squamous cell carcinoma (the most common malignancy of the head and neck) and adenocarcinoma. Reports on the association between adenocarcinoma of the ethmoid and the wood-working trade (especially hardwood exposure) began in 1965 in the UK [17,18]. The increased relative risk is similar to that for carcinoma of the bronchus in smokers, with a cumulative life-time risk of 1 in 120 and a 500–1,000 times greater risk than the general population of developing the condition. It became a recognized industrial disease in the UK in 1969.

Patients present with nasal symptoms, such as nasal obstruction and epistaxis. Orbital symptoms include swelling, diplopia and proptosis (see Fig. 15.3).

It is well recognized that, in the past, the poor prognosis associated with these tumors was a consequence of local recurrence engendered by inadequate resection. The realization that these tumors affect the inferior surface of the cribriform plate and roof of ethmoid (and hence are likely to have an intracranial component) led to the development of the combined skull base approach. This offered access and more rational, yet radical, resection choices, dependent on

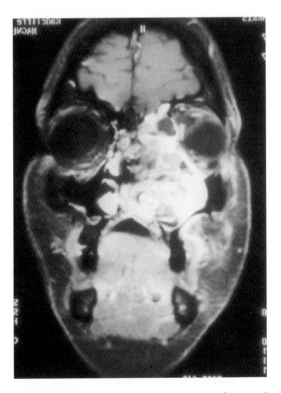

**Fig. 15.3.** Coronal MRI of patient with carcinoma of paranasal sinuses with involvement of the anterior cranial fossa.

anatomic considerations. Many patients with these tumors would be treated with a combination of craniofacial resection and radiotherapy.

In 1998, Lund et al. [19] published the results of a series of 209 patients undergoing craniofacial resection for sino-nasal neoplasia. The 5-year actuarial survival was 44%, falling to 32% at 10 years for malignant tumors. In the analysis of their results, it became clear that when disease affects the frontal lobe itself (as opposed to dural involvement alone), then there was a uniformly bad prognosis.

### Malignant Tumors of the Temporal Bone

Malignant tumors affecting the temporal bone account for only 0.05% of head and neck cancers [20]. Most are squamous cell carcinomas, arising in the external auditory canal and invading inward. Those arising within the middle ear/mastoid are often associated with the long-standing inflammation of chronic middle ear disease.

Patients present with discharge from the ear and associated bleeding and pain. In addition, alteration of facial nerve function should alert the clinician to the possibility of malignancy. In these circumstances, biopsy of any polyp or ulcer is mandatory.

Diagnosis is often made late. CT scan and MRI are used to assess the extent of the primary, and its relationship to the dura, brain, facial nerve and carotid artery. CT is more useful for detailing the intratemporal anatomy and showing the presence of bone erosion (and hence, by inference, presence of tumor). MRI is more useful to define tumor from brain and from the reactive/inflammatory changes that may occur, and gives information regarding ICA or sigmoid sinus patency by the presence or absence of flow void signals. Carotid angiography may, however, be necessary to establish unequivocally involvement of the carotid artery.

No coherent staging system exists and the lack of such a staging system means that comparing various treatment options described in the literature is impossible. Hence, there is great debate regarding an optimum treatment strategy.

In general, surgery and radiotherapy in combination are considered the treatment of choice. A number of surgical approaches are feasible that largely depend on the extent of the tumor.

Complete surgical resection with a clear microscopic margin is the preferred initial treatment objective. For small tumors, radiotherapy is an alternative.

The most widely accepted operative concept is to free the involved temporal bone from its surrounding venous sinuses, protect the internal carotid artery and brainstem and avoid injury to cranial nerves, if they are still functioning. Typically, the patient would also receive adjuvant radiotherapy. Although this approach has probably resulted in an improved quality of life for patients, the impact on survival is unknown.

# Surgical Approaches to the Skull Base

Careful planning, consideration of the aims of the surgery, detailed review of the radiology and an in-depth discussion with the patient and family are mandatory before any skull base approach is undertaken. The aim is to help, but this is invariably high-risk surgery and it is vital that the patient and the family understand what is being undertaken and why.

The surgical exposure of skull base lesions commonly involves extensive bone work. Exposure must be adequate and yet not excessive. Adequate exposure reduces the operating distance of deep lesions from the surgeon, reduces the need for brain retraction and provides space for manoeuvring. An adequately planned incision should take into account any previously existing incisions, the vascularity of the flap, cosmetic appearances and the course of the facial nerve. The exposure should also take into consideration proximal and distal control of major vessels. We would utilize electrophysiologic monitoring of the facial nerve in any case where its function could be compromised.

As in every other branch of surgery, there are a vast number of surgical approaches described for different areas of the skull base. We are limited to describing a small number of procedures and will therefore describe only techniques we have used and found "practical".

## Anterior Fossa

Anterior and anterolateral craniofacial resections (CFR) are designed to encompass tumors

along the anterior and middle cranial fossae. The interorbital compartment, limited by the medial walls of the orbits, the cribriform plate/ roof of ethmoid sinuses and the dura encompass the usual specimen removed during anterior CFR. Any lateral extension of the perimeter of excision would then constitute anterolateral CFR.

### Anterior Craniofacial Resection

Anterior CFR encompasses structures of the anterior mid-line and paramedian skull base (see Fig. 15.4). The ethmoid sinuses superiorly, the anterior wall of the sphenoid posteriorly, the frontal sinus anteriorly, and the nasopharynx inferiorly are included in the surgical perimeter of the anterior craniofacial resection.

*Indications*

- Resection of malignant tumors of the paranasal sinuses involving the ethmoid/ frontal sinus with proximity to or involvement of the ethmoid roof/ cribriform plate.
- Resection of benign tumors of the paranasal sinuses, meninges or skull base with involvement of, or extension through, the skull base.

*Surgical Steps*

The anterior CFR is performed through bicoronal and paranasal facial incisions. Following facial bone exposure, the medial walls of both orbits are explored, identifying and cauterising the anterior and posterior ethmoidal vessels. This establishes the lateral perimeter of the resection. Osteotomies can be performed at this point through the medial orbital wall of each orbit at the junction with the orbital floor. Anteriorly, a vertical cut can be made from the level of the lacrimal fossa to the level of the nasion, and a similar cut can be made posteriorly at the level of the posterior ethmoidal foramina.

At this point, a bifrontal craniotomy is performed. The bicoronal incision allows wide access to the frontal bone and, most importantly, preservation of pericranium [21] for use as a vascularized flap to repair the anterior fossa floor defect (it is raised in a rectangular shape with its base at the supraorbital region and receives its blood supply from supraorbital and

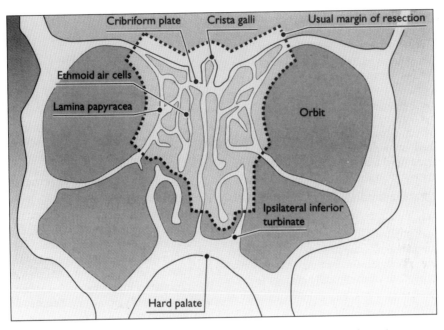

**Fig. 15.4.** Coronal anatomy, showing area of resection in anterior craniofacial resection.

supratrochlear vessels). A bi-frontal bone flap is then raised, either as a free flap or pedicled on temporalis. Care should be taken to keep the dura intact whilst opening the bone.

Exposure of the floor of the anterior fossa is best achieved by opening the dura on either side of the superior sagittal sinus as far anteriorly as possible. The sinus and underlying falx can then be divided between stay sutures. If a lumbar drain has been inserted, this can now be opened to allow CSF to drain. Diuretics may help provide good exposure without retraction of the frontal lobes.

Full exposure of the anterior cranial fossa floor invariably requires division of the olfactory tracts. Of course, if one or both can be protected, so much the better but, usually, patients with tumors requiring such an approach are anosmic.

The basal dura is reflected along the cribriform plate to the planum sphenoidale (if dura is involved, then it is mobilized more laterally and involved dura is resected with the tumor). Further cuts can then be made into the bone outside the tumor margins through the roof of the ethmoid/orbit laterally, through the planum sphenoidale into the sphenoid sinus posteriorly

and through the floor of the frontal sinus into the anterior ethmoid anteriorly (these cuts are often made from both above and below). The tumor specimen is then only attached by the perpendicular plate of the ethmoid (which forms the postero-superior part of the nasal septum), and this is divided using heavy scissors. The specimen can then be "rocked out" through the transfacial exposure, dividing any mucosal attachments that might still remain.

The resultant defect has as its anterior margin the anterior wall of the frontal sinus/nasion, posteriorly the remaining portion of the sphenoid sinus and optic nerves, and the periorbita laterally. Inferiorly, the defect is open to the nasopharynx. Reconstruction of the defect in the anterior cranial fossa floor involves use of the pericranial flap – it is "posted" back into the anterior fossa over the supraorbital bar of bone (and beneath the frontal bone when it is replaced at the end of the procedure). This vascularized graft is then sutured to the basal dura (and if sutures are too difficult to place, tissue glue is used) to provide a carpet-like resurfacing of the anterior cranial fossa. A second layer of free pericranium, placed intradurally, can then be used, again, glued into position. We have not found it necessary to replace bone and have had no problems with brain herniation. However, great care must be taken with this repair to achieve a water (CSF)-tight closure. The use of the lumbar drain post-operatively helps.

Often, the nasolacrimal duct is transected during this approach, and can be stented at the end of the procedure. The nasal cavity is then packed to help avoid a post-operative cerebrospinal fluid leak.

## Anterolateral Craniofacial Resection

Antero–lateral craniofacial resection also encompasses structures of the anterior mid-line and paramedian skull base but may also include the orbitomaxillary and infratemporal regions, as well as the floor of the middle cranial fossa.

### Indications

- As for anterior CFR, but with orbital involvement.
- Extensive maxillary tumors with orbital/ ethmoidal involvement.
- Extensive transcranial middle fossa tumors, e.g. meningiomas.

### Surgical Steps

This approach can be performed through a bicoronal scalp flap, especially if a dural graft is required to effect a repair. Alternatively, an extended pterional flap may be used.

The facial incisions are usually paranasal, with possible lip splitting and eyelid incisions. The precise shape of the craniotomy and the extent of any facial osteotomies depend on the size and site of the tumor. For a purely intra-orbital tumor, a pterional approach with extra-dural removal of lateral and superior orbital walls provides good access to the posterior part of the orbital cavity. Clearly, this would be inadequate for an extensive maxillary or ethmoidal lesion with orbital involvement, when a bi-frontal flap will allow far better access. As regards the facial osteotomies, in general, they are made within the orbit along the medial and lateral wall as well as across the zygoma.

For reconstruction, following dural repair, soft tissue may be brought into the area using either temporalis muscle or a free microvascular flap, depending upon the size of the defect.

## Middle Fossa

### Infratemporal–Middle Cranial Fossa Approach

This technique, pioneered by Fisch [22] and further developed by Sekhar [23] and Schramm [24], provides excellent access to regions previously characterized by difficult dissection and poor exposure. The entire middle cranial fossa, from the petrous ridge to the lesser wing of the sphenoid, can be exposed (see Fig. 15.5). Patients who require this approach present with a wide variety of disease processes. Tumors may be benign or malignant, and may originate intracranially from dura or calvarial bone or extracranially from the soft tissues that occupy the subcranial area. Most common among the intracranial neoplasms that extend extracranially are meningioma, chordoma, chondroma and chondrosarcoma. Among the extracranial tumors that extend intracranially are schwannoma (often of the trigeminal nerve); parotid tumors, especially of the deep lobe; and squamous cell carcinomas from the paranasal sinuses, nasopharynx and temporal bone.

### Surgical Steps

The approach is attained through a long incision, extending from the calvarial vertex to in front of the ear, then curving posteriorly under the lobule and into the neck, similar to the modified Blair incision for parotidectomy. The cutaneous flap is elevated anteriorly to a point from

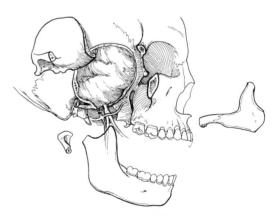

**Fig. 15.5.** Infratemporal fossa/middle cranial fossa approach. Removal of zygomatic arch (and possibly mandibular condylectomy), allowing access for craniotomy.

the angle of the mandible to the lateral orbital rim. The internal jugular vein and internal carotid artery are isolated in the neck and controlled with vascular loops.

The temporalis muscle, with a cuff of pericranium, is elevated to the zygomatic arch. Having fashioned a fronto-temporal craniotomy, the lateral orbital rim and zygomatic arch are removed in a single piece and stored for later reconstruction. This allows access to the infratemporal fossa, and this access can be improved, if required, by removing the mandibular condyle.

Once the zygomatic arch is removed, the temporalis muscle can be dissected down to its insertion on the coronoid process. This allows an exposure of the undersurface of the sphenoid and temporal bones. A subperiosteal dissection of the subcranial part of the middle cranial fossa is performed from the glenoid fossa posteriorly, to the base of the pterygoid plates anteriorly and is carried medially to the foramen spinosum and foramen ovale. These are the medial landmarks for the subsequent extension of the craniotomy.

The key to the exposure of the middle fossa and its immediate subcranial structures is an L-shaped craniotomy. This has a vertical component comprising the greater wing of the sphenoid and squamous part of the temporal bone, and a short horizontal component that ends at the foramen ovale and spinosum. The size of the craniotomy is determined by the extent of intracranial tumor. If exposure of the intrapetrous internal carotid is required, the craniotomy needs to be extended into the anterior part of the bony external auditory canal.

Extracranial and intracranial tumor can be removed simultaneously or in sequence. Closure of smaller resections may be achieved using the available temporalis muscle, but larger resections may once again require a microvascular free flap.

## Posterior Fossa

There are several posterior fossa craniotomies/craniectomies used to access the CPA. The retrosigmoid approach uses an opening in the suboccipital bone posterior to the sigmoid sinus, with dural exposure over the lateral cerebellar hemisphere; for details of this approach, see the section on cerebello-pontine tumors.

The three transtemporal approaches (retro-labyrinthine, translabyrinthine and transcochlear) expose the posterior fossa dura anterior to the sigmoid sinus, but through the posterior aspect of the petrous pyramid. The transtemporal craniotomies require removal of bone, 1–2 cm behind the sigmoid sinus, to allow posterior displacement of the sinus. In the retro-labyrinthine approach, bone is removed up to the semicircular canals. This provides a limited view of the posterior aspect of the CPA. In the translabyrinthine approach, the canals are also removed – a maneuvre that provides access to the IAC and enhances CPA exposure. In the transcochlear approach, the entire inner ear (i.e. semicircular canals and cochlea) is removed and the facial nerve is re-routed posteriorly from its intratemporal course, thus providing access to the anterior aspect of the CPA and the space ventral to the brainstem.

## Temporal Bone Resection

This procedure is employed for malignant disease of the external auditory canal and middle-ear cleft (this is most common squamous cell carcinoma). If the tumor has not involved more medial structures, a lateral temporal bone resection is employed (see Fig. 15.6) that removes the ear canal en bloc, with the tympanic membrane and lateral ossicles. A parotidectomy and/or neck dissection often supplements this procedure.

### Surgical Steps

At the beginning of this procedure, the ear canal is transected and closed. This closure is different from that used during lateral skull base surgery – simply sewing the tragal skin to the conchal margin permits resection of the skin of the entire ear canal.

After transection of the cartilaginous ear canal just beneath the meatus, an intact canal wall mastoidectomy is performed. The middle ear is opened by performing a posterior tympanotomy (opening into the middle ear from the mastoid between the upper vertical portion of the facial nerve and the chorda tympani). The incus is then removed and the descending portion of the facial nerve is skeletonized.

In order to isolate the ear canal as an en bloc specimen, bone must be removed from 360°

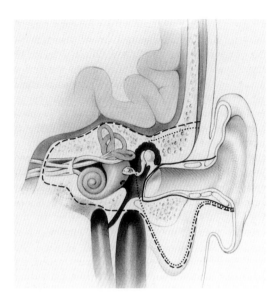

**Fig. 15.6.** Anatomy of the temporal bone in the coronal plane, showing the extent of the resection in a lateral temporal bone resection (outlined by the dotted line) and total petrosectomy (outlined by the dashed line).

around the ear canal. The posterior tympanotomy is extended to the posterior and inferior aspects of the middle ear. The front of the mastoid is removed between the inferior margin of the bony ear canal and the stylomastoid foramen. Superiorly, the root of zygoma and the posterior aspect of the glenoid fossa are removed.

Working between the floor of the middle cranial fossa and the roof of the ear canal, the root of zygoma is drilled away until the anterior middle ear has been opened into the glenoid fossa. After the ear canal has been isolated from above, behind and below, it remains attached only anteriorly. This bony attachment can then be "cracked" using an osteotome and the specimen removed. This specimen includes both the cartilaginous and bony ear canal, together with the tympanic membrane with the malleus attached.

## Approaches to the Clivus

Whether trying to access the upper, mid or lower clivus, careful planning of the approach is paramount. That said, for success, it is important that the approach is familiar and practiced.

In our unit, we have used, in principle, two routes to gain entry to this most difficult of areas:

- Extended pre-sigmoid translabyrinthine approach: this has been used for lesions involving the inner third of the petrous bone and upper half of the clivus.

- Far lateral approach: for access to the lower half of the clivus and the anterior aspect of the foramen magnum.

We shall now consider each of these routes in turn.

## Extended Presigmoid Translabyrinthine Approach

Space, or the lack of it, always seems to be the problem here. Certainly, at the beginning of most procedures, visualization of the important structures is difficult.

The principle of the approach is similar to the translabyrinthine route, but combined with a temporal craniotomy and division of the tentorium all the way down to the tentorial hiatus.

The procedure starts, therefore, with the patient in a park-bench position. Diuretics, antibiotics and anticonvulsants should be given. A question-mark-shaped incision is made, extending from just above the zygomatic process of the temporal bone down to below the mastoid process. The skin flap is reflected, leaving the temporalis fascia intact and extended all the way forward to the external auditory meatus.

Incisions are then made to elevate the temporalis muscle forwards on its blood supply, and to reflect the sub-occipital muscles inferiorly. This then allows a posterior fossa craniotomy to expose the straight and sigmoid sinuses, and a temporal craniotomy to expose the temporal lobe above the straight sinus and above the petrous bone. Great care must be taken to avoid injury to the sinuses.

The translabyrinthine exposure is then performed as previously described (see chapter on cerebellopontine angle tumors). This should be taken as far forward as possible and as low as possible towards the jugular bulb, to expose as much of the presigmoid dura as can be achieved. The exposure must include the undersurface of the temporal dura. Clearly, the amount of bone removed can be adapted to the specific requirements of the case.

Now, the dural cuts are performed to expose the surface of the temporal lobe and of the cerebellum. Usually, the posterior fossa dura is opened first. It may be possible to release some CSF early, which will slacken things off. The dural opening is T-shaped, crossing the superior petrosal sinus that always bleeds but is easily controlled. The secret to this is the opening of the dura over the temporal lobe. This must be long enough to allow safe access to the undersurface of the temporal lobe, so that the sinus can be approached from above and below. The vein of Labbe is at risk and must be protected at all times.

The final part of this approach is to divide the tentorium. Again, visualization both above and below allows this to be performed safely. Vessels coursing within the tentorium must be coagulated, the division being done using the microscope. Be careful not to lose direction and watch out for the fourth cranial nerve and the posterior cerebral artery. Division of the tentorium must be complete or access will always be restricted. Once complete, access to the upper clivus and inner petrous bone is possible with minimal retraction.

Closure must focus upon achieving a watertight seal. Meticulous attention to the petrous bone is the secret, with closure of the middle ear, if appropriate, by removal of the ossicles. Fibrin glue is a great help, as is the use of a lumbar drain for several days following the surgery.

### Far Lateral Approach

Again, the park-bench position is used. The usual preparations are made, the approach being made through an extended incision to allow access to the upper lateral aspect of the cervical spine. Exposure of the posterior fossa dura is like a retro-mastoid craniotomy for a CPA lesion. However, the sub-occipital muscles are reflected like the leaves of a book to define the transverse process and lamina of C1 and the upper aspect of C2. The vertebral artery courses over the arch of C1 before it enters the posterior fossa via the foramen magnum. Depending upon the extent of the exposure, the artery can be transposed to widen the amount of C1 arch that can be removed and, following that, the amount of the foramen magnum that is removed. Clearly, the further forward this is taken, the more of the condylar joint is removed and thus the greater the requirement for postoperative stabilization. However, failure to remove sufficient amounts of the joint will restrict visibility and access to the anterior part of the foramen magnum and the lower clivus. If exposure is limited, more bone can always be removed.

Once the bone work is completed, dural opening will allow exposure of the area. Within the dura at the foramen magnum lies a dural sinus that has to be divided. The dura is remarkably thick in this area, and the use of stitches to retract the dura may assist the opening process. Be prepared to use artery clips to stop the bleeding whilst completing the dural opening – getting haemostasis is then easier.

Closure of the dura will not be possible without insertion of a dural patch. Again, using a lumbar drain may reduce the incidence of CSF leakage.

## Conclusion

Skull base surgery is a challenging and exciting area that can offer hope to patients previously considered "inoperable". Any young neurosurgeon interested in this field needs to recognize that it requires a multi-disciplinary approach – one that can only be developed through mutual trust and respect for your colleagues. It is truly a "team effort" and, if you are going to go into the surgical "no man's land", you want to go with some good friends!

## Key Points

- *Skull base tumors are rare, probably accounting for less than 1% of intracranial tumors.*
- *Management options include a conservative approach with serial scans, conventional surgery or radiotherapy/stereotactic radiosurgery.*
- *Removal of adequate amounts of bone from the cranial base should provide sufficient access without the necessity to retract dura/brain.*
- *Surgery for these tumors is difficult because of problems with access, involvement of basal*

blood vessels/cranial nerves and the potential for post-operative cerebrospinal fluid leakage.

● *Skull base surgery requires a true multidisciplinary approach.*

# Self-assessment Questions

☐ Discuss the surgical difficulties of skull base surgery and how they may be overcome.

☐ Discuss the management of a 25-year-old woman presenting with unilateral proptosis and a diagnosis of fibrous dysplasia involving her anterior cranial fossa.

☐ A 30-year-old man presents with a 3-year history of anosmia. Nasal endoscopic examination reveals a right-sided nasal polyp and biopsy shows it to be an olfactory neuroblastoma. Describe his further management, including the surgical approach.

☐ A 77-year-old lady presents with left pulsatile tinnitus. Imaging confirms the diagnosis of a type B glomus jugulare. What are the management options available?

☐ Describe the surgical approaches to the clivus.

# References

1. Ketcham AS, Wilkins RH, Van Buren JM et al. A combined intracranial facial approach to the paranasal sinuses. Am J Surg 1963;103:698–703.
2. Uttley D, Moore A, Archer J. Surgical management of mid-line skull base tumors: a new approach. J Neurosurg 1989;71:705–10.
3. Sekhar LN, Janecka IP. Surgery of cranial base tumors. New York: Raven Press Ltd, 1993.
4. Donald PJ. Surgery of the skull base. Philadelphia: Lippincott-Raven Publishers, 1998.
5. Kveton JF, Brackman DE, Glasscock ME et al. Chondrosarcoma of the skull base. Otolaryngol Head Neck Surg 1986;94:23.
6. Robinson PJ, Woodhead P. Primary hyperparathyroidism presenting with a maxillary tumor and hydrocephalus. Journal of Laryngology & Otology 1988;162:1164–7.
7. Hug EB, Slater JD. Proton radiation therapy for chordomas and chondrosarcomas of the skull base. Neurosurgery Clinics of North America 2000;11(4):627–38.
8. Barnes L. Pathobiology of selected tumors of the skull base. Skull Base Surgery 1991;1:207.
9. Woodhead P, Lloyd GAS. Olfactory neuroblastoma, imaging by magnetic resonance, CT and conventional techniques. Clinical Otolaryngology 1988;13:387–94.
10. DulgerovP, Calcaterra T. Esthesioneuroblastoma: the UCLA experience 1970–1990. Laryngoscope 1992;102:843.
11. Eden BV, Debo RF, Larner JM. Esthesioneuroblastoma: long-term outcome and patterns of failure – the University of Virginia experience. Cancer 1994;73:2556.
12. Hirose T, Scheitauer BW, Lopes MDB et al. Olfactory neuroblastoma: an immunohistochemical, ultrastructural and flow cytometric study. Cancer 1995;76:4.
13. Schwaab G, Micheau C, LeGuillou C et al. Olfactory esthesioneuroma: a report of 40 cases. Laryngoscope 1988;98:872.
14. Harrison D, Lund VJ. Tumors of the upper jaw. Edinburgh: Churchill Livingstone, 1993.
15. Barnes L, Weber PC, Krause JR et al. Angiofibroma: a flow cytometric evaluation of 31 cases. Skull Base Surgery 1992;2:195.
16. Spector GJ, Ciralsky R, Maisel RH et al. Multiple glomus tumors in the head and neck. Laryngoscope 1975;85:1066.
17. Macbeth RG. Malignant disease of the paranasal sinuses. Journal of Laryngology & Otology 1965;79:592–612.
18. Hadfield EH. A studies of adenocarcinoma of the paranasal sinuses in woodworkers in the furniture industry. Annals of Royal College of Surgeons of England 1970;46:301–9.
19. Lund VJ, Howard DJ, Weui WI et al. Craniofacial resection for tumors of the nasal cavity and paranasal sinuses: a 17-year experience. Head Neck 1998;20:97–105.
20. Arena S, Keen M. Carcinoma of the middle ear and temporal bone. Am J Otolaryngol 1988;9:351–6.
21. Snyderman CH, Kanecka IV, Sekhar LN et al. Anterior cranial base reconstruction: role of galeal and pericranial flaps. Laryngoscope 1990;100:607–14.
22. Fisch U. Infratemporal fossa approach for extensive tumors of the temporal bone and base of the skull. In Silverstein H, Norrell H, editors. Neurological surgery of the ear. Birmingham, Alabama: Aesculapiul, 1977;34–53.
23. Sekhar LN. Operative management of tumors involving the cavernous sinus. In Schramm VL, Sekhar LN, editors. Tumors of the cranial base. New York: Futura, 1987; 393–419.
24. Scramm VL. Infratemporal fossa surgery. In Schramm VL, Sekhar LN, editors. Tumors of the cranial base. New York: Futura, 1987; 421–37.
25. Browne JD, Fisch U. Transotic approach to the cerebellopontine angle. Otolaryngol Clin North Am 1992;25:331–47.

# 16

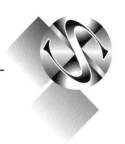

# Tumors: Cerebral Metastases and Lymphoma

Sepideh Amin-Hanjani and Griffith R. Harsh, IV

## Summary

This chapter focuses on two intracranial neoplasms: cerebral metastases and lymphoma. Cerebral metastases are the most common form of intracranial tumor and often require treatment with surgery and/or radiation. Improvement of neurological function occurs in 50–75% of patients. Primary lymphoma represents about 1% of intracranial tumors and is highly responsive to chemotherapy and whole brain radiotherapy.

## Introduction

This chapter will focus on two intracranial neoplasms of increasing prominence: cerebral metastases and lymphoma.

Cerebral metastases are the most common form of intracranial tumor. Although metastases usually convey a poor prognosis, their timely diagnosis and treatment can often palliate neurologic symptoms, prevent progression of brain disease and, less frequently, prolong patient survival. As the efficacy of treatment of systemic disease improves, cerebral metastases will become more prevalent and therapy for cerebral metastases will have an increasing impact on patient survival.

CNS lymphoma occurs either as metastatic disease from systemic primary tumor or as primary CNS lymphoma. Primary CNS lymphoma has become much more prevalent over the past two decades, as a result of an increase in the number of patients with immunosuppression arising from HIV infection or immunosuppressive therapy following organ transplantation. Vigilant surveillance of these two at risk populations is important to early detection and effective treatment of primary CNS lymphoma.

## Cerebral Metastases

Cerebral metastases represent the secondary involvement of the brain by neoplasms originating outside the central nervous system (CNS). Currently, cerebral metastases are the most common type of intracranial tumor [1]. The predilection for spread of systemic tumor to the CNS is highly dependent on its histologic type [1].

### Epidemiology

Improved neuroimaging has revealed that patients with cerebral metastases outnumber those with primary brain tumors. At autopsy,

25% of cancer patients harbor intracranial metastases [2]. Cerebral metastases – those involving the brain parenchyma itself – occur in about 15% of patients with solid systemic tumors [2]. This prevalence is likely to increase as the proportion of elderly in the population increases, as diagnostic neuroimaging becomes even more sensitive and as patients with cancer live longer.

The pattern of metastasis to the CNS varies with tumor type. Intracranial metastases include those to the skull, meningeal spaces and brain parenchyma. Many skull metastases originate from breast and prostate cancer [3]. Metastases to the pituitary gland are often from breast cancer.

Lung and breast cancer, followed by melanoma, genitourinary cancer and gastrointestinal cancer, are the most common histological types of cerebral metastasis (Table 16.1). The risk of developing cerebral metastasis is highest with malignant melanoma, followed by lung and breast cancer (Table 16.2). Among the types of lung cancer, small cell carcinoma and adenocarcinoma more frequently spread to the brain than does squamous cell carcinoma.

Most cerebral metastases spread to the brain hematogenously. Tumor cells distributed arterially commonly originate from the lung, either from a primary lung tumor or from an extrapulmonary primary that has metastasized to the lung. Less commonly, venous routes are taken. The anastomotic pelvic–vertebral venous plexus

**Table 16.1.** Primary sites of cancer in patients with cerebral metastases.

| Primary tumor | % of cases (total n = 210) |
|---|---|
| Lung | 40 |
| Breast | 19 |
| Melanoma | 10 |
| Genitourinary* | 7 |
| Gastrointestinal* | 7 |
| Female genital tract* | 5 |
| Sarcoma | 3 |
| Lymphoma | 1 |
| Other | 6 |
| Unknown | 2 |

\* Gastrointestinal: colorectal, esophagus, gastric, pancreas.
  Genitourinary: renal, testis, bladder, prostate.
  Female genital tract: ovary, uterus, cervix, choriocarcinoma.

Adapted from Posner JB. Neurologic complications of cancer. Contemporary Neurology series. Volume 45. Phildelphia: Davis, 1995.

described by Batson (termed Batson's plexus) is a potential path of spread of pelvic and retroperitoneal tumors. Tumors from these areas have a predilection for the posterior fossa.

Tumor cells carried arterially are commonly deposited at the junction of gray and white matter of the brain, particularly within watershed zones. Tumor cells are readily lodged within the end vessels of these regions, where vessel caliber changes rapidly. Otherwise, the likelihood of a particular brain region

**Table 16.2.** Frequency of intracranial metastases from systemic cancers.

| Primary tumor | Intracranial tumor at autopsy (%) | Intracerebral tumor at autopsy (%) |
|---|---|---|
| All sites | 24 | 15 |
| Melanoma | 72 | 40 |
| Lung | 34 | 21 |
| Breast | 30 | 10 |
| Leukemia | 23 | 3 |
| Lymphoma | 16 | 1 |
| Gastrointestinal* | 7 | 3 |
| Colon | 8 | 5 |
| Pancreas | 7 | 2 |
| Genitourinary* | 19 | 11 |
| Renal | 27 | 21 |
| Prostate | 31 | 0 |
| Ovary | 5 | 5 |

*Gastrointestinal includes colon, gastric and pancreatic tumors. Genitourinary includes renal, prostate, testis, cervix and ovarian tumors.

Adapted from Posner JB, Chernik NL. Intracranial metastases from systemic cancer. Advances In Neurology 1978; 19:579–92.

developing a metastasis reflects its tissue volume and rate of blood flow. Consequently, almost 90% of metatases are supratentorial and the frontal and parietal lobes are most commonly affected.

Approximately 50% of patients with secondary cerebral tumor have more than one lesion. This incidence of multiple metastasis is likely to increase as neuroimaging becomes more sensitive. Multiple lesions are common with melanoma and lung cancer, whereas patients with breast, abdominal and pelvic cancer more often have a single brain metastasis [3].

Cerebral metastases occur with equal frequency in men and women. The incidence of brain metastasis is the same for all races. Brain metastases are most likely to appear in people between 50 and 70 years of age. In children, CNS metastases are most commonly from leukemia, followed by lymphoma, sarcoma and germ cell tumor.

## Clinical Presentation

Brain metastases are most commonly discovered after a diagnosis of the primary tumor has been established; more than 80% of cerebral metastases present after discovery of the systemic source. Most appear at a late stage in the dissemination of the tumor. One exception is lung cancer, in which metastases often occur in the early stages of the disease and neurological symptoms secondary to metastases frequently antedate discovery of the primary tumor [3].

The clinical presentation of a metastasis reflects the location and size of the tumor [4]. The most frequent presenting symptoms are headache, focal deficits and behavioral or cognitive changes (Table 16.3). Headache, although non-specific, is the most common single symptom. In a patient with known cancer, new onset of headaches, especially those occurring in the early morning, warrants radiologic investigation. Behavioral changes are more common with multiple than with single metastases. They may be as subtle and non-specific as mild confusion, memory loss, depression or emotional lability. Symptoms such as headache, behavioral change and focal deficits are usually subtle in onset and slowly progress as the mass effect from the tumor increases.

Seizures, hemorrhage and infarction bring a more acute presentation. Seizures, focal or

**Table 16.3.** Presenting symptoms and signs of cerebral metastases.

| Symptom/sign | % of cases (total n = 284) |
|---|---|
| Headache | 24 |
| Focal weakness | 20 |
| Behavioral and cognitive changes | 14 |
| Seizures | 12 |
| Ataxia | 7 |
| Asymptomatic* | 7 |

Asymptomatic lesions discovered in the course of staging patients with known systemic cancer.

Adapted from Posner JB. Brain metastases: 1995. A brief review. J Neuro-oncol 1996;27:287–93.

generalized, are the presenting symptom in about 10% of patients. They, too, are more frequent in patients with multiple metastases [3]. Hemorrhage or infarction from a tumor embolus occurs in 5–10% of cases [3]. Hemorrhage is more common with metastases from melanoma, choriocarcinoma, renal cell carcinoma and bronchogenic carcinoma.

The differential diagnosis of the clinical presentation of metastasis includes other mass lesions (abscess, granuloma, resolving hematoma, radiation necrosis) demyelination and infarction (non-bacterial thrombotic endocarditis, cerebral venous occlusion) [4].

## Diagnosis

### Imaging

Thorough and accurate radiographic imaging is an essential aspect of managing patients with cerebral metastases. CT has been superceded by MRI with gadolinium contrast as the modality of choice [5].

CT is useful for screening for large or hemorrhagic metastases with acute presentations and for skull tumors. Most metastases are hypodense or isodense, well circumscribed masses on non-contrast images. Those with necrotic centers have hypodense interiors. Hyperdensity is seen with acute intratumoral hemorrhage, some melanomas, some densely cellular tumors (adenocarcinoma and small cell lung carcinoma) and rare calcified lesions [5]. Most metastases enhance brightly with intravenous contrast, particularly when given in double dose. CT is relatively insensitive in detecting very small lesions, particularly those in the posterior fossa, and leptomeningeal spread.

Diagnostic screening and treatment planning benefit greatly from the sensitivity, specificity and anatomic resolution (particularly in the posterior fossa) of MRI. Most metastases are isointense on T1-weighted images and hyperintense on T2-weighted images. Central necrosis, cysts and peripheral edema are all hypointense on T1 images and hyperintense on T2 images. The intensity pattern of hemorrhagic metastases varies with the age of the hematoma. Anomalies include melanomas that may be hyperintense on T1 images and adenocarcinomas, highly cellular tumors, and calcified lesions that may be hypointense on T2 images.

Metastases usually enhance brightly and homogeneously with gadolinium, except in their necrotic, cystic or hemorrhagic portions. Rim-enhancing metastases have a center of fluid or necrosis; the rim is more irregular than that of benign cysts, abscesses and resolving hematomas [6]. Metastases may sometimes be distinguished from malignant gliomas that also have nodular rim-enhancement by multiplicity and a circumferential pattern of T1 hypointense, T2 hyperintense edema that is less likely to involve the cortex or corpus callosum [5]. Higher doses of contrast (0.3 mmol/kg) significantly increase the sensitivity of detecting small lesions. Diffuse leptomeningeal disease, carcinomatous meningitis, appears as sulcal enhancement on post-gadolinium T1 scans and as hyperintense linearities on flair sequences.

## Biopsy

Biopsy of a brain mass to obtain histologic verification of metastasis is rarely required when there are multiple parenchymal brain lesions in a patient with known active systemic malignancy, particularly if there are metastases to other organs. In contrast, biopsy is almost always indicated when the brain lesion is solitary (the patient's only known tumor) and nonsurgical treatment is planned. The need for biopsy of a single brain lesion in a patient with known systemic cancer depends on several factors. Although one study of biopsy results found that 11% of single brain lesions thought to be metastases based upon enhanced CT were a different pathology [7], current high resolution MRI is often quite specific. Systemic disease in recession (a primary histology that infrequently spreads to the brain) and an atypical radiographic appearance favor biopsy. Active systemic disease, a primary histology that commonly spreads to the brain and a typical radiographic appearance mitigate the need for biopsy. Current stereotactic biopsy techniques permit retrieval of diagnostic tissue in approximately 95% of cases, with a morbidity from hemorrhage, seizure, worsened neurologic deficit and infection of 3% and a mortality of 0.6% [8]. A highly vascular appearance on neuroimaging and a primary histology associated with a tendency for brain metastases to bleed is a relative contraindication to biopsy.

## Treatment

Cerebral metastases generally carry a very poor prognosis when not treated. The median survival for patients with symptomatic brain metastases that are not treated is 4–6 weeks. The optimal treatment of brain metastases must consider several factors, including the patient's neurologic and general medical condition, the number, location and size of the lesions, and the histology, the extent, the prior treatment and the response to treatment of the systemic disease. Two current trends in the approach to cerebral metastasis are evident: a shift from mere palliation of symptoms to tumor eradication, in an effort to improve survival, and an increased emphasis on the patient's quality of life. Three main modalities of treatment are used for brain metastases: radiation, surgery and chemotherapy.

## Medical Therapy

Corticosteroids often markedly improve neurologic symptoms by reducing peritumoral vasogenic edema. Generalized symptoms, such as headache and lethargy, respond more consistently than do focal symptoms and signs. The clinical response is usually apparent within a day and peaks by 7 days. Dexamethasone, which has the benefit of lacking mineralocorticoid effect, is the steroid used most frequently. Steroids are considered palliative treatment that is used transiently, while other, more definitive therapy is planned or delivered. Treatment with steroids alone results in a median survival of

8–10 weeks. The dose of steroid medication should be tapered and discontinued when clinically possible, to avoid side effects such as myopathy, psychiatric change (agitation, delirium, and psychosis), gastric disturbances (ulceration with bleeding or perforation) and opportunistic infections.

Prophylactic anticonvulsants are not indicated unless there is a history of seizure.

## Radiation

Radiotherapy is indicated for almost all patients with cerebral metastasis. The optimal method of delivery, dose and regimen varies with the individual patient. In many cases, these are controversial. Radiation can be administered either as fractionated external radiotherapy to the whole brain (WBRT), the region of the tumor (local fractionated radiotherapy) or both (WBRT with a local boost), as single exposure radiosurgery or as interstitial brachytherapy.

Fractionated whole-brain radiotherapy has been the standard treatment for brain metastases for almost half a century. WBRT increases the median duration of survival of patients to 3–6 months from 1–2 months (10–15% survive for at least 1 year) [7,9]. Treatment improves neurologic function in 50–75% of patients [9]. Large retrospective studies reveal that 50% of the patients treated with WBRT die from systemic cancer, rather than from progressive brain disease. The dosing regimen most commonly employed is 30 Gy over 2 weeks in ten daily 3.0 Gy fractions. This regimen is as effective as those with higher doses or more extended fractionation.

Prognostic factors favoring survival include age less than 60 years, Karnofsky performance score of at least 70, control of the primary tumor and absence of extracranial metastases. Radiation cell sensitizers such as nitroimidazoles are not beneficial. Although certain types of tumor, such as renal cell carcinoma and melanoma, are relatively radioresistant, the duration of patient survival following radiotherapy of cerebral metastases is similar for most tumor types [9].

Radiation therapy has significant risk of acute and long-term complications. Acutely, fatigue, headache, nausea and vomiting may occur during and shortly after treatment and neurologic deficits may be exacerbated. Steroid therapy is often required. Chronically, side effects, such as dementia, ataxia and urinary incontinence, occur in at least 5% of patients who survive longer than 1 year [10]. In one study, 50% of patients surviving for more than 2 years after surgical resection and WBRT developed leukoencephalopathy or atrophy-induced hydrocephalus ex vacuo. More prolonged fractionation schemes and more focal treatment are strategies designed to decrease the risk of dementia. Patients expected to survive longer than 6–12 months are often treated with 40 Gy in 2 -Gy fractions over 4 weeks. In an attempt to spare normal brain, fractionated local radiotherapy has been used for single metastases, but the relative effectiveness of focal and whole-brain therapy has not been studied. Additional local dose can also be administered as a boost to the lesion following WBRT.

Radiosurgery involves single-session high-dose irradiation of a stereotactically defined target. In that radiosurgery intends inactivation of all tissue within a targeted volume, it is a non-invasive alternative to surgical excision. Multiple techniques (Linac, Gamma Knife, Cyber Knife, and Proton Beam) are able to deliver the conformal radiation required. Since the likelihood of controlling tumor growth and the risk of radiation injury to surrounding tissue both increase with increasing dose and the risk of radiation injury increases with increasing target volume, there is an interdependence of tumor volume, dose, tumor control rate and complication rate. Empirically defined relationships specify an inverse relationship between two variables (e.g. tumor size and dose) after two parameters have been established (e.g. minimal acceptable rate of tumor control and maximal acceptable rate of complication). For example, if one posits that at least 15 Gy is required to achieve a 90% rate of tumor control at 1 year and that the acceptable risk of complication is 1%, then the maximal tumor volume that can be safely and effectively treated is 10 cm$^3$. In other words, given such specifications for safety and efficacy, there is an ideal dose for each tumor volume. In general, stereotactic radiosurgery is an effective treatment for intracranial metastases of less than 10 cm$^3$ in volume (2.5–3.0 cm in diameter).

Radiosurgery is indicated for surgically inaccessible lesions and is an acceptable alternative to surgery for many accessible ones. Although it is occasionally used in the patient with more than three lesions, it is usually reserved for patients with single or, at most, several metastases. Median duration of patient survival following radiosurgery for an intracranial metastasis is 7–12 months, similar to that for surgical resection [11]. Randomized studies comparing radiosurgical and surgical treatments for single brain metastases have not yet been completed.

Whether WBRT is needed in addition to radiosurgery for single metastases is controversial. Much of the radiosurgical data was accumulated in patients who also received WBRT and, given the conformal nature of the radiosurgical treatment volume, it is unlikely that the addition of WBRT to radiosurgery significantly increases the risk of radiosurgery. Nonetheless, given the inefficacy and toxicity of WBRT and the ability to detect and to treat new lesions conformally with radiosurgery, radiosurgery alone may be appropriate initial treatment for most metastases of appropriate size. Essentially, stereotactic radiosurgery and WBRT can be viewed as complementary: radiosurgery focally targets one to three tumors of 1–10 cm$^3$ in volume, whereas WBRT intends to control higher numbers of small tumors or microscopic spread throughout the brain. Radiosurgery alone is most strongly indicated for a single metastasis from systemic tumor that is indolent or well controlled (and thus not an immediate threat to survival) and of a histologic type prone to single brain metastases (e.g. breast and non-small cell lung carcinoma) or relatively refractory to fractionated radiotherapy (e.g. melanoma, renal cell carcinoma and sarcoma). WBRT is likely needed in addition to radiosurgery when there are multiple cerebral tumors, especially those with histologies prone to disseminated brain metastases and high sensitivity to fractionated radiation (e.g. small cell lung carcinoma, testicular carcinoma and lymphoma). In many patients with these histologies, WBRT is given first and radiosurgery is reserved for tumors that subsequently resume growth. When brain metastases are multiple and systemic disease is refractory to treatment, WBRT alone is given as palliation.

Interstitial brachytherapy (the temporary or permanent placement of radioactive seeds within a tumor) and interstitial radiosurgery (the transient stereotactic placement of the tip of a miniature generator of X-rays within a tumor) also achieve high-dose focal irradiation of brain metastases. Their invasiveness, with the concomitant risks of infection and hemorrhage, and their limited conformity are disadvantages relative to radiosurgery. However, they do offer an additional treatment option for single, surgically inaccessible tumors that are too large to be treated safely and effectively with radiosurgery.

## Surgery

In patients with cerebral metastases and well controlled systemic disease, the former becomes a more significant determinant of survival. It is within this subgroup of patients that aggressive treatment, including surgery, is considered. Resection of single brain metastases was initially advocated for patients with good prognoses because of the low rates of long-term tumor control (40% at 1 year) with conventional WBRT [6]. Prospective randomized trials have firmly established the superiority of surgical resection followed by WBRT to WBRT alone for a single cerebral metastasis [6]. The median duration of survival is 10–14 months rather than 4–6 months. As noted above, although direct comparisons of surgery and radiosurgery for a single metastasis have not yet been completed, radiosurgery is often an acceptable alternative to craniotomy. Also, a surgically inaccessible location, multiple brain metastases or extensive systemic disease usually contraindicate resection. An exception is the need to resect a tumor from a location, such as the posterior fossa, in which it is immediately life threatening, even if the patient has multiple metastases and significant systemic disease.

The utility of surgery for multiple cerebral metastases is controversial. Modern surgical series show that early post-operative mortality and morbidity following resection of multiple metastases is comparable to those following resection of a single metastasis. One study found a significantly shorter duration of survival (5 vs 12 months) of patients who had multiple metastases resected compared to those undergoing surgery for a single metastasis. However, gross resection of all tumors was not achieved in the majority of patients with multiple lesions. Another study reported a median duration of survival of 14 months for patients with two or three metastases that were totally resected – a result similar to that achieved for patients with single metastases. These studies support surgical removal of one to three metastases, particularly those too large to be treated by radiosurgery [12].

Historically, most patients have received WBRT post-operatively – even those whose tumors were totally removed. Currently, however, many consider WBRT to be relatively contraindicated by its chronic sequelae in patients expected to live longer than 6 months. Although some studies have found that post-operative WBRT lengthens median survival, several others have found no significant difference between patients treated with surgical resection alone and those receiving resection and post-operative WBRT. Post-operative WBRT, however, did yield other benefits: improved control of local tumor, decreased risk of distant tumor, increased time to neurological recurrence and decrease in the percentage of patients dying of neurologic disease [13]. Post-operative radiosurgery, in addition to WBRT, may be indicated in cases of incomplete removal of a metastasis. As an alternative to post-operative WBRT, it is likely to improve control of local tumor but not affect the incidence of distant metastases.

## Chemotherapy

Unfortunately, chemotherapeutic agents which are effective against primary solid tumors are seldom as effective against brain metastases. The blood–brain barrier is partly responsible but other factors are likely to contribute, as lipid soluble agents are also ineffective, the blood–brain barrier around most metastastic lesions is deficient and intrathecal or intraventricular injection does not significantly improve outcome. However, chemotherapy of cerebral metastases of some histologies, including breast cancer, small cell lung carcinoma and choriocarcinoma, can effect remission, stabilize neurologic deficits and prolong median survival. The current role for chemotherapy of cerebral metastases is limited to adjuvant treatment of such chemosensitive tumors. Improvements in the delivery of drugs to the CNS and new multi-agent regimens may broaden the role of chemotherapy in the future.

## Recurrent Metastases

Many of the principles of treating brain metastases at their original presentation apply to treatment of recurrent disease, with the proviso that the effects of the previous therapy must be considered. Local recurrence of a previously treated tumor has different implications from the appearance of distant failure. Surgery, stereotactic radiosurgery, focal radiotherapy, interstitial radiosurgery and brachytherapy are options for local recurrences, depending on the size and location of the lesion. In one study, among patients with a single recurrent tumor and well controlled systemic disease, two-thirds improved neurologically after tumor resection and the median duration of survival was 9 months [14].

Diffuse distant metastases probably warrant WBRT if it has not been given. For tumors recurrent after WBRT, an additional 20 Gy of fractionated radiation may improve the neurologic function of selected patients but does not significantly lengthen survival [15]. In one study, among patients with well controlled systemic disease and a good response to their initial radiation, fewer than half had neurologic improvement after additional radiotherapy and the median duration of survival was 5 months [15].

## Summary

The selection of a treatment plan for an individual patient must consider multiple factors. These include the number, location and size of the metastases, the histology, extent and prior treatment of the systemic disease, and the patient's neurologic status, medical condition and personal preference. In general, radiosurgery is the treatment of choice for most patients with one to three brain metastases. Surgical resection is indicated for one or two accessible lesions larger than 2–3 cm in diameter and for those threatening cerebral herniation; adjuvant radiosurgery to any residual tumor or the resection bed is likely warranted. WBRT is indicated when there are more than a few metastases, when the histology predicts disseminated metastasis or radiosensitivity or when the patient has a particularly poor prognosis. Table 16.4 summarizes general recommendations for the treatment of metastases, taking these factors into consideration. The

**Table 16.4.** Recommendations for management of cerebral metastases.

| Systemic disease (median survival) | 1–3 (< 10 cc) accessible | 1–3 (< 10 cc) inaccessible | 1–3 (> 10 cc) accessible | 1–3 (> 10 cc) inaccessible | > 3 |
|---|---|---|---|---|---|
| Absent/Stable (> 6 months ) | Surgery or radiosurgery +/- WBRT* | Radiosurgery +/- WBRT* | Surgery +/- WBRT | Fractionated focal radiation | WBRT |
| Slowly progressive (4–6 months) | Surgery or radiosurgery + WBRT | Radiosurgery + WBRT | Surgery + WBRT | **WBRT + fractionated boost** | **WBRT** |
| Moderately progressive (2–4 months) | WBRT | WBRT | WBRT | WBRT | WBRT |
| Rapidly progressive (< 2 months) | None | None | None | None | None |

*Given the potential for long-term complications in patients with prolonged survival, noncomitant WBRT is less desirable in these groups of patients.

guidelines propose treating patients with well controlled systemic disease aggressively, by offering treatments that are effective for one to three lesions.

# Lymphoma

Lymphoma is a malignant lymphocytic neoplasm that can occur in the central nervous system (CNS), either primarily or as a secondary manifestation of systemic disease. Lymphoma of the brain or spinal cord not involving other areas, except for ocular structures, is termed "primary CNS lymphoma" (PCNSL). The incidence of CNS lymphoma has increased significantly over the last two decades.

# PCNSL

PCNSL has been referred to within the literature as reticulum cell sarcoma, perivascular sarcoma, immunoblastic sarcoma, microgliomatosis and malignant reticulosis. The disease most frequently appears as solitary or multi-focal lesions of the cerebrum of middle-aged adults. The immunologic competency of the patient affects the neurologic presentation. Immunodeficiency is a well recognized risk factor for the disease.

## Epidemiology

Primary CNS lymphoma represents about 1% of intracranial tumors. The incidence of primary CNS lymphoma has been increasing steadily for the past two decades [16]. This increase is partially attributable to an increased prevalence of immunodeficient patients secondary to acquired immune deficiency syndrome (AIDS) and immunosuppressive treatment after organ transplantation. However, the incidence of the disease among immunocompetent persons has also increased. According to surveillance by the National Cancer Institute, the annual incidence of PCNSL increased from 2.7 cases/ten million persons in 1973–75 to 7.5 cases/ten million persons in 1982–84, even after exclusion of never married men as a relatively high-risk group for AIDS. Continuation of this trend produced an incidence of 30 cases/ten million persons in 1991–92 [17]. Although some of the increase may result from improved radiographic and immunologic detection, the trend antedates the widespread use of such technologies. Other etiologies for the observed increase in incidence of primary CNS lymphoma, such as environmental factors, remain speculative.

For immunocompetent patients, the sixth decade of life is the most common age of diagnosis of PCNSL [16,18]. The median age for presentation in the immunocompromised population falls within the fourth decade. Childhood disease is rare and is usually associated with congenital or acquired immunodeficiency.

In the immunocompetent population with primary CNS lymphoma, 60% of patients are male and 40% are female [16]. This is similar to the gender distribution of patients with systemic lymphoma. The immunocompromised population with PCNSL is even more disproportionately male because of the male predominance in the AIDS epidemic.

Several risk factors for developing PCNSL have been identified (Table 16.5). Given its etiologic role in other lymphoproliferative disorders among immunosuppressed patients, the Epstein–Barr virus (EBV) may contribute to the development of primary CNS lymphoma in immunocompromised patients. EBV RNA has been found in CNS lymphoma tissue obtained from immunocompromised patients. Primary CNS lymphoma also occurs as a second malignancy after treatment of other malignancies, such as Hodgkin's lymphoma, non-Hodgkin's lymphoma and colon, breast and thyroid cancer. It is unclear whether this phenomenon reflects an underlying predisposition to cancer among these patients or it results from exposure to agents used to treat the initial malignancy.

## Pathology

Primary CNS lymphoma, like systemic lymphoma, arises from lymphocytes. The source of the pre-malignant lymphocytes is controversial as the CNS lacks lymphoid tissue and lymphatics. The perivascular distribution of cerebral tumor suggests that it may originate from systemic neoplastic lymphocytes that selectively infiltrate CNS tissue. This selectivity may depend on adhesion molecules within the CNS vasculature and parenchyma specific for the malignant cells.

The macroscopic appearance of deposits of PCNSL within the brain varies. They may be leptomeningeal, parenchymal, subependymal or a combination of these. Primary CNS lymphoma may be unifocal or multicentric. In either case, it can appear to be relatively well circumscribed or irregularly margined. In the leptomeningeal variant of PCNL, tumor exclusively infiltrates the leptomeninges, cranial nerves and spinal nerve roots. Primary parenchymal CNS lymphoma softens affected brain tissue and turns it yellow–brown. There may be areas of focal hemorrhage or necrosis.

Microscopically, diffuse infiltration of tumor into brain parenchyma well beyond the macroscopic borders of the tumor is common. Neoplastic lymphocytes aggregate perivascularly and infiltrate the walls of small blood vessels (Fig. 16.1). This perivascular cuffing is most prominent at the tumor margins. Tumor cells also commonly extend in the subpial plane or in the subarachnoid space. An astrocytic reaction can be prominent, especially in the peripheral parts of the tumor. An infiltrate of T lymphocytes is typically present at the tumor margins and occasionally within the tumor itself.

The tumor has histological features similar to those of systemic non-Hodgkin's lymphoma. Hodgkin's lymphoma is almost never seen as a primary CNS tumor. The great majority of PCNSLs are monoclonal B cell lymphomas. T cell lymphomas of the CNS are exceptionally rare and must be differentiated from B cell lymphomas with a prominent reactive T-cell

**Table 16.5.** Risk factors for primary CNS lymphoma.

| | |
|---|---|
| Acquired immunodeficiency | AIDS |
| | Immunosuppressive therapy for transplant or autoimmune conditions |
| Congenital immunodeficiency | Wiskott–Aldrich syndrome |
| | Severe combined immunodeficiency syndrome |
| | IgA deficiency |
| | Ataxia–telangiectasia |
| | X-linked lymphoproliferative syndrome |
| | Chediak–Higashi syndrome |
| Autoimmune diseases | Rheumatoid arthritis |
| | Sjögren's syndrome |
| | Idiopathic thrombocytopenic purpura |
| | Systemic lupus erythematosis |
| | Sarcoidosis |
| Viral infections | Epstein–Barr virus |

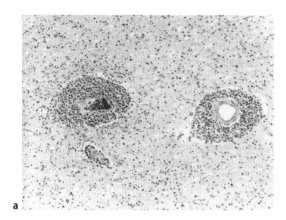

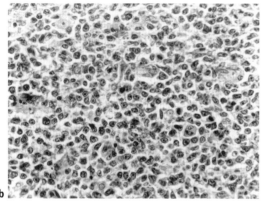

**Fig. 16.1. a** Perivascular aggregation of neoplastic lymphoid cells typical for primary CNS lymphoma. **b** Malignant lymphoid cells with cytologically atypical nuclei.

**Table 16.6.** Frequency of presenting symptoms.

| Symptom | % of cases |
| --- | --- |
| Personality change | 24 |
| Cerebellar signs | 21 |
| Headache | 15 |
| Seizures | 13 |
| Motor dysfunction | 11 |
| Visual changes | 8 |

Adapted from Hochberg FH, Miller DC. Primary central nervous system lymphoma. J Neurosurg 1988; 68:835–53.

changes and altered affect are relatively common modes of presentation, given the relatively frequent involvement of the frontal lobes (Table 16.6). Seizure was a first presenting symptom in 13% of one series of 66 patients [16]. The time elapsing between onset of symptoms and diagnosis is often short – on the order of 2–3 months. The constellation of symptoms is not noticeably different between immunocompetent and immunocompromised patients.

Murray et al. found the majority of lesions to be solitary and supratentorial (52.1%), with the most frequent sites of involvement being frontal (26%), temporal (15%) and parietal (14%) [18]. Diencephalic and infratentorial lesions, particularly in the cerebellum (11%), were also seen. The tumor is solitary almost twice as often as it is multifocal. Diffuse meningeal disease has also been described and accounted for 12% of cases in the Massachusetts General Hospital (MGH) series of 66 patients [16].

component. The relative incidences of B-cell subtypes among PCNSLs differ from those found systemically. Unlike systemic lymphomas, which are typically follicular B cell lymphomas, most PCNSLs are diffuse large cell or large cell immunoblastic in type [18]. Immunological markers help to distinguish B cell lymphomas from other tumors such, as gliomas and small cell carcinomas (antibody against CD45, a leukocyte marker), and from T-cell lymphomas (antibodies against CD20 and CD79a, both B cell markers).

## Clinical Features

Primary CNS lymphoma typically presents with symptoms and signs of increased intracranial pressure or cortical dysfunction, depending upon the location of the lesions. Personality

## Diagnosis

### Imaging

CT reveals an isodense or moderately hyperdense lesion that enhances strongly and homogeneously with contrast. Mild or moderate edema is typical. Tumors in immunocompromised patients in particular may show a ring enhancing pattern. The periventricular area is a common location; most tumors abut the ependyma.

Primary CNS lymphomas are usually isointense or slightly hypointense on T1-weighted MR images and isointense or slightly hyperintense on T2-weighted images (Fig. 16.2). The enhancement pattern in immunocompetent patients is usually dense and homogeneous, but can be heterogeneous (Figs 16.2 and 16.3).

TUMORS: CEREBRAL METASTASES AND LYMPHOMA

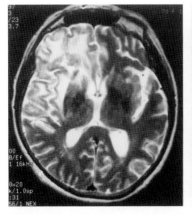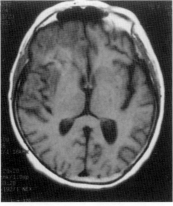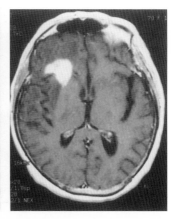

**Fig. 16.2.** Axial T2-weighted images (left) and T1-weighted images without (center) and with (right) gadolinium enhancement in an immunocompetent patient with primary CNS lymphoma. The right frontal mass appears heterogeneously isointense and hyperintense on T2-weighted images, with surrounding hyperintense edema . On T1-weighted images, the isointense mass enhances densely and homogeneously, following contrast administration.

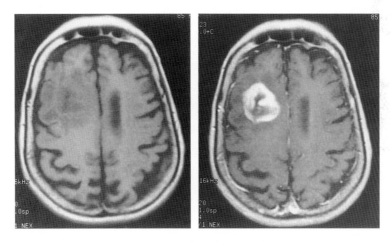

**Fig. 16.3.** Axial T1-weighted images without (left) and with (right) gadolinium enhancement in an immunocompetent patient with primary CNS lymphoma. The ring enhancing lesion could also be metastasis, malignant glioma or even abscess.

Non-enhancing tumors have been seen, but are rare. In patients with AIDS-associated PCNSL, enhancement may be heterogeneous and is frequently rim-enhancing (Fig. 16.4). Radiographic evidence of hemorrhage and necrosis may be seen.

In patients with AIDS, CNS lymphoma may be very difficult to distinguish radiographically from other common intracranial pathologies, such as toxoplasmosis. Positron emission tomography and thallium SPECT have been proposed as more sensitive imaging modalities for distinguishing lymphoma from infectious lesions. Some authors claim that the combination of increased uptake on thallium SPECT and EBV DNA in CSF has 100% sensitivity and specificity for CNS lymphoma and obviates the need for biopsy [19].

The typical CSF profile with primary CNS lymphoma is elevated protein, low glucose and pleocytosis. CSF cytology showing a monomorphic population of abnormal lymphocytes is diagnostic, but only 10% of patients undergoing CSF analysis at the time of presentation have positive cytologic findings. Furthermore, lumbar puncture may be contraindicated by

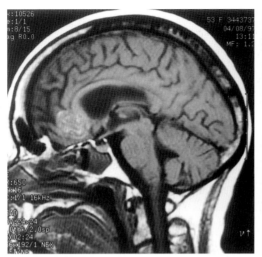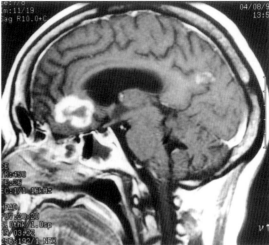

**Fig. 16.4.** Sagittal T1-weighted images without (left) and with (right) gadolinium enhancement in a patient with AIDS, demonstrating the typical heterogeneous rim enhancement seen with primary CNS lymphoma in this population of patients.

increased intracranial pressure in many patients. Definitive diagnosis usually requires tissue. Biopsy is more likely to yield diagnostic tissue if it is performed prior to the administration of corticosteroids, which, by lysing the malignant tumor cells, may obscure the diagnosis [16].

Once a diagnosis of CNS lymphoma is established, the need for investigations to exclude systemic lymphoma with secondary cerebral involvement is controversial. In immunocompetent patients, spread of systemic lymphoma to the CNS is uncommon. When it does occur, it is usually late in the course of the disease and the leptomeninges are predominantly affected. In general, investigations should be limited to determining the extent of disease within the CNS [20]: cranial MRI with contrast, ophthalmologic examination, spinal MRI with contrast (for patients with neck or back pain or myelopathy) and lumbar puncture (if not contraindicated). For patients with AIDS, systemic lymphoma has a greater propensity to involve the CNS secondarily. In these patients, screening for systemic disease with bone marrow aspiration and chest, abdominal and pelvic imaging is advisable. Because of the association between PCNSL and AIDS, testing for HIV is also indicated for patients first found to have primary CNS lymphoma.

## Treatment and Outcome

The options for treating PCNSL have evolved significantly during the last decade (Table 16.7). Radiotherapy and chemotherapy, separately and in combination, have significantly increased the survival of many immunocompetent patients with PCNSL. The prognosis for AIDS-related primary CNS lymphoma, however, remains poor, with a median duration of survival of less than 3 months, despite treatment [21].

### Radiotherapy

Primary CNS lymphoma is highly radiosensitive. Early reports indicated an increase in median survival from 3.3 to 15.2 months for patients receiving radiotherapy. Subsequent reports confirmed this benefit to survival. Despite a high initial response rate, radiotherapy alone rarely leads to long-term survival; only 7% of patients are alive 5 years after treatment [22].

The optimal dose of radiation is controversial. Retrospective data suggest that total doses of 40–50 Gy to the primary tumor improve survival [6]. No additional survival benefit follows higher doses. The Radiation Therapy Oncology Group (RTOG) failed to improve outcome with

**Table 16.7.** Recent trials of combined therapy for primary CNS lymphoma.

| Reference | No. of pts | Chemotherapy | Radiotherapy | Median survival | Median survival RT only [d] | Major toxicities |
|---|---|---|---|---|---|---|
| **Pre-irradiation chemotherapy** | | | | | | |
| Bessell, 1991 | 10 | BVAM (MTX 1.5 g/m$^2$) | WBRT 45 Gy Boost 10 Gy Spine 35 Gy* | 10 | – | Myelosuppression |
| Liang, 1993 | 9 | CHOP MTX IT (12 mg) | WBRT 36 Gy Boost 18 Gy | 30 | – | Leukoencephalopathy |
| LaChance, 1994 | 6 | CHOP | WBRT 45 Gy Boost 10.8 Gy Spine 30 Gy | 8.5 | – | – |
| Glass, 1994 | 25 | MTX (3.5 g/m$^2$) | WBRT 30–44 Gy Boost 0- 23.4 Gy | 33 | – | Mucositis Myelosuppression Leukoencephalopathy |
| Glass, 1996 | 18 | MCHOD (MTX 3.5g /m$^2$) | WBRT 30 Gy Boost +/- | 25.5 | – | Myelosuppression Leukoencephalopathy |
| Schultz, 1996 | 52 | CHOD | WBRT 41.4 Gy Boost 18Gy | 16.1 | 11.6 | Myelosuppression |
| Brada, 1998 | 31 | MACOP B (MTX 0.4–2 g/m$^2$) | WBRT 30–45 Gy, Boost 15–25 Gy Spine 30–35 Gy* | 23 | 16** | Myelosuppression Mucositis Hepato/nephrotoxicity |
| Abrey, 1998 | 31 | MTX IV (1 g/m$^2$) MTX IT (12 mg) Ara-C (post-RT) | WBRT 40 Gy Boost 14.4 Gy | 42 | 21.7*** | Leukoencephalopathy |
| Hiraga, 1999 | 29 | MTX (0.1 g/kg) | WBRT 30 Gy Boost 10–20 Gy | 39.3 | – | Myelosuppression Leukoencephalopathy |
| **Post-irradiation chemotherapy** | | | | | | |
| Shibamato, 1990 | 10 | VEPA | WBRT 30–40 Gy Boost 20–30 Gy | 16+ | 7 | Leukoencephalopathy/necrosis |
| Chamberlain, 1992 | 16 | Hydroxyurea, PCV | WBRT 55–62 Gy | 41 | 13**** | Myelosuppression |
| Rosenthal, 1993 | 6 | CHOP | WBRT 45 Gy Boost 10 Gy | 25+ | 18 | Myelosuppression |
| **No initial irradiation** | | | | | | |
| Neuwelt, 1991 | 17 | CMPD (MTX 2.5 g IA) BBB disruption | None (at relapse) | 44.5 | – | Seizure Myelosuppression |
| Cher, 1996 | 19 | MTX (3.5–8 d/m$^2$), or MCHOD | None (at relapse) | 51 | – | Nephrotoxicity |
| Freilich, 1996 | 13 | MTX (1–3.5 g/m$^2$), P +/- V,T,ara-C | None (at relapse) | 30.5 | – | Leukoencephalopathy |
| Sandor, 1998 | 14 | MTX (1.5 g/m$^2$), V,T | None (at relapse) | 30+ | – | Myelosuppression Neurocognitive decline |

MTX, methotrexate; BVAM, BCNU, vincristine, cytosine arabinoside, methotrexate; IT, intrathecal;;CHOP, cyclophosphamide, doxorubicin, vincristine, prednisone; MCHOD, methotrexate, cyclophosphamide, doxorubicin, vincristine, dexamethasone; CHOD, cyclophosphamide, doxorubicin, vincristine, dexamethasone; MACOP-B, methotrexate, doxorubicin, cyclophosphamide, vincristine, prednisone, bleomycin; IV, intravenous; Ara-C, cytosine arabinoside; VEPA vincristine, doxorubicin, cyclophosphamide, prednisolone; PCV, procarbazine, CCNU, vincristine; CMPD, cyclophosphamide, methotrexate, procarbazine, dexamethasone; IA, intra-arterial; BBB, blood–brain barrier; P, procarbazine; V, vincristine; T, thiotepa.
[d] Historical controls.
*Only patients with proven CSF disease treated with full craniospinal irradiation.   ** From Brada, 1990.
*** From DeAngelis , 1992.   ****From Chamberlain, 1990.
Note: median survival times not supplied by the reference were calculated from Kaplan–Meier analysis of individual survival times reported within the text.

60 Gy (40 Gy to the whole brain, 20 Gy boost to the tumor and its margin) [23].

The optimal extent of radiation is also controversial. Radiation may be administered to the involved field, the whole brain or the entire cranio–spinal axis. Historically, whole-brain irradiation has been the standard treatment, even though its advantage relative to other protocols has never been definitively established [6,22]. In fact, one review reports a median survival of 40 months for local treatment and 25.3 months for whole-brain irradiation, although this difference may merely reflect selection bias [22]. Radiating the entire cranio–spinal axis prophylactically is not warranted. The potential for radiation toxicity and the fact that the survival of most patients with spinal disease is determined by control of cerebral tumor argue against using prophylactic spinal radiation. Spinal irradiation is reserved for patients with spinal disease, demonstrated radiographically or by CSF cytology.

Radiation therapy yields both clinical and radiographic response in AIDS-related primary CNS lymphoma, but the median survival in this population remains poor, ranging from 2 to 5.5 months [24]. Younger age and higher Karnofsky performance status at the time of treatment correlate with better outcome.

The complications of radiation therapy for primary CNS lymphoma are the same as those seen with radiation in any setting. The acute toxicities include headaches, nausea/vomiting and local skin reactions. Chronic complications include cognitive impairment and radiation necrosis of brain tissue. The risk of late neurologic sequelae increases with higher radiation dose and with age.

## Chemotherapy

The use of chemotherapy for PCNSL is expanding [26–41] (Table 16.7). Patients receiving chemotherapy and radiotherapy live longer than those receiving radiotherapy alone [36, 41–44]. The median survival following combinations of radiation and chemotherapy has ranged from 16 to 44.5 months; the 5-year survival rate is 20–30%. Long-term follow-up in one group of 31 patients revealed frequent relapse (15 of 29 patients) and a high rate of late neurologic toxicity, especially in patients

older than 60 years [32]. Patients with AIDS-associated disease, selected for good performance status, lack of active comorbid disease and high CD4 counts, may also benefit from chemotherapy [45].

Differences among chemotherapy regimens for primary CNS lymphoma are numerous: the agents used, the timing of administration (before or after radiotherapy) and the method of delivery (intravenous, intrathecal, or intra-arterial). The chemotherapeutic agents used are those with demonstrated efficacy against systemic lymphomas: corticosteroids, methotrexate, vinca alkaloids and alkylating agents. Corticosteroids lyse tumor cells and induce radiographic and clinical remission, but their effects are often brief. Methotrexate penetrates the intact blood brain barrier. It has demonstrated impressive efficacy against primary CNS lymphoma [46]. Although agents such as cyclophosphamide have been used with success against systemic lymphomas, they have not proven as efficacious against CNS disease, probably because of poor penetration of the blood–brain barrier.

Toxicity depends on the drug used. In general, acute systemic effects include mucositis, myelosuppression, nausea, vomiting and alopecia. Cognitive impairment is the feared late complication. Methotrexate administered after radiotherapy has been implicated in a higher incidence of this problem.

The rationale for administering chemotherapy before radiotherapy is twofold: (1) since radiotherapy often results in complete radiographic remission, administering it first prevents assessment of the effect of chemotherapy on measurable disease, and (2) the neurologic toxicity of some chemotherapeutic agents, including methotrexate, is less frequent and less severe when the drug is given prior to, rather than after, radiation. Intrathecal injection and intra-arterial delivery following blood–brain barrier disruption have been used to improve the penetration of these agents into the brain parenchyma [37].

Chemotherapy alone, with radiotherapy reserved for failure, has shown promise in uncontrolled trials [38–40]. The high initial response rates and the avoidance of radiation induced toxicity of this strategy warrant its further study.

## Surgery

The role of surgery in the management of primary CNS lymphoma is limited. Surgical management is usually restricted to tumor biopsy for diagnosis. Rarely, shunting is needed for obstructive hydrocephalus. Craniotomy for tumor resection does not confer a survival benefit [6, 41].

## Recurrent Disease

Relapse eventually occurs in almost all cases of primary CNS lymphoma, even despite newer and more aggressive multimodality treatment [37, 44]. Relapse can be intracerebral, spinal, ocular or even systemic. Approximately 90% of relapses occur within the brain [23]. Treatment is primarily palliative, although additional chemotherapy, usually with different agents, is often appropriate for younger patients, with good performance status.

# Secondary CNS Lymphoma

Systemic lymphoma spreads to the CNS in about 10% of cases, most commonly in the setting of advanced or relapsing disease [47]. Certain sites of systemic disease are more likely to seed the CNS: the testis, bone marrow, bone, orbit, peripheral blood and paranasal sinuses. Propensity to spread to the CNS also varies with histologic subtype. Low-grade lymphomas rarely metastasize to the brain. Most metastases are diffuse large-cell or high-grade lymphomas. High-grade histology, elevated LDH levels, advanced disease and symptoms such as fever, sweats and weight loss are predictive of CNS relapse.

CNS involvement by secondary lymphoma is usually leptomeningeal; the parenchyma is rarely involved. The clinical presentation of secondary CNS lymphoma reflects the predominantly leptomeningeal disease. Symptoms and signs typically include headache, altered mental status, meningismus and cranial or spinal neuropathy.

Leptomeningeal involvement by lymphoma is best visualized with contrast-enhanced MRI. Given the common meningeal involvement in secondary CNS lymphoma, CSF cytology is more frequently positive than in primary CNS lymphoma. CSF may be positive in up to 70% of cases [47]. The combination of abnormal brain imaging and CSF findings in the setting of progressive or relapsing systemic lymphoma makes biopsy for diagnosis unnecessary.

Choice of therapy for secondary cerebral lymphoma must consider both the systemic and cerebral disease. Frequently, the combination of systemic and intrathecal chemotherapy is chosen. Whole-brain radiation and the drugs given for primary CNS lymphoma are also used frequently. Response to therapy, as reflected by clinical remission of CNS disease, is a favorable prognostic sign [47].

The prognosis for patients with secondary cerebral lymphoma is poor. Fewer than 15% survive for 1 year. Progressive systemic disease is the usual cause of death. Cerebral involvement is often used as an indicator of the extent of systemic disease. It rarely independently worsens the outcome.

Patients at high risk for CNS involvement, such as those with high-grade lymphomas, warrant prophylactic treatment. Intrathecal methotrexate (the agent most frequently used) reduces the incidence of cerebral metastasis [48].

# Conclusion

Cerebral lymphoma, specifically PCNSL, is increasing in incidence. The role of surgery is usually limited to stereotactic biopsy for diagnosis. Multimodality therapy, combining chemotherapy and whole-brain radiotherapy, has improved the survival of patients with primary CNS lymphoma, but long-term relapse-free survival is still rare. Currently, a number of clinical trials are evaluating single-modality treatment protocols, in an effort to lengthen patient survival without incurring late neurologic toxicity.

# Key Points

- *Cerebral metastases represent the most common intracranial tumour.*
- *The selection of a treatment plan for an individual patient must consider multiple factors.*
- *Radiotherapy is indicated for almost all patients with cerebral metastases, with the*

*method of delivery, dose and regimen indi-vidual to each patient.*

● *Lymphoma can occur as either metastatic to the brain or as primary CNS lymphoma.*

● *The majority of primary CNS lymphomas are monoclonal B-cell lymphomas.*

# References

1. Johnson JD, Young B. Demographics of brain metasta-sis. Neurosurg Clin N Am 1996;7:337–44.
2. Posner JB, Chernik NL. Intracranial metastasis from systemic cancer. Advances in Neurology 1978;19:579–92.
3. Posner JB. Neurologic complications of cancer. Contemporary Neurology series. Volume 45. Phildelphia: Davis, 1995.
4. Das A, Hochberg FH. Clinical presentation of intracra-nial metastases. Neurosurg Clin N Am 1996;7:377–91.
5. Schaefer PW, Budzik RF, Gonzalez GG. Imaging of cere-bral metastases. Neurosurg Clin N Am 1996;7:393–423.
6. Murray K, Kun L, Cox J. Primary malignant lymphoma of the central nervous system: results of treatment of 11 cases and review of the literature. J Neurosurg 1987;65:600–7.
7. Patchell RA, Tibbs PA, Walsh JW et al. A randomized trial of surgery in the treatment of single metastases to the brain. NEJM 1990;322:494–500.
8. Chin L, Zee C, Apuzzo M. Special considerations in point stereotactic procedures. In: Apuzzo M, editor. Brain surgery. New York: Churchill Livingstone, 1993;414–25.
9. Cairncross JG, Kim J, Posner JB. Radiation therapy for brain metastases. Ann Neurol 1980;7:529–41.
10. Paleologos NA, Imperatu JP, Vick NA. Brain metastasis: effects of radiotherapy on longterm survivors. Neurology 1991;41(Suppl. 1):129.
11. Alexander E III, Moriarity TM, Davis RB, Wen PY, Fine HA, Black PM et al. Stereotactic radiosurgery for the definitive nininvasive treatment of brain metastases. J Natl Cancer Institute 1995;87:34–40.
12. Lang FF, Sawaya R. Surgical management of cerebral metastases. Neurosurg Clin N Am 1996;7:459–84.
13. Patchell RA, Tibbs PA, Regine WF, Dempsey RJ, Mohiuddin M, Kryscio RJ et al. Postoperative radio-therapy in the treatment of single metastases to the brain: a randomized trial. JAMA 1998;280:1485–9.
14. Sundaresan N, Sachdev VP, DiGiacinto GV, Hughes JEO. Reoperation for brain metastases. J Clin Oncol 1988;6:1625–9.
15. Cooper JS, Steinfeld AD, Lerch IA. Cerebral metastases: value of reirradiation in selected patients. Radiology 1990;174:883–5.
16. Hochberg FH, Miller DC. Primary central nervous sys-tem lymphoma. J Neurosurg 1988;68:835–53.
17. Corn BW, Marcus SM, Topham A et al. Will primary central nervous system lymphoma be the most frequent brain tumor diagnosed in the year 2000? Cancer 1997;79:2409–13.
18. Miller DC, Hochberg FH, Harris NL et al. Pathology with clinical correlations of primary central nervous system
non-Hodgkin's lymphoma: the Massachusetts General Hospital experience 1958–1989. Cancer 1994;74:1383–97.
19. Antoniri A, De Rossi G, Ammassari A. Value of com-bined approach with thallium-201 single-photon emis-sion computed tomography and Epstein–Barr virus DNA polymerase chain reaction in CSF for the diagno-sis of AIDS-related primary CNS lymphoma. J Clin Onc 1999;17:554–60.
20. DeAngelis LM. Current management of primary central nervous system lymphoma. Oncology 1995;9:63–71.
21. Remick SC, Diamond C, Migliozzi JA et al. Primary cen-tral nervous system lymphoma in patients with and without the acquired immune deficiency syndrome: a retrospective analysis and review of the literature. Medicine 1990;69:345–60.
22. Leibel SA, Sheline GE. Radiation therapy for neoplasms of the brain. J Neurosurg 1987;66:1–22.
23. Nelson DF, Martz KL, Bonner H et al. Non-Hodgkin's lymphoma of the brain: can high dose, large volume radiation therapy improve survival? Report on a prospective trial by the Radiation Therapy Oncology Group (RTOG): RTOG 8315. Int J Radiat Oncol Biol Phys 1992;23:9–17.
24. Goldstein JD, Dickson DW, Moser FG et al. Primary cen-tral nervous system lymphoma in acquired immune deficiency syndrome: a clinical and pathologic study with results of treatment with radiation. Cancer 1991;67:2756–65.
25. Bessell EM, Punt J, Firth J et al. Primary Non-Hodgkin's lymphoma of the central nervous system: Phase II study of chemotherapy (BVAM) prior to radiotherapy. Clin Oncol 1991;3:193–8.
26. Liang BC, Grant R, Junck L et al. Primary central ner-vous system lymphoma: treatment with multiagent sys-temic and intrathecal chemotherapy with radiation therapy. Int J Oncol 1993;3:1001–4.
27. LaChanceDH, Brizel DM, Gockerman JP et al. Cyclophosphamide, doxorubicin, vincristine, and pred-nisone for primary central nervous system lymphoma: short duration response and multifocal intracerebral recurrence preceding radiotherapy. Neurology 1994;44:1721–7.
28. Glass J, Gruber ML, Cher L, et al. Preirradiation methotrexate chemotherapy of primary central nervous system lymphoma: long term outcome. J Neurosurg 1994;81:188–95.
29. Glass J, Shustik C, Hochberg FH, et al. Therapy of pri-mary central nervous system lymphoma with pre-irra-diation methotrexate, cyclophosphamide, doxorubicin, vincristine, and dexamethasone (MCHOD). J Neuro-oncol 1996;30:257–65.
30. Schultz C, Scott C, Sherman W, et al. Preirradiation chemotherapy with cyclophosphamide, doxorubicin, vincristine, and dexamethasone for primary CNS lym-phomas: intial report of radiation therapy oncology group protocol 88–06. J Clin Onc 1996;14:556–64.
31. Brada M, Hjiyiannakis D, Hines F, et al. Short intensive primary chemotherapy and radiotherapy in sporadic primary CNS lymphoma (PCL). Int J Radiat Oncol Biol Phys 1998;40:1157–62.
32. Abrey LE, DeAngelis LM, Yahalom J. Long-term sur-vival in primary CNS lymphoma. J Clin Onc 1998;16:859–63.

33. Hiraga S, Arita N, Ohnishi T, et al. Rapid infusion of high-dose methotrexate resulting in enhanced penetration into cerebrospinal fluid and intensified tumor response in primary central nervous system lymphomas. J Neurosurg 1999;91:221–30.

34. Shibamoto Y, Tsutsui K, Dodo Y, et al. Improved survival rate in primary intracranial lymphoma treated by high-dose radiation and systemic vincristine–doxorubicin–cyclophosphamide–prednisolone chemotherapy. Cancer 1990;65:1907–12.

35. Chamberlain MC, Levin VA. Primary central nervous system lymphoma: a role for adjuvant chemotherapy. J Neuro-oncol 1992;14:271–5.

36. Rosenthal MA, Sheridan WP, Green MD et al. Primary cerebral lymphoma: an argument for the use of adjunctive systemic chemotherapy. Aust N Z J Surg 1993;63:30–2.

37. Neuwelt EA, Goldman DL, Dahlborg SA et al. Primary CNS lymphoma treated with osmotic blood-brain barrier disruption: prolonged survival and preservation of cognitive function. J Clin Onc 1991;9:1580–90.

38. Cher L, Glass J, Harsh GR et al. Therapy of primary CNS lymphoma with methotrexate-based chemotherapy and deferred radiotherapy: preliminary results. Neurology 196;46:1757–9.

39. Freilich RJ, Delattre JY, Monjour A et al. Chemotherapy without radiation mtherapy as initial treatment for primary CNS lymphoma in older patients. Neurology 1996;46:435–9.

40. Sandor V, Stark-Vancs V, Pearson D et al. Phase II trial of chemotherapy alone for primary CNS and intraocular lymphoma. J Clin Oncol 1998;16:3000–6.

41. Pollack IF, Lunsford LD, Flickinger JC et al:. Prognostic factors in the diagnosis and treatment of primary central nervous system lymphoma. Cancer 1989;63: 939–47.

42. Brada M, Dearnaley D, Horwich A et al. Management of primary cerebral lymphoma with initial chemotherapy: preliminary results and comparison with patients treated with radiotherapy alone. Int J Radiat Oncol Biol Phys 1990;18:787–92.

43. Chamberlain MC, Levin VA. Adjuvant chemotherapy for primary lymphoma of the central nervous systyem. Arch Neurol 1990;97:1113–6.

44. DeAngelis LM, Yahalom J, Thaler H et al. Combined modality therapy for primary CNs lymphoma. J Clin Onc 1992;10:635–43.

45. Chamberlain MC. Long survival in patients with acquired immune deficiency syndrome related primary central nervous system lymphoma. Cancer 1994;73: 1728–30.

46. Blay J-Y, Conroy T, Chevreau C et al. High-dose methotrexate for the treatment of primary cerebral lymphomas: an analysis of survival and late neurologic toxicity in a retrospective series. J Clin Onc 1998;16:864–71.

47. Liang RH S, Woo EKW, Yu Y et al. Central nervous system involvement in non-Hodgkin's lymphoma. Eur J Clin Onc 1989;25:703–10.

48. Perez-Soler R, Smith TL, Cabanillas F. Central nervous system prophylaxis with combined intravenous and intrathecal methotrexate in diffuse lymphoma of aggressive histologic type. Cancer 1986;57:971–7.

# 17

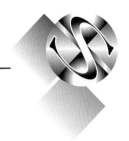

# Pediatric Neuro-oncology

Kevin L. Stevenson, J. Russell Geyer and
Richard G. Ellenbogen

## Summary

Tumors of the CNS are, as a group, the
second most frequent malignancy of childhood and the most common solid tumor
in this age group. In this chapter, the epidemiology, clinical presentation, surgical
considerations, chemotherapy and radiation
therapy options regarding pediatric brain
tumors will be reviewed. In addition, we will
specifically focus on several of the major categories of pediatric CNS malignancy and the
late effects resulting from current treatment
regimens.

## Introduction

Tumors of the CNS are, as a group, the second
most frequent malignancy of childhood and the
most common solid tumor in this age group. In
general, children with brain tumors have not
shared in the remarkable improvement in prognosis that has characterized other childhood
malignancies. In this chapter, the epidemiology,
clinical presentation, surgical considerations,
chemotherapy and radiation therapy options
regarding pediatric brain tumors will be
reviewed. In addition, we will specifically focus
on several of the major categories of pediatric
CNS malignancy and the late effects resulting
from current treatment regimens. In conclusion, the future directions in pediatric brain
tumor management will be discussed.

## Epidemiology

CNS tumors represent approximately 17% of all
malignancies in the pediatric age range, including adolescents. Approximately 2,000 children
younger than 20 years of age are diagnosed
annually with tumors of the CNS [1]. Brain
tumors in childhood are a heterogeneous group.
Astrocytomas are the most frequent, accounting
for approximately 52%, while primitive neural
epidermal tumors account for approximately
21%, ependymomas 9% and other tumor types
represent the remaining 15%. While in older
children and adults the most frequent site of
malignant brain tumors is supratentorial, young
children have a relatively high occurrence of
tumors in the cerebellum and brain stem. The
incidence of CNS tumors is greater in those
children younger than 8 years of age – approximately 35 cases per million children – than it is
in children from 8 to 17 years of age – approximately 20 per million [1].

Over the last two decades, CNS cancer incidence in children appears to have increased.
While this has provoked concern that there may
be changes in environmental exposures responsible for this increasing incidence, epidemio-
logic evidence to support this hypothesis is
lacking. Alternatively, the increase in incidence

299

could be related to improving diagnostic technology. There are several known risk factors predisposing to the development of CNS tumors in childhood. Therapeutic doses of radiation utilized in the treatment of leukemia or previous brain tumors are clearly implicated as a risk factor. Patients with several inherited genetic conditions have greatly increased risk of brain tumors, specifically neurofibromatosis, tuberous sclerosis and the Li–Fraumeni syndrome. Taken as a whole, these known risk factors account for a small percentage of pediatric brain tumors; for the great majority of brain tumors in childhood, there is no specific risk factor known to be related to their incidence.

# Medulloblastoma/Primitive Neuroectodermal Tumor

PNETs of the CNS are a group of embryonal tumors that histologically comprise poorly differentiated neural epithelial cells. These tumors occur predominantly, though not exclusively, in childhood and constitute approximately 20–30% of all childhood brain tumors [1]. This group of tumors shares the biologic propensity of dissemination throughout the subarachnoid space, in addition to recurrence or progression at the primary site.

Tumors of this histology are most common in the posterior fossa and, in this location, are commonly called medulloblastomas (Fig. 17.1a). However, tumors that histologically appear identical to those found in the posterior fossa can occur in other locations throughout the CNS, where they are referred to as supratentorial PNETs, pineoblastomas in the pineal region and retinoblastomas in the eye [2]. While PNETs of the posterior fossa and of other sites share a common histologic appearance and a similar propensity for a pattern of metastases, the issue of whether these tumors share a common origin in biology remains quite controversial [2]. Recent studies examining the

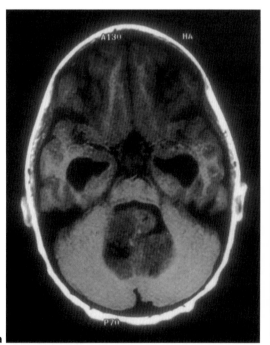
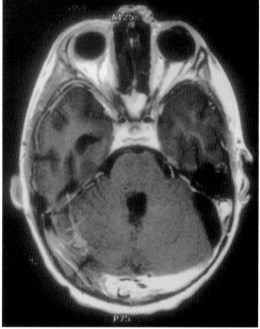

**Fig. 17.1. a** Axial MRI (T1), showing moderately sized medulloblastoma. Typical of medulloblastomas, this tumor involves the roof of the fourth ventricle, without invading the floor. Also note the markedly enlarged temporal horns of the lateral ventricles. **b** Post-operative axial gadolinium-enhanced MRI (T1), showing resection of the fourth ventricular tumor, as well as resolution of hydrocephalus.

molecular biology of these tumors suggest that there may be differences, in spite of the common histologic appearance. Nonetheless, treatment strategies over the last decade have combined supratentorial PNETs and medulloblastomas.

## Clinical Presentation

The vast majority of children with medulloblastomas present with signs and symptoms of hydrocephalus: headache, nausea, vomiting and lethargy. It should be kept in mind that this symptom triad is not unique to medulloblastomas; any posterior fossa tumor can produce this symptom complex. Headaches tend to be worst in the morning upon awakening, and are often accompanied by nausea. Vomiting will often temporarily decrease or eliminate the headache, perhaps due to hyperventilation-induced hypocarbia. It is not uncommon for children to have several months of headache, nausea and/or vomiting prior to diagnosis. During this time, more common etiologies of these symptoms are often investigated, including migraines, primary gastrointestinal disorders, and even psychiatric disorders. In addition to hydrocephalus, etiologies of lethargy in medulloblastoma include dehydration and direct brainstem compression/invasion by the primary lesion. Other common signs and symptoms of medulloblastomas include papilledema, ataxia, dysmetria and diplopia. As 15–20% of children with medulloblastomas will have spinal disease ("drop metastases") at the time of diagnosis [3], back pain may uncommonly be the initial complaint.

## Surgery

Despite advances in the non-surgical management of medulloblastomas, surgical resection remains the primary initial treatment of these tumors. In addition to providing histologic diagnosis and relief of tumor burden, surgical resection of medulloblastomas can provide immediate relief of neurologic signs and symptoms due to hydrocephalus and direct brainstem compression. Because 90% of children present with hydrocephalus, and up to 30% will require chronic CSF diversion [4], an EVD is inserted prior to tumor resection, regardless of the degree of hydrocephalus present on

imaging. More recently, endoscopic third ventriculostomy may be another appropriate approach to relieving the block of CSF flow at the level of the aqueduct of Sylvius. Typically arising from the roof of the fourth ventricle, medulloblastomas invade the floor of the ventricle in up to 36% of cases [5]. Unlike ependymomas (discussed later), tumor residual in the brainstem does not adversely affect outcome [6] and most pediatric neurosurgeons will resect the tumor flush with the floor of the fourth ventricle, without entering the brainstem (Fig. 17.1b). Adjuvant technology, such as the operating microscope, intraoperative cranial nerve/SSEP monitoring and post-resection intraoperative ultrasound are essential in our institution for achieving the goal of radical resection of these tumors. For staging purposes, a lumbar puncture can be performed with the child still anesthetized. In these authors' experiences, immediate lumbar puncture after tumor resection does not lead to false-positive results.

## Radiation Therapy and Chemotherapy

Recognition that metastatic failure throughout the sub-arachnoid space was second only to local recurrence as a site of failure in children with medulloblastoma led to the use of cranio–spinal radiation as adjuvant treatment by the mid-1950s. Several clinical studies demonstrated a dose–response relationship in regard to the dose of radiation required to control disease at the primary site, with doses of less than approximately 5,000 cGy resulting in higher rates of failure [7]. Until recently, however, the cranio–spinal dose–response relationship was unclear, but, by convention, most children received doses from 3,000 to 3,600 cGy. Following surgical resection and cranio–spinal radiation at these doses, durable survival was reported in approximately 30–50% of children by the mid-1970s.

Two large co-operative trials treating children with medulloblastoma were conducted in the late 1970s: one by the Children Cancer Group (CCG), in the USA, and one by the Society of International Pediatric Oncology (SIOP), conducted in Europe [8,9]. In both studies, patients were randomly assigned to receive irradiation alone or irradiation plus adjuvant chemotherapy, which, in both studies, consisted of vincristine and lomustine. More than 500 patients were accrued between the two studies and the 5-year-of-entry survivals of approximately 50% in both studies were very similar. Overall, neither study demonstrated survival advantages of the use of adjuvant chemotherapy. However, chemotherapy did show a benefit in subgroups of patients in both the CCG and SIOP studies. Those with partial resection brainstem involvement and large tumors and the other patients with extensive disease, i.e. large tumors and sub-arachnoid metastases, had superior survival when treated with adjuvant chemotherapy in addition to irradiation. These studies delineated a group of patients at higher risk for disease progression, i.e. those with larger partially resected tumors and those with metastatic disease at diagnosis, and confirmed the value of adjuvant chemotherapy for this high-risk group. As a result of these studies, post-surgical staging of the subarachnoid space, initially with myelogram and more recently with gadolinium-enhanced MRI has become standard, as has the use of adjuvant chemotherapy in the patients at high risk.

The issue of appropriate dose of neuraxis irradiation was addressed in a prospective study conducted by the Pediatric Oncology Group (POG) and the CCG in the mid-1980s [10]. In this study, children with medulloblastoma without high-risk features were randomly assigned to receive either standard-dose irradiation to the neuraxis (3,600 cGy) or reduced-dose irradiation (2,300 cGy). All children received a total dose of posterior fossa irradiation of 5,400 cGy. In the final analysis, eligible patients receiving standard-dose neuraxis irradiation had a 67% event-free survival at 5 years, while those patients receiving reduced neuraxis had only a 52% event-free survival at 5 years. Thus, at least when used as the only adjuvant treatment modality, the dose of cranio–spinal irradiation has been defined as 3,600 cGy. Unfortunately, this same study demonstrated that, at least for those children younger than 8 years, treatment with the higher dose of neuraxis radiation resulted in greater intellectual morbidity than those treated with the lower dose. Efforts to develop treatment approaches that allow a lower dose of radiation to be administered to the neuraxis continue to be investigated.

As noted above, the first randomized studies demonstrated that the addition of adjuvant chemotherapy to neuraxis radiation was of benefit for those patients at higher risk of tumor progression, i.e. those with significant residual post-operative tumor and those with metastatic disease. A number of single-arm studies, as well as randomized studies, have been conducted in an effort to optimize adjuvant chemotherapy. In a single-institutional study, children with medulloblastoma and high-risk features were treated with standard-dose cranio–spinal irradiation, as well as with CCNU, vincristine and cisplatin. The 5-year progression-free survival was greater than 70% [11]. A randomized trial in the CCG compared adjuvant therapy with CCNU, vincristine and prednisone with a multiple-drug regimen, which included vincristine, CCNU and cisplatin. Overall, the study demonstrated a 5-year progression-free survival in patients with non-metastatic disease of greater than 70% but those children with metastatic disease had an approximately 40% event-free survival at 5 years [12]. In addition, in this study, the complex regimen was clearly inferior to the two-drug regimen. In an attempt to improve survival outcome for children with average-risk medulloblastoma, as well as to effectively utilize reduced-dose neuraxis irradiation, a study treated children with average-risk disease with reduced-dose radiotherapy (2,300 cGy), as well as vincristine, cisplatin and CCNU.

The 5-year event-free survival from this study was approximately 80%, suggesting that reduced-dose neuraxis radiation can be safely employed if combined with adjuvant chemotherapy [13]. An ongoing, randomized trial in the Childrens Oncology Group (COG) is comparing two regimens of chemotherapy, both in the context of reduced-dose neuraxis radiation for those children with average-risk medulloblastoma.

The survival outcome of children with high-risk medulloblastoma, particularly those with metastatic disease, remains poor. Ongoing trials are investigating the role of high-dose chemotherapy with stem cell rescue in combination with standard irradiation. Another trial is investigating the concomitant addition of carboplatin with the radiation in an attempt to radiosensitize the tumor.

Successful treatment of children with recurrent medulloblastoma remains problematic, with the 2-year survival rate following initial relapse being less than 10% in most studies [12]. High-dose chemotherapy with stem cell rescue has shown promise in limited studies as a salvage regimen for those children with local recurrence; this appears to be of limited benefit in those with sub-arachnoid metastatic recurrence.

# Astrocytomas

Astrocytomas account for approximately 50% of CNS tumors in childhood. Of these, approximately 10–20% are high-grade astrocytomas and thus the majority are low-grade astrocytomas.

## High-grade Astrocytomas

High-grade astrocytomas represent a rare group of primary brain tumors in children. While the majority of pediatric astrocytomas occur in the posterior fossa, the minority are high-grade, representing 4–8% of all cerebellar astrocytomas [14,15]. Supratentorial astrocytomas, while less common than those in the infratentorial space, are more likely to be pathologically high-grade, with 20% of all hemispheric tumors being high-grade gliomas [16]. Anaplastic (WHO Grade III) gliomas histologically show

marked nuclear pleomorphism, anaplasia and hyperchromasia, with variable degrees of mitoses and endothelial proliferation, while glioblastoma multiforme (WHO Grade IV) displays similar characteristics, with areas of necrosis.

## Low-grade Astrocytomas

The low-grade astrocytomas of childhood can be further sub-divided into pilocytic astrocytomas, which account for approximately 75% of the group of low-grade astrocytomas, and other histologies, including fibrillary, protoplasmic and gemistocytic tumors, make up the remaining 25%. Pilocytic astrocytomas are histologically composed of fusiform astrocytes, loosely interwoven in a fine fibrillary background. These tumors frequently have a microcystic component, Rosenthal fibers and large macrocysts. While the most common location of pilocytic astrocytomas is in the cerebellum (Fig. 17.2), they can be found in other locations within the CNS, notably the visual pathway and optic chiasm, the brain stem and the cerebral cortex. The biologic behavior of these pilocytic tumors can be quite indolent and, in fact, spontaneous cessation of growth, as well as regression without treatment, has been observed. More commonly, however, these tumors progress slowly and present with symptoms

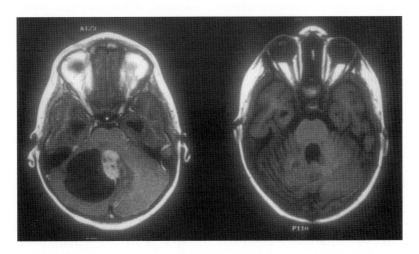

**Fig. 17.2.** (Left) Axial gadolinium-enhanced MRI (T1), showing a vermian juvenile pilocytic astrocytoma. Typical of pilocytic astrocytomas, the majority of the mass effect is due to the large cyst, while the enhancing solid portion contributes much less. (Right) Post-operative axial MRI (T1) after gross total resection of the solid portion of the astrocytoma. As the cyst wall is not composed of tumor cells, it is unnecessary, and potentially morbid, to resect the cyst wall.

characteristic of their site of origin, i.e. hydro-cephalus and ataxia for those of the posterior fossa and visual abnormalities associated with those tumors of the visual pathway, including the optic chiasm.

## Management

In general, complete resection of pilocytic astro-cytomas results in long-term disease control in the great majority of patients. For example, resection of cerebellar pilocytic astrocytomas has resulted in more than 95% of the patients being free of disease 5 years from the time of surgical intervention in most series. Therefore, adjuvant therapy following gross total resection of these tumors is not indicated. The natural history of pilocytic astrocytomas was the subject of a recent large co-operative group trial. In this study, patients with low-grade astrocy-tomas, principally pilocytic astrocytomas, who underwent a complete surgical resection were observed. The progression-free survival at 5 years was 85%. Those patients who were unable to undergo a complete resection were observed and did not, in most instances, receive either adjuvant radiation or chemotherapy. The 5-year progression-free survival for this group of patients was 60%. Thus, while progression fol-lowing a subtotal resection, or no resection, of pilocytic astrocytomas occurs much more frequently than is observed following gross total resection, it is by no means inevitable. Therefore, achieving a gross total resection at the expense of significant morbidity is not indi-cated in the management of these tumors. Furthermore, given that a substantial propor-tion of patients do not inevitably progress, even following limited or no resection, it is not clear that adjuvant radiation or chemotherapy is required for these patients. In the asymptomatic patient, serial observations, including neu-roimaging, is often employed, withholding adjuvant therapy for clear evidence of either neurologic or radiographic progression. Should progression of subtotally resected or unre-sectable pilocytic astrocytomas occur, a number of studies have demonstrated the value of involved field radiation in the long-term control of these tumors [17]. In one study, 5-year progression-free survival was greater than 90%, as was 10-year progression-free survival. Thus, involved field radiation therapy remains

important adjuvant therapy for the treatment of progressive pilocytic astrocytomas.

Inasmuch as these tumors often occur at a very young age, particularly those tumors originating in the visual pathway and chiasm, concern over the late effects of radiation therapy has led to investigation of alternative modalities of treatment, when required. Initial trials of chemotherapy with vincristine and dactino-mycin were modeled on treatment protocols utilized for non-CNS low-grade tumors and demonstrated tumor stabilization and, in some cases, initial tumor regression in patients with tumor recurrence after radiation therapy and subsequently in newly diagnosed patients with progressive disease prior to radiation therapy. Subsequent protocols have utilized other alter-native chemotherapeutic regimens. The largest data set exists for the use of carboplatin and vin-cristine. In a prospective study of these agents in children with progressive low-grade astrocy-tomas (primarily of the visual pathway), the 3-year progression-free survival was over 50% [18]. Subsequent resumption of tumor growth after several years is not uncommon and radia-tion can be then employed, but it is hoped that delaying radiation therapy for even several years in a very young child might ameliorate late toxicities. Currently, a randomized trial comparing carboplatin and vincristine to a multi-drug regimen consisting of vincristine, procarbazine, thioguanine and CCNU is being evaluated within the COG. While the utility of delaying radiation therapy in the younger child is reasonably clear, the benefits of such an approach in adolescents are less obvious. Nonetheless, utilization of chemotherapy either as front-line or salvage therapy in the instance of progression of low-grade astrocytoma in the adolescent should be considered. Children with low-grade astrocytomas, particularly those with pilocytic histology, can have a chronic course, requiring multiple interventions. A principle guiding therapeutic intervention should be that of minimizing morbidity. Therefore, avoid-ing adjuvant therapy in the asymptomatic patient without demonstrated progression, utilizing the modality of treatment with the least long-term morbidity initially (i.e. chemother-apy) and avoiding rapid institution of a therapy change based on minimal changes in imaging studies are important strategies. The long-term outcome in terms of survival for these tumors is good but the potential for significant morbidity, both as a result of progressive disease, i.e. visual loss in the case of those patients with visual pathway tumors, or morbidity related to therapy, is considerable and requires ongoing management by an experienced neuro-oncology team. Non-pilocytic low-grade astrocytomas, such as those with fibrillary histology, are less frequent in childhood and outcome is somewhat less predictable. A similar approach to that described above for pilocytic astrocytomas is reasonable.

# Ependymoma

Approximately 10% of childhood brain tumors are ependymomas [1]. This tumor is most frequent in young children, with approximately half of the cases occurring before age 5 years. This tumor type appears to be approximately twice as common in males as in females, with an incidence rate of approximately 3.5 per million amongst males and 1.8 per million amongst females. Histologically, ependymomas are composed predominantly of neoplastic ependymal cells, where there is great variability of morphologic appearance. The WHO grading system recognizes four tumor types: subependymoma and myxopapillary ependymoma (Grade I tumor), low-grade ependymoma (Grade II tumor) and anaplastic ependymoma (Grade III tumor) [19]. However, there is great variability in the classification of ependymomas within these grades and the recognition of the malignant variant is not easily reproducible. Reports in the literature in terms of frequency of the anaplastic variant show wide variation. Several reports using the WHO classification had failed to link poor histologic grade with poor outcome. Thus, the prognostic significance of histology in ependymoma remains unclear.

## Management

The pattern of recurrence of ependymoma is primarily local, with less than 10% of relapses occuring distant from the primary site. Furthermore, most recent series have demonstrated complete resection to be the most important favorable prognostic sign [20,21]. Therefore, aggressive surgery is the primary modality in the treatment of ependymomas (Fig. 17.3). So important is total tumor resection that serious consideration should be given to

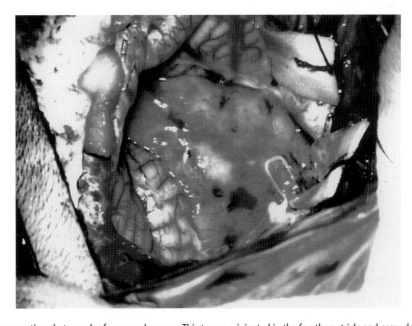

**Fig. 17.3.** Intraoperative photograph of an ependymoma. This tumor originated in the fourth ventricle and grew dorsally into the cisterna magna, as well as laterally to encase cranial nerves IX, X and XI on the right.

radical resection, including the tumor infiltrating the brainstem. While this approach offers a significantly greater chance of long-term survival, it also significantly increases the risks of serious and permanent neurologic disability; the risks of such an aggressive approach must be thoroughly discussed with the family.

Although several small series have suggested that some patients with ependymoma treated only by gross tumor resection are long-term survivors [22], most clinicians have followed surgical resection with radiation therapy. Several single-institution studies have shown durable progression-free survival in greater than 50% of patients receiving focal radiotherapy following gross total resection, while children with significant post-surgery residual tumor have considerably worse survival, even with radiotherapy [23].

While several chemotherapeutic agents have demonstrated activity in ependymoma, no randomized trials have shown that the addition of chemotherapy to post-operative radiotherapy improves prognosis. When an aggressive chemotherapeutic protocol was used without radiation therapy in the treatment of infants with ependymoma, the 5-year progression-free survival was 34% [24]. Thus, the role of chemotherapy in the treatment of ependymoma has yet to be defined. A study soon to open in the COG will evaluate the use of chemotherapy in patients with incompletely resected tumors to render these tumors resectable at second-look surgery.

# Germ Cell Tumors

Germ cell tumors originate in the primordial germ cells, which may undergo either germinomatous or embryonic differentiation. They are biologically diverse and range from benign teratomas to the malignant germinomas and non-germinomatous germ cell tumors. These tumors are located primarily in the midline, with the majority occurring outside the CNS. Approximately 5% of germ cell tumors in children occur within the CNS, most frequently in the pineal and suprasellar regions [1] (Fig. 17.4). Germinomas account for approximately 60% of these tumors, teratomas 30% and the malignant embryonal carcinoma, choriocarcinomas and endodermal sinus tumors approximately 10%. The non-germinomatous malignant germ cell tumors are often characterized by secretion of either beta HCG, alphafetoprotein or both. Significant elevation of one or both of these tumor markers, in association with a tumor located in the characteristic region, are sufficient to make a diagnosis. However, in the absence of such tumor marker elevation, tumor biopsy is required.

## Surgery

Surgical resection of the benign teratomas is the only treatment required in the majority of cases. On the other hand, germinomas require adjuvant treatment to effect a cure. In fact, these

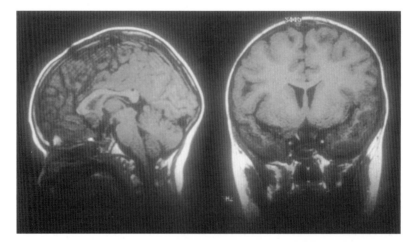

**Fig. 17.4.** Sagittal (left) and coronal (right) MRI (T1), showing a suprasellar germinoma. Typically located in the midline, the pineal region is also a common location for germinomas.

tumors are highly radiation and chemotherapy sensitive and the surgical approach should be limited to obtaining diagnostic tissue; aggressive resection is contraindicated. In the setting of co-existant hydrocephalus, a combined endoscopic third ventriculostomy (ETV) with tumor biopsy can be attempted if the tumor resides within the third ventricle. Although an attractive approach, this strategy is not uniformly successful due to the difficuty in reaching the tumor from the standard ETV trajectory. We have successfully utilized both flexible endoscopy and a more anterior burr hole for our rigid endoscope to achieve the goal of endoscopic third-ventricle fenestration and biopsy. An alternate approach is an image-guided stereotactic approach to biopsy of presumed germinomas, treating the hydrocephalus in a second stage, if needed.

The role of resection in malignant non-germinomatous germ cell tumors is controversial. While most series suggest that obtaining a complete response with the use of combined modality treatment, including surgery, is necessary to achieve long-term disease control, these tumors are often locally invasive and initial complete resection not feasible. While these tumors are less chemo- and radiosensitive than are germinomas, significant and even complete responses have been obtained utilizing chemotherapy; this modality should be employed prior to definitive attempt at resection, in preference to a radical initial approach if there is significant likelihood of morbidity [25].

## Radiation Therapy

There is no established role for adjuvant radiation therapy in the management of the resected teratoma. On the other hand, germinomas are highly radiosensitive and radiation therapy is curative in the majority of patients. Subarachnoid dissemination of germinomas is well recognized but, in the absence of dissemination at diagnosis, subarachnoid spread occurs infrequently and the role of cranio–spinal irradiation is controversial.

Malignant non-germinomatous germ cell tumors are much less radiosensitive and the use of radiation therapy as a stand-alone adjuvant modality results in tumor recurrence in the majority of cases. However, combination therapy with radiation and chemotherapy has resulted in long-term disease control in the majority of patients in several recent series [25].

## Chemotherapy

As is the case with non-CNS malignant germ cell tumors, tumors in the CNS are quite responsive to chemotherapy, particularly cisplatin-based treatment. Complete responses occur in the majority of patients with germinomas and in a high percentage of patients with non-germinomatous malignant germ cell tumors of the CNS [26]. However, chemotherapy without radiation therapy for both germinomas and non-germinomatous malignant germ cell tumors has resulted in tumor recurrence in the majority of patients [26]. Recognizing the activity of chemotherapy in germinomas, as well as the potential toxicity of radiation therapy, several recent studies have investigated the use of chemotherapy and reduced-volume and dose-of-radiation therapy in the treatment of germinomas, with good results [27]. The definitive role of chemotherapy in the treatment of germinomas of the CNS remains controversial. As noted above, radiation therapy alone is insufficient to effect a cure in the majority of patients with malignant non-germinomatous germ cell tumors of the CNS. Several recent studies combining platinum-based chemotherapy with radiation therapy and, often, second-look surgery have significantly improved the prognosis of patients with these tumors, such that over 50% long-term progression-free survival has been reported [25].

# Other CNS Tumors of Childhood
# Craniopharyngioma

Despite benign histopathology and their relative rarity (6–9% of all pediatric brain tumors), craniopharyngiomas often prove one of the most difficult pediatric tumors to cure without significant neurologic morbidity. Due to their intimate association with the ventricular system, visual pathways, hypothalamus and pituitary, craniopharyngiomas commonly present with signs and symptoms of hydrocephalus, visual disturbance (occasionally blindness) and/or endocrine dysfunction. While some degree of endocrine dysfunction is noted in up to 90% of newly diagnosed patients, only a minority come to medical attention secondary to their endocrinopathy, most commonly short stature, diabetes insipidus and hypothyroidism. The most common histology seen in pediatric craniopharyngioma is the adamantinomatous type, composed of epithelial cells, keratin, microcalcification and cholesterol clefts. Grossly, and on imaging, craniopharyngiomas can be primarily cystic, primarily solid or, most commonly, a mixture of the two (Fig. 17.5) and it is not uncommon for a rim of calcium to be seen on CT scan.

## Surgery

Craniopharyngioma is primarily a surgical disease. Gross total resection is reported in up to 70%, with 90% of this group going on to enjoy a surgical cure [28]. Because of their sellar/parasellar location and the tendency for the tumor to adhere to adjacent structures (optic apparatus, hypothalamus, pituitary stalk), postoperative neurologic morbidity can be as high as 30%, panhypopituitarism develops in up to 90% and overall operative mortality reaches 12% [28]. Operative mortality associated with recurrent craniopharyngioma surgery has been reported to be as high as 42% in the best of hands [29], including late mortality related to chronic endocrinopathy and shunt malfunction.

By limiting surgical resection, neurologic morbidity decreases, as does tumor control. In light of the significant morbidity and mortality associated with craniopharyngioma resection, many pediatric neurosurgeons have used minimally invasive techniques to effectively treat these lesions, with far fewer operative complications. Endoscopic endonasal transphenoidal techniques have been successfully employed in a select patient population, with promising results, primarily in patients with sella-based lesions. Increasingly, stereotactic techniques are being used, with excellent results in cystic craniopharyngiomas. Stereotactic intracavitary irradiation with $^{32}P$ or $^{90}Y$ has shown complete cyst resolution in 80% of patients, while installation of bleomycin can provide adequate tumor control in approximately 70%. Finally, stereotactic radiosurgery has shown to be effective treatment for the non-cystic craniopharyngiomas, either as initial treatment or for treatment of the solid portion of mixed tumors following intracavitary treatment and cyst involution. Tumor control rates of 90% have been achieved when combined intracavitary and stereotactic irradiation are used as first-line therapy, and tumor control rates of approximately 60% have been shown in recurrent craniopharyngiomas using stereotactic radiosurgery alone. Given the low rate of post-operative complications, these minimally invasive techniques offer new options in the surgical management of this tumor.

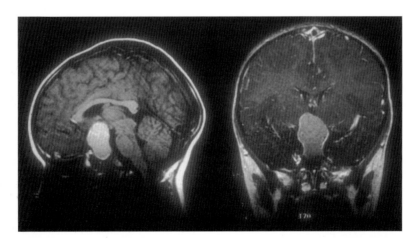

**Fig. 17.5.** Sagittal (left) and coronal (right) gadolinium-enhanced MRI (T1), showing a craniopharyngioma. This example is entirely cystic in appearance, with pronounced enhancement of the wall.

## Radiation Therapy

Subtotal, or planned, limited resections of craniopharyngiomas without post-operative radiation therapy will lead to recurrence and growth of the tumor, residual in the majority of cases. Conventional radiation therapy for residual craniopharyngioma consists of fractionated therapy to 5,500 cGy at 180 cGy/fraction. At doses of more than 5,400 cGy, the recurrence rate after fractionated radiation therapy is 15%, and doses greater than 6,100 cGy are associated with unacceptably high complications, making 5,500 cGy an acceptable dose.

# Brainstem Gliomas

Brainstem gliomas account for approximately 10–20% of childhood CNS malignancies. Of these tumors, 64–75% are intrinsic to the brainstem, centered in the pons and histologically low-grade – the so-called "diffuse brainstem glioma". These tumors tend to present after a rapid course of subtle, progressive ataxia and cranial nerve dysfunction, most commonly V, VI, VII, IX and X. Focal tumors of the brainstem are much less common than diffuse brainstem tumors in the pediatric population and tend to be slowly progressive in nature. Signs and symptoms are related to the involved brainstem region, and low-grade lesions far outnumber high-grade malignancies in this group. A subtype of focal brainstem tumor is the tectal glioma. Typically coming to neurosurgical attention due to late-onset hydrocephalus due to acquired "aqueductal stenosis", these children typically have an essentially normal brain on imaging, with the exception of obstructive hydrocephalus. A third category of brainstem tumor is the dorsally exophytic tumor. Arising from the subependyma of the fourth ventricle and growing dorsally, these patients present similarly to patients with medulloblastomas and ependymomas of the posterior fossa: headache, nausea and vomiting due to hydrocephalus. These tumors grow primarily into the fourth ventricle, rather than invading the brainstem, and are most commonly pilocytic astrocytomas on pathological examination (Fig. 17.6). Exophytic tumors that grow laterally and/or ventrally are more likely to be high-grade in

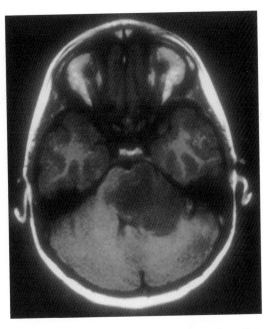

**Fig. 17.6.** Axial MRI (T1) of an exophytic brainstem glioma. Note the paucity of mass effect, edema and hydrocephalus, typical of these indolent lesions.

nature, and typically present after a shorter course of neurologic symptoms.

## Summary

The role of surgery in the intrinsic brainstem glioma is limited to the occasional necessity for permanent CSF diversion. Biopsy has not proven to add important information which will alter therapy and, given the high potential for morbidity, is not recommended. On the other hand, focal lesions of the brainstem can often be approached surgically (Fig. 17.7). In most cases, a subtotal resection is all that can be safely accomplished. Even in the absence of post-operative adjuvant treatment, generous central debulking of focal brainstem tumors can provide significant disease control and surgical success should be based on neurologic outcome from surgery, rather than the amount of tumor resected. Exophytic tumors of the brainstem should be approached like other fourth-ventricular tumors until the fourth ventricle is free of tumor. A decision to enter the brainstem should only be made after confirmation of low-grade histology and then surgery should proceed as described above for focal brainstem tumors.

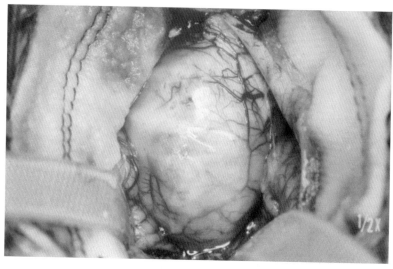

**Fig. 17.7.** Intraoperative photograph of a focal brainstem glioma arising from the pons and growing into the fourth ventricle.

## Radiation Therapy

The only modality that is demonstrated effective for intrinsic brainstem gliomas, albeit transiently, involves field radiation therapy of doses exceeding 50 GY. Use of this modality often results in symptomatic improvement but, in the vast majority of children, progression occurs despite completion of radiation therapy. Radiation therapy for focal brainstem lesions results in a high degree of disease control, which is not surprising given that the majority of these tumors are pilocytic in histology. Radiation therapy can be employed should there be progression after surgical resection or in those instances in which the risk of severe neurologic compromise is sufficiently high from re-operation.

## Chemotherapy

Intrinsic brainstem gliomas are quite refractory to chemotherapy. Responses in phase II trials have been infrequent and, in the only randomized trial comparing radiation and chemotherapy with radiation therapy alone, no survival advantage was demonstrated for the use of chemotherapy.

Recent approaches have attempted to improve the activity of radiation therapy by utilizing concomitant chemotherapy but, as yet,

these approaches have not resulted in demonstrable improvement in survival.

## Choroid Plexus Tumors

Neoplasms of the choroid plexus account for approximately 3% of brain tumors in children and are much more common during the first year of life. The majority of these tumors originate in the lateral ventricles (specifically the trigone), but they can occur in the fourth, and rarely the third, ventricle as well. Choroid plexus papillomas are slow-growing tumors and complete resection, possible in the majority of patients, is generally curative. The choroid plexus carcinoma is an anaplastic choroid plexus neoplasm and constitutes approximately 15% of choroid plexus neoplasms. This histology is much more invasive than the papilloma and has propensity for sub-arachnoid metastasis. Long-term survival following complete resection has been well documented but survival following incomplete resection, in spite of the use of either radiation, chemotherapy or both, is infrequent. The role of chemotherapy as an adjuvant therapy is unclear, although several series have documented the utility of chemotherapy in the incompletely resected choroid plexus carcinoma, in an attempt to improve the resectability at second-look surgery by decreasing vascularity and size of the tumor.

# Rhabdoid Tumors

Rhabdoid tumors of the CNS, also called atypical teratoid tumors, are recently described neoplasms characterized by monosome 22. These tumors are likely related to the renal rhabdoid tumor of infancy. The majority of these tumors occur in children of less than 2 years of age and more than half are supratentorial in location. These tumors are locally aggressive and approximately 25% of cases will display sub-arachnoid metastasis. Long-term survival is infrequent, even with the use of aggressive adjuvant chemotherapy and, in the absence of complete resection, extremely unlikely. The role of radiation therapy is unclear and the young age of these children has precluded aggressive radiation therapy approaches.

# Late Effects

Survivors of childhood brain tumors are at risk for long-term complications, both from their tumors and their therapies. In fact, significant evolution of therapy over the last two decades has been an attempt to reduce the morbidity of treatment. Of principal concern is the effect of radiation therapy on the developing CNS. It is quite clear that impairment of cognitive function can result from cranial irradiation. Volume (i.e. whole-brain vs focal irradiation), age (i.e. young children vs older children) and total dose of radiation all play roles in predicting a higher likelihood of significant neurocognitive sequelae [30]. This has led to ongoing attempts at reducing radiation doses, at times by substituting chemotherapy, or at decreasing the volume of radiation with new radiotherapy techniques characterized by recent and ongoing investigations. Those children who have received cranial irradiation require careful neurocognitive follow-up and involvement with the educational process. Cranial irradiation can also result in multiple endocrine abnormalities, principally growth hormone and thyroid deficiencies. Fortunately, replacement therapy can ameliorate many of the long-term consequences but it is imperative that these children receive timely evaluation by an endocrinologist experienced in the management of these problems. Second malignant neoplasms are well described, particularly following radiation therapy for both CNS and other malignancies. Such second malignancies are often high-grade astrocytomas and quite refractory to salvage therapy.

# Conclusion and Future Directions

Significant improvement in the diagnosis and management of pediatric CNS tumors has occurred over the last several decades and the majority of children with CNS tumors will be long-term survivors. Nonetheless, improvements in prognosis and quality of life for many children with CNS tumors has been less dramatic than that seen for other childhood malignancies. This lack of progress probably has several causes. Although CNS tumors in childhood constitute the most common solid tumor as an aggregate, the multiple histologies involved make any single tumor type relatively infrequent. The need for enrolment of every eligible patient in co-operative group trials if at all possible is imperative, given the relative infrequency of these tumors. The lack of understanding of the basic biology of these tumors has been hampered by inadequacies of tissue availability. As new molecular techniques have become available for further understanding the basic genetic abnormalities of CNS tumors, the necessity for obtaining tumor tissue from as many patients as possible for evaluation in ongoing biologic studies is critical. Care of children with CNS tumors is complex, requiring multimodality treatment, with experts in a range of medical and supportive areas. Improvement in outcome has been demonstrated in studies in which a dedicated pediatric neuro-oncology team is available to provide expertise in diagnosis, management and long-term follow-up care.

# References

1. Ries L, Kosary C, Hankey B. SEER cancer statistical review, 1973–1994. National Cancer Institute, SEER Program NIH Publication Number 97-2789, 1997.

2. Rorke LB, Gilles FH, Davis RL, Becker LE. Revision of the World Health Organization classification of brain tumors for childhood brain tumors. Cancer 1985; 56:1869–86.
3. O'Reilly G, Hayward R, Harkness W. Myelography in the assessment of children with medulloblastoma. Br J Neurosurg 1993;7:183–8.
4. Albright A. Medulloblastomas. In: Albright A, Pollack I, Adelson P, editors. Principles and practice of pediatric neurosurgery. New York: Theime, 1999; 591–608.
5. Park T, Hoffman H, Hendrick B, Humphreys R, Becker L. Medulloblastoma. Clinical presentation and management: experience at the Hospital For Sick Children, Toronto, 1950–1980. J Neurosurg 1983;58:543–52
6. Albright AL, Wisoff JH, Zeltzer PM, Boyett JM, Rorke LB, Stanley P. Effects of medulloblastoma resections on outcome in children: a report from the Children's Cancer Group. Neurosurgery 1996;38:265–71.
7. Hughes EN, Shillito J, Sallan SE, Loeffler JS, Cassady JR, Tarbell NJ. Medulloblastoma at the joint center for radiation therapy between 1968 and 1984: the influence of radiation dose on the patterns of failure and survival. Cancer 1988;61:1992–8.
8. Evans AE, Jenkin RD, Sposto R, Ortega JA, Wilson CB, Wara W et al. The treatment of medulloblastoma: results of a prospective randomized trial of radiation therapy with and without CCNU, vincristine, and prednisone. J Neurosurg 1990;72:572–82.
9. Tait DM, Thornton-Jones H, Bloom HJ, Lemerle J, Morris-Jones P. Adjuvant chemotherapy for medulloblastoma: the first multi-centre control trial of the International Society of Paediatric Oncology (SIOP I). Eur J Canc 1990;26:464–9.
10. Thomas PR, Deutsch M, Kepner JL, Boyett JM, Krischer J, Aronin P et al. Low-stage medulloblastoma: final analysis of trial comparing standard-dose with reduced-dose neuraxis irradiation. J Clin Oncol 2000;18:3004–11.
11. Packer RJ, Sutton LN, Elterman R, Lange B, Goldwein J, Nicholson HS et al. Outcome for children with medulloblastoma treated with radiation and cisplatin, CCNU, and vincristine chemotherapy. J Neurosurg 1994;81: 690–8.
12. Zeltzer PM, Boyett JM, Finlay JL, Albright AL, Rorke LB, Milstein JM et al. Metastasis stage, adjuvant treatment, and residual tumor are prognostic factors for medulloblastoma in children: conclusions from the Children's Cancer Group 921 randomized phase III study. J Clin Oncol 1999;17:832–45.
13. Packer RJ, Goldwein J, Nicholson HS, Vezina LG, Allen JC, Ris MD et al. Treatment of children with medulloblastomas with reduced-dose craniospinal radiation therapy and adjuvant chemotherapy: a Children's Cancer Group Study. J Clin Oncol 1999;17:2127–36.
14. Steinbok P, Mutat A. Cerebellar astrocytomas. In: Albright AL, Pollack IF, Adelson PD, editors. Principles and practice of pediatric neurosurgery. New York: Thieme, 1999.
15. Wisoff JH, Boyett JM, Berger MS, Brant C, Li H, Yates AJ et al. Current neurosurgical management and the impact of the extent of resection in the treatment of malignant gliomas of childhood: a report of the Children's Cancer Group trial Number CCG-945. J Neurosurg 1999;90:1147–8.
16. Pollack IF. Brain tumors in children. N Engl J Med 1994;331:1500–7.
17. Shaw EG, Daumas-Duport C, Scheithauer BW, Gilbertson DT, O'Fallon JR, Earle JD et al. Radiation therapy in the management of low-grade supratentorial astrocytomas. J Neurosurg 1989;70:853–61.
18. Packer RJ, Ater J, Allen J, Phillips P, Geyer R, Nicholson HS et al. Carboplatin and vincristine chemotherapy for children with newly diagnosed progressive low-grade gliomas. J Neurosurg 1997;86:747–54.
19. Kleihues P, Burger P, Scheithauer B. Histological typing of tumors of the central nervous system: WHO International Histological Classification of Tumors. 2nd Edition. Berlin: Springer-Verlag, 1993.
20. Duffner PK, Krischer JP, Sanford RA, Horowitz ME, Burger PC, Cohen ME et al. Prognostic factors in infants and very young children with intracranial ependymomas. Pediatr Neurosurg 1998;28:215–22.
21. Healey EA, Barnes PD, Kupsky WJ, Scott RM, Sallan SE, Black PM et al. The prognostic significance of postoperative residual tumor in ependymoma. Neurosurgery 1991;28:666–71.
22. Hukin J, Epstein F, Lefton D, Allen J. Treatment of intracranial ependymoma by surgery alone. Pediat Neurosurg 1998;29:40–5.
23. Perilongo G, Massimino M, Sotti G, Belfontali T, Masiero L, Rigobello L et al. Analyses of prognostic factors in a retrospective review of 92 children with ependymoma: Italian Pediatric Neuro-oncology Group. Med Pediat Oncol 1997;29:79–85.
24. Geyer R: , 2002.
25. Robertson PL, DaRosso RC, Allen JC. Improved prognosis of intracranial non-germinoma germ cell tumors with multimodality therapy. J Neuro-oncol 1997;32: 71–80.
26. Balmaceda C, Heller G, Rosenblum M, Diez B, Villablanca JG, Kellie S et al. Chemotherapy without irradiation. A novel approach for newly diagnosed CNS germ cell tumors: results of an international cooperative trial. The First International Central Nervous System Germ Cell Tumor Study. J Clin Oncol 1996;14:2908–15.
27. Allen JC, Kim JH, Packer RJ. Neoadjuvant chemotherapy for newly diagnosed germ-cell tumors of the central nervous system. J Neurosurg 1987;67:65–70.
28. Hoffman HJ, DeSilva M, Humphreys RP, Drake JM, Smith ML, Blaser SI. Aggressive surgical management of craniopharyngiomas in children. J Neurosurg 1992; 76:47–52.
29. Yasargil MG, Curcic M, Kis M, Siegenthaler G, Teddy PJ, Roth P. Total removal of craniopharyngiomas: approaches and long-term results in 144 patients. J Neurosurg 1990;73:3–11.
30. Duffner PK, Cohen ME. Long-term consequences of CNS treatment for childhood cancer. Part II: clinical consequences. Pediat Neurol 1991;7:237–42.

# 18

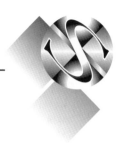

# Management of Spinal Tumors

Karl F. Kothbauer, George I. Jallo and
Fred J. Epstein

## Summary

This chapter describes the treatment approach to patients with intradural spinal tumors, with the most common being nerve sheath tumors and meningiomas, representing a combined 55%. The remaining 45% of intradural tumors are intramedullary. Surgical management of these tumors may include the application of the Cavitron ultrasonic aspirator and the laser. Many intramedullary tumors are amenable to gross total resection using an aggressive approach. Techniques for surgical resection and monitoring techniques are discussed.

## Introduction

The first successful resection of an intramedullary spinal cord tumor was performed in 1907 in Vienna, by Anton von Eiselsberg [1]. The first publication appeared in 1911 in New York, by Charles Elsberg [2]. He developed a strategy for a two-stage operation: a myelotomy was performed at the first surgery and, by the second surgery (about a week later), the tumor had already partly extruded itself from the cord substance, facilitating further resection. The first intradural extramedullary tumor resections are credited to William Macewen in 1883 and Victor Horsley [3].

After the work of these pioneers, the neurological risk of surgery for intramedullary neoplasms was considered unacceptably high. This led to the development of a conservative treatment concept with biopsy, dural decompression and subsequent radiation therapy, regardless of the histological diagnosis. Intradural–extramedullary tumors were commonly regarded as surgically resectable tumors.

The microscope and microsurgery have revolutionized all neurosurgery and also opened the door to innovation in the treatment of spinal cord tumors. CT and particularly MRI have dramatically improved pre-operative planning and significantly contributed to the development of modern treatment strategies of both intra- and extramedullary spinal cord tumors. In particular, the conservative treatment strategy for intramedullary tumors changed to an aggressive approach. Since the large majority of these tumors are histologically benign, complete or near complete, resection results in long-term progression-free survival, with acceptable neurological morbidity [4–7]. More recently, the application of intraoperative neurophysiological monitoring techniques has made a significant impact on the treatment management of both intra- and extramedullary tumors [8,9].

This chapter describes the treatment approach to patients with intradural spinal tumors.

# Epidemiology and Pathology

Intradural spinal cord tumors have a prevalence of 3–10 per 100,000 per year. They predominantly occur in the middle third of life. The most common tumors are nerve sheath tumors, which account for about 30%, and meningiomas, which account for another 25%. The remainder includes sarcomas, epidermoids and dermoids. Intramedullary tumors are rare – approximately 20–35% of all intradural neoplasms, with a higher percentage (55% of all intradural neoplasms) in children [10]. The most common intramedullary tumors are astrocytomas and ependymomas. Hemangioblastomas, cavernomas, epidermoids and lipomas are rare.

## Intradural Extramedullary Tumors

*Nerve sheath tumors* (Fig. 18.1) usually arise from the dorsal roots. They are relatively avascular, globoid and without calcification. The dorsal root of origin is most often intimately adherent to the tumor and can rarely be preserved during surgical resection. In patients with neurofibromatosis, these tumors are multiple and occur at numerous levels of the spinal canal. When located in the area of the intervertebral foramen, they may assume a characteristic dumbbell configuration, with an extra- and an intradural component (Fig. 18.1).

*Meningiomas* [11] (Fig. 18.2), unlike nerve sheath tumors, arise from arachnoid cluster cells and thus are usually separate from the nerve roots. These tumors tend to have a lateral or ventrolateral location relative to the spinal cord. They may arise in any age group, mostly occurring between the fifth and seventh decades of life, and are seen more frequently in women. They are most often located in the thoracic spine.

## Intramedullary Tumors

*Astrocytomas* (Fig. 18.3) are the most common intramedullary tumors. They can occur at any age but are most frequent in the first three decades. The majority of these neoplasms are benign, being either low-grade fibrillary or pilocytic astrocytomas. They usually are not well demarcated from the surrounding neural tissue and they may contain cystic areas, as well as adjacent, non-neoplastic cysts.

*Gangliogliomas* (Fig. 18.4) are benign neoplasms, mostly occurring in children and young

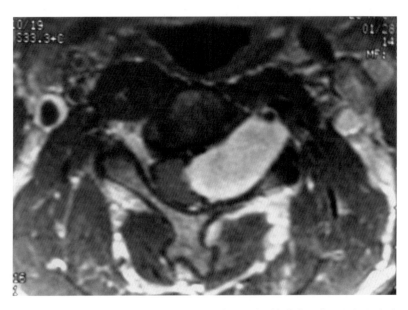

**Fig. 18.1.** Axial T1-weighted MRI after contrast administration shows a dumbbell-shaped cervical spinal schwannoma.

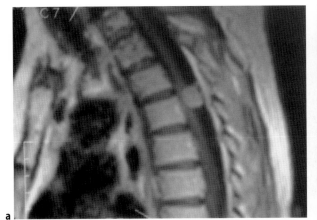

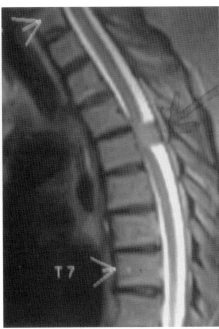

**Fig. 18.2. a** Sagittal T1- and **b** T2-weighted images of a typical thoracic spinal meningioma.

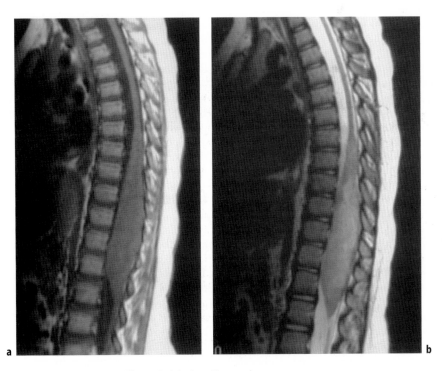

**Fig. 18.3.** Spinal cord low-grade astrocytoma.

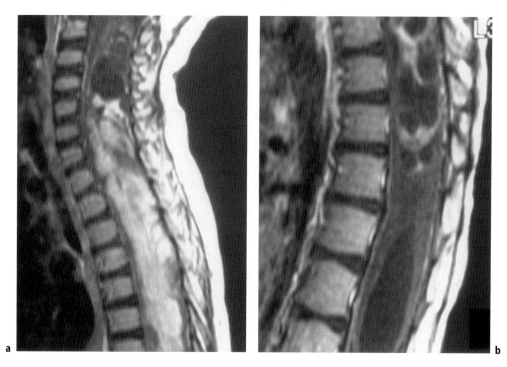

**Fig. 18.4.** Large spinal cord ganglioglioma involving the entire cord with **a** the solid and **b** the cystic portion.

adults. They consist of well differentiated neo-plastic neurons and astrocytes. The neurons have characteristic nuclear and nucleolar fea-tures, abundant cytoplasm and argyrophilic neuritic processes. Their expression of neuronal markers like synaptophysin and neurofilament proteins also serves to identify these abnormal neurons. Most gangliogliomas grow slowly and have an indolent course.

*Ependymomas* (Figs 29.5 and 29.6) are the most common intramedullary neoplasms in adults [12,13], while in children they account for only 12% of all intramedullary tumors. Ependymomas typically have a central location in the cord. They occur throughout the spinal axis. They are well delineated from the sur-rounding spinal cord and often have rostral and caudal non-neoplastic cysts that cap the tumor poles. Virtually all of them are histologically benign.

*Myxopapillary ependymomas* (Fig. 18.7) are a subgroup of ependymomas with characteristic microcystic histologic features. Their typical location is the conus-cauda region [14]. Located in the filum, they may grossly enlarge the filum

and displace the nerve roots laterally and anteriorly. In spite of their benign histology, a small percentage of them tend to sub-arachnoid dissemination.

*Hemangioblastomas* account for 3–7% of intramedullary spinal cord tumors. They occur throughout the spinal canal. Spinal cord heman-gioblastomas are mostly sporadic, but up to 25% of the patients have von Hippel–Lindau disease.

## Clinical Presentation

Intramedullary spinal cord tumors may remain asymptomatic for a long time and may increase to a considerable size before they are detected. The onset of symptoms is often insidious and they may be present for months or even years before the diagnosis is established. Symptoms may also appear at the time of a trivial injury. Not infrequently, exacerbations and remis-sions occur. A common early symptom is back or neck pain, occurring in up to two-thirds of patients. The pain may be either diffuse, in

# MANAGEMENT OF SPINAL TUMORS

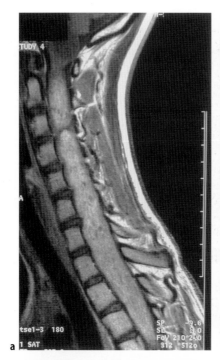

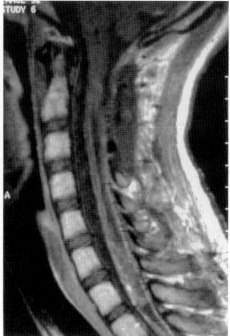

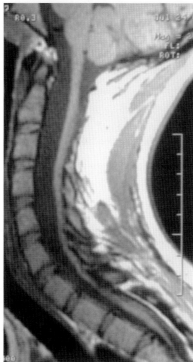

**Fig. 18.5. a** Pre-operative, **b** immediate post-operative and **c** 3-year follow-up sagittal T1 contrast-enhanced images of a large cervical intramedullary ependymoma.

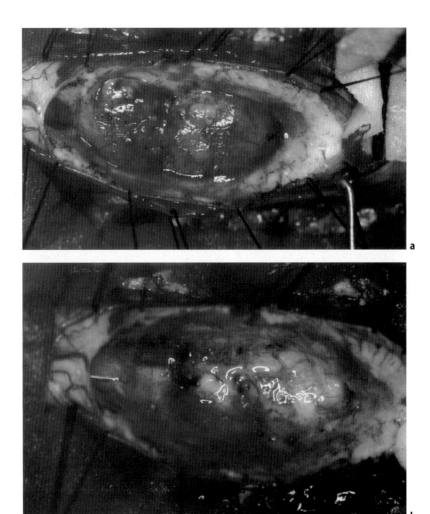

**Fig. 18.6.** Intraoperative view of an ependymoma **a** before and **b** after resection.

which case an intramedullary tumor is the more likely cause, or it may have a radicular distribution, which is more common in intradural extramedullary lesions [15]. Young children may even present with abdominal pain as a non-specific symptom that makes finding the correct diagnosis particularly difficult. Pain is characteristically more severe in the horizontal position, thus causing nighttime pain.

Motor function appears to be affected early [5,16] in younger children: this may manifest as motor regression, i.e. refusal to stand or crawl after having learned to walk, or as gait abnormality. Young adults present with lower-extremity weakness, clumsiness or frequent

falls. On examination, the majority of these patients show some mild to moderate motor deficit, as well as upper motor neuron-type findings, such as spasticity, hyperreflexia and clonus.

About one-third of the patients have some degree of spinal deformity, most of them with tumors in the thoracic region. Paraspinal pain is common in this group and attributed to the scoliosis. Torticollis was seen in about one-fifth of the pediatric patients.

Sensory symptoms, mostly dysesthesias, described as unpleasant hot or cold sensations, are also found in about 20% of the patients. In glial tumors, as opposed to ependymomas, the

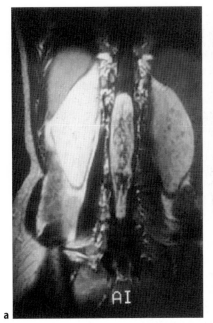

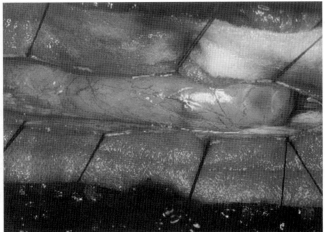

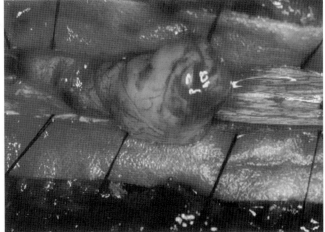

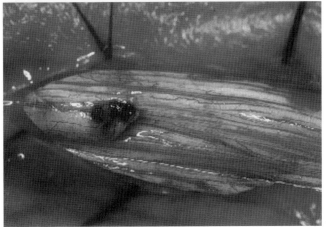

**Fig. 18.7.** Myxopapillary ependymoma of the filum on **a** MRI and **b** and **c** during resection.

sensory symptoms are frequently asymmetric. Sphincter dysfunction is present late in the clinical course, except for tumors located in the conus medullaris. Malignant intramedullary gliomas are rare [7,16–18]; their symptomatology is similar, but with a significantly shorter history.

Almost all patients with extramedullary tumors have pain, which most commonly has a radicular distribution. The number of patients with mild motor deficits at presentation is high, but only a minority are severely impaired [11].

## Hydrocephalus

Hydrocephalus has been reported to occur in as many as 15% of patients with intramedullary tumors. The mechanisms for hydrocephalus include an increased concentration of protein in the cerebrospinal fluid, arachnoidal fibrosis and sub-arachnoid dissemination. The incidence of hydrocephalus is substantially higher in patients with malignant tumors (approximately 35%) than in those with low-grade tumors (approximately 15%). Patients with cervical tumors are more likely to develop hydrocephalus, probably secondary to obstruction of the fourth ventricle outlets.

# Diagnostic Studies

## MRI

MRI is the study of choice to identify both intra- and extramedullary spinal cord neoplasms [4]. Extramedullary lesions are readily identified as such and their relation to the cord, attachment to dura and displacement of the cord are visualized.

MRI scans should be performed before and after intravenous administration of contrast agents (gadolinium diethylene-triamine-pentacetic acid), with T1-weighted images in multiple planes [19]. These images demonstrate the solid tumor component. T2-weighted images optimally show the cerebrospinal fluid and tumor-associated cysts. While MRI does not allow for a certain histologic diagnosis pre-operatively, the more common tumors have typical patterns of imaging appearance.

Ependymomas usually enhance brightly and homogeneously (Fig. 18.5), frequently have rostral and caudal cysts and, not uncommonly, a hemosiderin "cap" at their poles. On axial view, they are usually seen in the center of the cord. Astrocytomas (Fig. 18.3) and gangliogliomas (Fig. 18.4), on the other hand, enhance less frequently and, if enhancement is seen, it is more often heterogeneous. On axial images, these neoplasms are more frequently found to be eccentric in the cord. They may cause asymmetric enlargement of the cord. Hemangioblastomas (Fig. 18.8) characteristically show bright enhancement of a tumor nodule and associated cysts, often with significant cord edema adjacent to it. Meningiomas (Fig. 18.2) and nerve sheath tumors (Fig. 18.1) may have similar appearance on MRI and they commonly enhance brightly. Schwannomas sometimes show large cysts, while meningiomas often can be identified by a broad dural attachment.

## Plain Radiographs

Spinal X-rays should be taken, particularly in patients who present with scoliosis. These films serve as a baseline for the future management of the spinal deformity. Intradural extramedullary tumors can thin or cause sclerosis of the pedicles. A tumor that extends through a neural foramen enlarges that foramen, which can be seen on oblique films. Intramedullary neoplasms may show a diffusely widened spinal canal, with associated erosion of the pedicles and scalloping of the vertebrae.

## Myelography and CT

Myelography with water-soluble contrast agent combined with CT was used extensively in the evaluation of suspected intraspinal lesions [7]. Today, CT–myelography is reserved for the rare cases where MRI may be impossible to perform (e.g. due to metallic implants) or impossible to interpret due to image distortion from metallic artifacts.

## Angiography

Angiographic evaluation of the vascular supply and venous drainage is strongly recommended before the removal of a spinal cord hemangioblastoma (Fig. 18.8) is attempted.

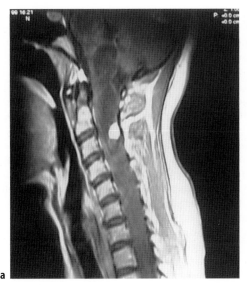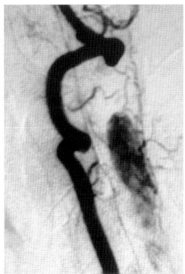

**Fig. 18.8. a** Intramedullary hemangioblastoma with bright enhancing nodule and cyst on the sagittal T1-weighted image. **b** The angiogram depicts the vascular anatomy of the lesion.

# Surgical Management of Intradural Tumors

## Surgical Instruments

Suction and bipolar cautery are used, together with a set of specialized instruments that aid in minimizing surgical trauma to normal neural tissue. Some of these specialized instruments have become essential for the microsurgical resection of spinal cord tumors.

### Ultrasonic Aspirator

The application of the Cavitron ultrasonic aspirator (CUSA) system was a significant advancement in the removal of spinal cord tumors. It uses high-frequency sound waves to fragment the tumor tissue, which is then aspirated by the suction apparatus at the tip of the device. This allows much easier and quicker removal of a bulk of tumor tissue, with less manipulation of the adjacent neural tissue as compared to the suction–cautery technique.

### Laser

The laser is an excellent surgical adjunct for spinal cord surgery. We prefer the Nd:YAG Contact Laser™ System (SLT, Montgomeryville, PA) to other available laser technologies. This system has a handpiece and contact probes, and can be used as a microsurgical instrument. The laser is particularly useful as a scalpel to perform the myelotomy, demarcate the glial–tumor interface and remove residual tumor fragments. Firm lesions, such as meningiomas, neurofibromas or rare types of intramedullary tumors, can only be removed with reasonable safety when the laser is available. These lesions cannot be manipulated with the bipolar and scissors because of inevitable manipulation of the adjacent spinal cord tissue, and they are too firm for the CUSA for internal debulking. For the rare spinal cord lipoma, the microsurgical laser is the instrument of choice for vaporization of fat and internal debulking.

## Surgical Technique

Surgery is performed with the patient in a prone position. A rigid head-holder (Sugita or Mayfield) is utilized for cervical and cervicothoracic tumors, to secure the head in a neutral position. The horseshoe headrest should be avoided because it does not secure a neutral neck position.

A laminectomy or osteoplastic laminotomy [20] is performed with a high-power drill using the craniotome attachment, round burr and rongeurs. The bone removal must always expose the solid tumor but not the rostral or caudal cysts. The cysts usually disappear after the neoplasm is resected, since the cyst walls of "capping" cysts are usually composed of non-neoplastic glial tissue.

Intraoperative sonography (Fig. 18.9) visualizes the full extent of the tumor and its relation to the bone removal, as well as cysts and displacement of the cord [21]. If the bone removal is not sufficient, the laminectomy is extended to expose the entire solid tumor prior to opening the dura.

The dura is then opened in the midline. The spinal cord is frequently expanded and it may even be rotated and distorted. The asymmetric expansion and rotation of the spinal cord may make identification of the midline raphe difficult. However, it is important to localize this raphe because this is the most frequent approach into the spinal cord. An alternative approach for extremely asymmetrical tumors is to enter the spinal cord through the dorsal root entry zone. This is an approach used sometimes when an asymmetric deficit is present; thus, it is essential to preserve the "good" arm and hand while the other upper extremity is already severely impaired, and deafferentation adds little morbidity.

If the tumor is not visible on the surface, the microsurgical laser is used to perform the myelotomy, with minimal neural injury. The various types of intramedullary tumors have different macroscopic appearances. Ependymomas (Fig. 18.6) are red or dark gray in color and have a clear margin from the spinal cord. This interface can be separated with the plated bayonet or the microsurgical laser. One pole of the tumor is identified and the cleavage plane separated in an axial direction. The ventral aspect of ependymomas is adherent to the anterior median raphe because the feeding vessels originate from the anterior spinal artery. It is essential to preserve this vessel. The majority of these tumors can be removed en bloc [6].

Astrocytomas or gangliogliomas have a gray–yellow glassy appearance. They must be removed from the inside out, until the glial–tumor interface is recognized by the change in color and consistency of the tissue. Rarely, a true plane between tumor and normal spinal cord exists, and futile efforts to define this interface result in hazardous manipulation of normal spinal cord tissue [18]. Their resection is usually started at the midportion rather than at the

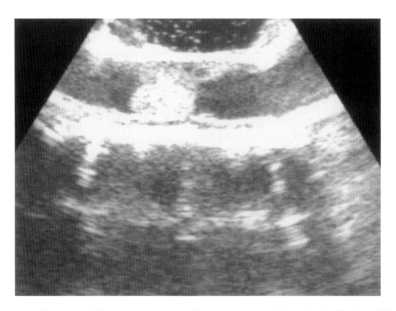

**Fig. 18.9.** The intraoperative sonographic view of an intramedullary ependymoma allows for identification of the solid and cystic components.

poles. The rostral and caudal poles are the least voluminous and manipulation there may be dangerous to the normal tissue.

Intramedullary lipomas appear well demarcated from the adjacent spinal cord, but they are intimately adherent to the normal tissue. Therefore, total removal is impossible without incurring neurological deficits and should not be attempted. The microsurgical laser is the instrument of choice for debulking a spinal cord lipoma. The laser vaporizes fatty tissue without surgical trauma to the spinal cord. The debulking of the lipoma may result in improvement of pain but rarely in improvement of neurological function. Further growth of a lipoma is unlikely or at least very slow. However, in adolescence, probably due to endocrine factors, lipomas of the cord may increase in size and may, at that time, cause progressive neurological dysfunction.

Following tumor removal, hemostasis is obtained with saline irrigation and local application of microfibrillar collagen (Avitene(r), C. R. Bard, Inc., 730 Central Avenue, Murray Hill, NJ). The dura is closed primarily in a watertight fashion. If an osteoplastic laminotomy was performed, the segments of bone are replaced and secured with a non-absorbable suture on each lamina bilaterally. One tissue layer must be closed in a cerebrospinal fluid (CSF)-tight fashion. The muscle and fascial closure must not be under tension. A subcutaneous drain is placed in large incisions, and particularly in re-operations, or when the patient had undergone prior radiation therapy. The skin is closed with running, locked sutures. Patients who have had previous surgery and received radiation therapy are at higher risk for wound dehiscence and CSF leak.

The resection of extramedullary tumors follows these same lines. The vast majority of them are tackled with a posterior approach. Dorsolateral approaches are rarely needed and anterior approaches are only required in the exceptional case. After laminectomy or laminotomy, adequate bony exposure and location of the lesion are assured with the intraoperative ultrasound. Depending upon their individual locations, schwannomas, meningiomas or myxopapillary ependymomas can be removed in toto. Large tumors, particularly when located ventrally or ventrolaterally, may require piecemeal resection. Firm texture of the tumor,

particularly in meningiomas, requires use of the microsurgical laser. We have found the use of this instrument to be by far the safest way to resect firm tumor attached to the cord. Manipulation of a firm mass with forceps, scissors or the CUSA may cause significant injury to the cord. The dural attachment of meningiomas need not be resected [11]; extensive coagulation of the dural layer after excision of the tumor bulk appears to be associated with the same small recurrence rate.

The most important strategy for the resection of completely intradural schwannomas is to sacrifice the nerve root that they are arising from. This greatly facilitates their resection and does not usually result in a significant neurological deficit.

In toto, resection of myxopapillary ependymomas of the filum should be attempted whenever the tumor has not yet spread into the arachnoid space (Fig. 18.7). Only disseminated ependymomas need to be resected in a piecemeal fashion, mostly using bipolar and suction. In this situation, there is invariably some residual tumor tissue left on the pia or the nerve root epineurium.

# Intraoperative Neurophysiological Monitoring

Intraoperative monitoring with motor evoked potentials (MEPs) is a direct motor tract monitoring technique which is now the most important monitoring tool for spinal cord surgery [8,9]. Motor potentials are evoked with transcranial electrical stimulation of the motor cortex in two ways: a single-stimulus technique and a multipulse technique (Fig. 18.10). With a single stimulus, a single volley of signals in fast conducting corticospinal axons is generated, which is then recorded with an electrode placed on the spinal cord, usually in the epidural space. This signal is called a D-wave, because it results from *D*irect activation of these fast-conducting axons. The D-wave's amplitude is a relative measure of the number of fast-conducting corticospinal fibers (Fig. 18.11). The multipulse or train stimulus technique [21] evokes a muscle response in target muscles (thenar, anterior

MOTOR EVOKED POTENTIALS

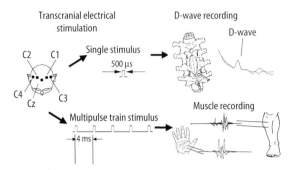

**Fig. 18.10.** Principles of MEP monitoring. MEPs are elicited with transcranial electrical stimulation (left) using two distinct stimulus techniques. The single-stimulus technique allows recording of D-waves (top), and the multipulse technique allows recording of muscle responses.

DECREASE OF D-WAVE AMPLITUDE

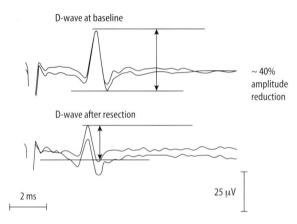

**Fig. 18.11.** The amplitude of D-waves is a measure of the number of fast-conducting fibers in the corticospinal tract. This amplitude is the primarily monitored parameter for intraoperative assessment of the functional integrity of the motor system in the spinal cord. A decrease of up to 50% from the baseline amplitude is associated with intact motor control in all instances.

tibialis). These muscle MEPs are interpreted in an all-or-none fashion. Their presence indicates intact functional integrity of the voluntary motor system in the spinal cord. Their absence indicates jeopardized functional integrity of the motor pathways, highly associated with an at least temporary disruption of voluntary motor control. The stimulation and recording of D-waves and muscle MEPs can be repeated every second. Therefore, the feedback information is provided in real time. Figure 29.4 summarizes the technique of stimulation and recording.

D-waves and muscle MEPs must be interpreted together. Loss of muscle MEPs during a spinal cord tumor resection indicates at least a temporary disruption of motor function of the spinal cord. The more incremental change of the D-wave amplitude then allows further interpretation of the motor outcome. A loss of muscle MEPs is highly associated with a temporary motor deficit in the lower extremities, even if the D-wave amplitude is unchanged. In the majority of cases, this is even side specific. As long as the D-wave amplitude remains above a cut-off value of about 50% of its baseline value, this motor deficit is temporary, with the patient recovering to pre-operative strength within hours to days, or sometimes weeks. A further decline in D-wave amplitude or its loss is associated with a long-term severe motor deficit [9].

The short-term neurological morbidity of intramedullary tumor surgery is about 30%. The combined use of epidural and muscle MEP recording has been shown to intraoperatively detect all post-operative motor deficits [8]. Most importantly, the combination of epidural and muscle MEPs allows for the neurophysiological identification of a reversible motor deficit. Thus, MEPs are giving information about injury to the motor system *before* this injury results in permanent, irreversible neurological deficit.

In particular, the resection of ventrally located intradural–extramedullary lesions requires some degree of spinal cord retraction. With the use of motor monitoring, this can be done safely, as the degree of retraction that is tolerated "functionally" can be assessed. This allows resection of anteriorly located extramedullary lesions via a simple posterior approach.

Somatosensory evoked potential (SEP) recording is of use to assess the functional integrity of the sensory system. The correlation of SEPs with post-operative motor function, however, is poor and, particularly in intramedullary surgery, SEPs tend to disappear when the midline myelotomy is performed and are then of no further use for the critical assessment of the motor system.

Electromyographic mapping of nerve roots, that is direct electrical stimulation of exposed nerves with a handheld probe and recording from lower extremity and sphincter ani muscles, is useful during resection of tumors in the conus/cauda equina region.

Continuous monitoring of the bulbocavernosus reflex (BCR) provides information on the functional integrity of oligosynaptic reflex arches involved in sphincter control. This has been shown to be feasible during general anesthesia, and there is good correlation of BCR data to post-operative sphincter control.

# Surgical Complications

## Functional Outcome

The feared complication after intraspinal and, in particular, intramedullary tumor surgery is paralysis. The incidence of this occurrence is related to the pre-operative functional status. Patients who have no or minimal pre-operative motor deficits have less than 3% incidence for this complication. On the other hand, patients who already have a significant motor deficit are more likely to deteriorate post-operatively [9].

While complete resection of extramedullary tumors should be attempted and is possible in almost all cases, the resection radicality in intramedullary surgery is lower. In fact, complete removal, particularly of the last fragments of tumor tissue, has a high risk of resulting in major neurological deficits. In the senior author's experience of intramedullary tumors, a gross total resection was feasible in about 70–80% of cases and a subtotal (80–97%) in the remainder. There was no surgical mortality. The short-term deterioration of motor function is significant. One-third of patients experience a transient motor deficit, which resolves within hours to days [8]. The long-term functional motor outcome is much better and directly related to the pre-operative neurological function [9]. Therefore, it is advisable that patients with intramedullary tumors undergo surgery before the development of significant neurological deficits.

Impaired joint position sense may be a serious functional disability and is more commonly seen after ependymoma rather than astrocytoma resection. Patients who have impaired proprioception may require extensive physical therapy to learn to compensate for this deficit. In addition, patients may experience a variety of pain syndromes, autonomic symptoms and decreased strength for prolonged physical activity.

## Post-operative Spinal Deformity

Another potential problem is spinal deformity. Scoliosis and kyphosis may evolve after surgery [22]. This is particularly important for the pediatric patients, of whom about one-third with a significant deformity eventually require a stabilizing orthopedic operation. Several surgeons recommended osteoplastic laminotomy for all children, to reduce the incidence of spinal deformity [20]. In a study of 58 patients younger than 25 years of age who underwent multi-level laminectomy for various conditions, deformity occurred in 46% of patients younger than 15 years, and in 6% of children older than 15 years. In this series, 100% (nine of nine) of children who had a cervical laminectomy developed a post-operative deformity as compared to 36% for thoracic laminectomy, and none of six patients after lumbar laminectomy. It is therefore essential that children be followed particularly closely with plain radiographs and receive orthopedic evaluation. Surgical indications for spinal fusion should be regarded as more urgent in these patients than in those with idiopathic deformity. Furthermore, patients who develop progressive deformity should also undergo a new MRI to rule out tumor recurrence.

A spinal deformity may also be a result of radiation therapy used to treat epidural tumors. Mayfield et al. reported that 32 of 57 children with neuroblastoma treated with radiation therapy and chemotherapy developed significant spinal deformities. A higher rate of deformity was associated with younger age at time of radiation, doses greater than 20 Gy and asymmetrical radiation fields. This emphasizes that radiation therapy cannot be regarded as a "noninvasive" alternative to surgically treatable spinal cord tumors.

## Cerebrospinal Fluid Leakage

This complication is very rare in patients who have not previously been operated on or received radiation therapy. However, after radiation therapy and/or previous surgery, there is a significant risk for wound dehiscence and CSF leak. Experiences with wound-healing problems revealed that meningitis resulted in the utilization of plastic surgical techniques with bilateral mobilization of the spinal muscles for wound closure. The fascia must be closed in a watertight fashion, without tension. Relaxing incisions laterally may be necessary to provide a tension-free closure. A sub-fascial or subcutaneous drain must be placed for several days to allow healing of the wound.

## Oncological Outcome

It must be emphasized that in intramedullary tumor surgery, despite gross total resections, residual microscopic fragments are left in the resection bed. This residual tissue (in particular for glial neoplasms) may remain dormant or

may involute over time. The clinical significance of these small fragments remains to be determined.

Long-term survival is better for low-grade neoplasms when compared to the high-grade group. The 5- and 10-year survival rates were 88 and 82%, respectively, for the low-grade neoplasms in the senior author's series. The cause of death in these patients was progression of disease and systemic complications after chemotherapy. The patients with high-grade neoplasms fared poorly, with an 18% 5-year survival, despite surgery and adjuvant therapy.

Intradural extramedullary tumors generally have a very favorable prognosis, with low recurrence rates (6%) after complete, and even after incomplete (17%), resection [11], unless the patient has neurofibromatosis [23].

## Adjuvant Therapy

The deleterious effect of radiation has been mentioned above and no study has convincingly demonstrated a beneficial effect of radiation therapy on survival or neurological function for low-grade tumors. Although some authors still recommend radiotherapy for intramedullary spinal cord tumors, no study has been performed comparing the effects of radiation therapy for intramedullary neoplasms. Thus, these tumors should be recognized as a surgical disease, both at presentation and at time of recurrence. Stein also did not recommend radiotherapy for adult patients with low-grade intramedullary neoplasms, regardless of the extent of removal, and emphasized the deleterious effects of radiation on the spinal cord tissue adjacent to the tumor site. The results are similar to others who have reported myelopathy in children who have received doses of 30 Gy. Thus radiation therapy is reserved for patients with malignant tumors, those with documented post-operative rapid tumor regrowth or for those with substantial residual tumor who are not candidates for further surgery. Intramedullary ependymomas should be resected and radiotherapy is not an option for these patients.

We employ total neuraxis radiation for the malignant tumors. Unfortunately, it has been shown that glioblastomas invariably progress. Despite aggressive radiotherapy and chemotherapy, patients with these neoplasms have a median survival of 12 months.

Adjuvant therapy is usually not used for patients with intradural extramedullary tumors. However, for instance, patients with meningiomas of the rare clear-cell variant should be radiated after resection of a recurrent tumor [24]. Radiotherapy for the recurrent and non-resectable meningioma must also be considered.

# Key Points

- *The strategy for intramedullary tumors has changed from a conservative to an aggressive approach with the improvement in pre-operative planning.*
- *Intramedullary spinal cord tumors may remain asymptomatic for a long time and may increase to considerable size before they are detected.*
- *MRI is the study of choice to identify both intra- and extramedullary spinal cord neoplasms.*

# References

1. Eiselsberg Av, Marburg O. Zur Frage der Operabilität intramedullärer Rückenmarkstumoren. Arch Psychiatr Nervenkr 1917;59:453–61.
2. Elsberg CA, Beer E. The operability of intramedullary tumors of the spinal cord: a report of two operations with remarks upon the extrusion of intraspinal tumors. Am J Med Sci 1911;142:636–47.
3. Gowers WR, Horsley V. A case of tumour of the spinal cord: removal and recovery. Med-Chir Trans 1888;53: 377–428.
4. Brotchi J, Dewitte O, Levivier M, Baleriaux D, Vandesteene A, Raftopoulos C et al. A survey of 65 tumors within the spinal cord: surgical results and the importance of preoperative magnetic resonance imaging. Neurosurgery 1991;29:651–6; discussion 656–7.
5. Epstein FJ, Epstein N. Surgical treatment of spinal cord astrocytomas of childhood. J Neurosurg 1982;57:685–9.
6. Greenwood J. Surgical removal of intramedullary tumors. J Neurosurg 1967;26:276–82.
7. Guidetti B, Mercuri S, Vagnozzi R. Long-term results of the surgical treatment of 129 intramedullary spinal gliomas. J Neurosurg 1981;54:323–30.
8. Kothbauer KF, Deletis V, Epstein FJ. Motor evoked potential monitoring for intramedullary spinal cord tumor surgery: correlation of clinical and neurophysio-logical data in a series of 100 consecutive procedures. Neurosurg Focus 1998;4:Article 1 (http://www.aans.org/journals/online_j/may98/4-5-1).
9. Morota N, Deletis V, Constantini S, Kofler M, Cohen H, Epstein FJ. The role of motor evoked potentials during surgery for intramedullary spinal cord tumors. Neurosurgery 1997;41:1327–36.
10. Yamamoto Y, Raffel C. Spinal extradural neoplasms and intradural extramedullary neoplasms. In: Albright AL, Pollack IF, Adelson PD, editors. Principles and practice of pediatric neurosurgery. New York: Thieme Medical Publishers, 1999; 685–96.
11. Solero CL, Fornari M, Giombini S, Lasio G, Oliveri G, Cimino C et al. Spinal meningiomas: review of 174 operated cases. Neurosurgery 1989;25:153–60.
12. Fischer G, Mansuy L. Total removal of intramedullary ependymomas: follow-up study of 16 cases. Surg Neurol 1980;14:243–9.
13. McCormick PC, Torres R, Post KD, Stein BM. Intramedullary ependymoma of the spinal cord. J Neurosurg 1990;72:523–32.
14. Schweitzer JS, Batzdorf U. Ependymoma of the cauda equina region: diagnosis, treatment, and outcome in 15 patients. Neurosurgery 1992;30:202–7.
15. Murovic J, Sundaresan N. Pediatric spinal axis tumors. Neurosurg Clin North Am 1992;4:947–58.
16. Constantini S, Miller DC, Allen JC, Rorke LB, Freed D, Epstein FJ. Radical excision of intramedullary spinal cord tumors: surgical morbidity and long-term follow-up evaluation in 164 children and young adults. J Neurosurg (Spine) 2000;93:183–93.
17. Cohen AR, Wisoff JH, Allen JC, Epstein F. Malignant astrocytomas of the spinal cord. J Neurosurg 1989; 70:50–4.
18. Epstein FJ, Farmer J-P, Freed D. Adult intramedullary astrocytomas of the spinal cord. J Neurosurg 1992; 77:355–9.
19. Goy AMC, Pinto RS, Raghavendra BN, Epstein FJ, Kricheff II. Intramedullary spinal cord tumors: MR imaging, with emphasis of associated cysts. Radiology 1986;161:381–6.
20. Raimondi AJ, Gutierrez FA, Di Rocco C. Laminotomy and total reconstruction of the posterior spinal arch for spinal canal surgery in childhood. J Neurosurg 1976;45:555–60.
21. Taniguchi M, Cedzich C, Schramm J. Modification of cortical stimulation for motor evoked potentials under general anesthesia: technical description. Neurosurgery 1993;32:219–26.
22. Yasuoka S, Peterson HA, MacCarty CS. Incidence of spinal column deformity after multilevel laminectomy in children and adults. J Neurosurg 1982;57:441–5.
23. Klekamp J, Samii M. Surgery of spinal nerve sheath tumors with special reference to neurofibromatosis. Neurosurgery 1998;42:279–90.
24. Jallo GI, Kothbauer KF, Silvera VM, Epstein FJ. Intraspinal clear cell meningioma. Diagnosis and management: report of two cases. Neurosurgery 2001;48: 218–22.

# 19

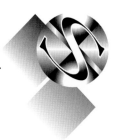

# Management of Extradural Spinal Tumors

David A. Lundin, Charlie Kuntz and
Christopher I. Shaffrey

## Summary

The pathology and pathophysiology of both primary bony tumors and metastatic lesions that commonly invade the axial skeleton of the spinal canal and involve the spinal column are examined. A detailed description of possible lesions, diagnostic evaluation and treatment paradigms is included.

## Introduction

There are a large number of tumors that involve the spinal column, spinal cord or the peripheral nerves near the axial skeleton. Despite the extensive differential diagnosis, there are factors such as age, location, incidence and pathology that provide important clues in correctly diagnosing each specific condition. The ability to effectively treat lesions involving the spinal column or spinal cord has increased dramatically over the past 15 years, if an early and accurate diagnosis is achieved.

For lesions involving the bony spinal column, younger patients tend to present with benign bone tumors more frequently than do those over 30 years of age. Adults, especially the elderly with spinal column lesions, are much more likely to have a malignancy. Malignant lesions involving the spinal column (whether primary tumors or metastases) occur more often in the vertebral body. Benign tumors usually originate in the spinous processes, laminae or the pedicles of the vertebrae. The incidence of skeletal metastases outweighs the incidence of primary malignant bone tumors by a margin of 25–40:1 [1–6].

A variety of parameters can be used to narrow the differential diagnosis for spinal cord and peripheral nerve tumors. Intramedullary tumors are much more common in children and represent approximately half of the intradural tumors. In adults, less than one-third of intradural tumors are in an intramedullary location. Taken as a whole, approximately two-thirds of spinal cord tumors are extramedullary and one-third are intramedullary. Intramedullary tumors are typically of glial origin – predominantly astrocytoma and ependymoma. In children, astrocyomas are more common, but in adults, ependymomas predominate. Extramedullary tumors are then divided into those which are intradural and those which are extradural. Intradural lesions are twice as frequent as extradural lesions, and primarily consist of nerve sheath tumors and meningiomas. Here, we will concentrate on those tumors arising in the extradural space. These consist of primary bone neoplasms and metastatic disease to the spine.

# Primary Bony Neoplasms

Primary bony neoplasms of the spine can be either benign or malignant, and optimal management depends upon a precise diagnosis. Unfortunately, many of these lesions are located in poorly accessible places and the approaches for direct or percutaneous biopsy can have substantial risks. When approaching spinal neoplasms, the principles of tumor staging and oncologic resection should be considered. In general, patients presenting with a short duration of symptoms and a rapid progression of neurological findings are more likely to have a malignancy than are those with the slow onset of symptoms. Typically, benign lesions are found in the posterior elements of younger patients, whereas lesions found in the vertebral body in older patients are worrisome for malignancy. One study found that 75% of primary bony tumors involving the vertebral body were malignant, as opposed to 35% when the posterior elements alone were involved. This same study found that 80% of primary tumors were malignant in patients older than 18 years and only 32% were malignant when the patient was younger than 18 years [5].

## Benign Tumors of the Spinal Column

Benign tumors of the axial skeleton are most commonly found in children and adolescents. When they occur in adults, they are generally found in individuals between 20 and 30 years of age, in a posterior location. The more common types of benign lesions – osteochondroma, osteoid osteoma and osteoblastoma – have a lower incidence of recurrence if a complete excision can be obtained. Unlike malignant tumors that require resection of a wide margin of normal tissue surrounding the lesion, resection of the benign tumor itself is usually curative. There are other "benign" tumors that can be associated with systemic disease, occur in multiple locations or are locally aggressive, including eosinophilic granulomas, giant cell tumors, aneurysmal bone cysts and hemangiomas, respectively.

*Osteochondroma* is a cartilage-capped, bony protuberance that is thought to develop from an adjacent physis or a cartilaginous remnant of the physis. Osteochondromas are the most common of the benign bone tumors. Over 50% of symptomatic spinal lesions occur in the cervical region, and they almost always involve the posterior elements. Osteochondromas can be a manifestation of multiple hereditary osteochondromatosis, which is one of the more common skeletal dysplasias. Clinical presentation varies from individuals reporting a dull backache (smaller tumors) to decreased motion or deformity (larger tumors). Neurological compromise is rare; however, when present, the cervical spine, followed by the thoracic spine, are the most common lesion locations, with resultant myelopathic symptoms. Plain radiographs demonstrate a protruding lesion, with well demarcated borders in the posterior elements. Treatment for this condition is usually observation, because the natural history is of very slow progression. On rare occasions, pain, neurological deficit or an accelerated growth pattern may necessitate surgical removal. Prognosis is usually excellent when complete curettage of the affected periosteum and surrounding cartilage is performed. Osteochondromas will occasionally degenerate into malignant chondrosarcomas (usually in patients with multiple lesions) [2–4].

*Osteoid osteoma* and osteoblastoma share a common pathologic origin but differ in size and incidence of spinal involvement. These tumors are thought to be a chronic inflammatory reaction rather than true neoplasms. Osteoid osteoma accounts for 2.6% of all excised primary bone tumors and up to 18% of axial skeletal primary lesions. By definition, osteoid osteomas are less than 2 cm in size; otherwise, the lesions are classified as osteoblastomas. Approximately 40% of spinal osteoid osteomas occur in the lumbar region, and the majority occur in the posterior elements. Most patients with symptomatic lesions are young and male. Half of all symptomatic lesions present in the second decade of life. On clinical presentation, patients report a dull ache, which is exacerbated at night. This condition is believed to be the result of prostaglandin production by the tumor – thus, the classic pain relief with aspirin. Neurological deficits are rare but osteoid osteoma is the most common lesion of painful scoliosis in adolescents. Radiologically, a radiolucent area with a central nidus and an appropriate degree of surrounding sclerosis

MANAGEMENT OF EXTRADURAL SPINAL TUMORS

characterizes the lesion. The treatment is excision. Instrumentation and fusion may be required if there is severe scoliosis, although minor deformities will resolve with resection alone. Overall, there is an excellent prognosis, with marginal recurrence rates related to inadequate excision of the nidus [1–4,6].

*Osteoblastomas* differ from osteoid osteomas in their attaining greater size (more than 2 cm). Histologically, the two lesions cannot be differentiated. Less common than osteoid osteomas, osteoblastomas represent less than 2% of primary benign bone tumors, but have a greater propensity for axial skeletal involvement. Approximately 30–40% of osteoblastomas involve the axial skeleton. The lesions are distributed throughout the longitudinal axis of the spine, occur most commonly in the posterior elements and have a propensity to produce spinal deformity (Fig. 19.1). In 90% of cases, osteoblastomas present in patients of 30 years of age or younger; these lesions have a male to female predominance of 2:1. Clinical presentation characteristically involves a higher incidence of neurological deficit, secondary to lesion size. Treatment is en-bloc resection, usually with resolution of scoliotic deformity. Prognosis is favorable with adequate removal. Long-term recurrence rates approach 10% [1–4,6].

*Giant cell tumors* (GCTs) are benign lesions of unknown cell origin. These aggressive tumors carry some malignant potential and a high incidence of local recurrence. They are responsible for 21% of all primary benign bone tumors and affect the spinal axis in 8–11% of all cases. They most commonly occur in the sacral region, when the spinal column is involved. Unlike the majority of primary bone tumors, GCTs are generally found in individuals in the third and fourth decades of life, with decreasing frequency in later years. Women are affected slightly more commonly than are men. Plain radiographs demonstrate cortical expansion, with little reactive sclerosis or periosteal reaction. MR images reveal homogeneous signals, while CT studies can better delineate the degree of vertebral bone involvement and define surgical margins. Because of the non-distinct histological characteristics of GCTs, a thorough evaluation, including radiographic investigation coupled with histopathology, is important, to differentiate this condition from other primary bone tumors. Treatment is usually an aggressive en-bloc resection, with consideration of adjuvant radiation therapy. There is a relatively poor prognosis because of the high recurrence rates (50%). These tumors have the potential for malignant transformation, especially after local radiation if surgical margins were inadequate [1–4].

*Aneurysmal bone cysts* (ABCs) are benign, non-neoplastic proliferative lesions. Although only responsible for approximately 1–2% of all primary bone tumors, ABCs affect the axial skeleton in 12–25% of all reported cases. The pathogenesis is unclear, but accepted theories include an underlying tumor or traumatic arteriovenous malformation, with subsequent development of a cyst. Histologically, ABCs contain fluid-filled spaces, separated by fibrous septa. The incidence of ABCs is greater in the thoracolumbar region. As in the majority of benign osseous lesions, posterior location predominates, with 60% of spinal aneurysmal bone cysts occurring in the posterior elements. ABCs typically present in young patients who are in their second decade of life, with a slight predominance in women. Radiographic imaging with MRI and CT demonstrates a multiloculated, expansile, highly vascular osteolytic lesion with a thin, well demarcated, eggshell-like cortical rim (Fig. 19.2). Multiple-level vertebral involvement may occur in up to 40% of cases. Treatment involves pre-operative embolization and surgical resection, or embolization alone

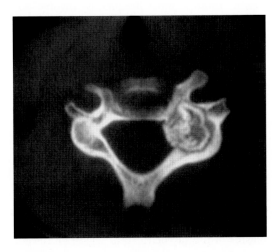

**Fig. 19.1.** Axial CT scan of an osteoblastoma. The patient is an 11-year-old male with a 6-month history of progressive neck pain.

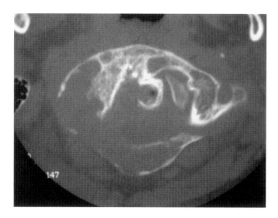

**Fig. 19.2.** Axial CT scan of an ABC. The patient is a 7-year-old female with a 3-month history of neck pain and torticollis.

*Eosinophilic granuloma* (EG) is the solitary osseous lesion in a continuum of disorders (histiocytosis X, Letterer–Siwe and Hand–Schuller–Christian diseases) characterized by an abnormal proliferation of Langerhans cells. EGs are uncommon lesions of the axial skeleton, occurring most frequently in the vertebral body. Most EGs occur in the pediatric population, with a peak incidence at between 5 and 10 years of age. MRI and CT are the investigative procedures of choice, with ultimate diagnosis relying on biopsy. Treatment is somewhat controversial but commonly includes surgical curettage. Adjuvant radiotherapy or chemotherapy is reserved for disseminated versions of this uncommon disease of the axial skeleton [1–4,6,9].

for areas of the spine that are difficult to approach surgically. Post-operative radiation may have a role if inadequate margins were obtained during surgical resection. Recurrence rates vary from 6 to 70%, depending on the extent of surgical resection and administration of post-operative radiation [1–4,6,7].

*Hemangiomas* are benign tumors of vascular origin and are probably the most common benign tumor of the spine. General autopsy studies have found hemangiomas of the axial skeleton in 10–12% of cases. Characterized by slow growth and a female predominance, vertebral hemangiomas occur most commonly in the thoracolumbar spine and have a predilection for the vertebral body. Symptomatic vertebral hemangiomas are exceedingly rare but, when they do present, the most common initial symptom is back pain, with or without radiation into the lower extremities. There is a loose relationship between pregnancy and expansile vertebral hemangiomas that produce a neurological deficit. This is believed to be the result of the physiological volume increase of the circulatory system during pregnancy, which results in expansion of a previously asymptomatic lesion. Diagnosis of symptomatic lesions is best made with MRI, while asymptomatic lesions are discovered incidentally during other radiographic investigations. Treatment for symptomatic lesions involving the spine incorporates a combination of embolization, surgical resection and possibly radiotherapy, and is generally performed in cases of pathological fracture or neural impingement [1–4,6,8].

## Malignant Tumors of the Axial Skeleton

Malignant tumors of the axial skeleton can either be primary (arising from the bony skeleton itself) or metastatic. The most common metastatic spinal column tumors are breast, lung and prostate malignancies, while multiple myeloma, chordoma, chondrosarcoma, osteogenic sarcoma and Ewing's sarcoma are the more common primary malignant axial skeletal neoplasms. Metastasis can result from direct extension or hematogenous spread. Primary malignant axial skeletal neoplasms and metastatic tumors most frequently involve the vertebral body. Malignant tumors of the spinal column are 25–40 times more likely to be metastatic than primary [1–4,6].

*Chordomas*, originally described by Virchow, are tumors originating from the primitive notochord. Being tumors of the axial skeleton and the skull base, chordomas account for 1–2% of all skeletal sarcomas. Chordomas are histologically low-grade, locally invasive tumors; however, metastases may occur in 5–43% of chordoma cases. More than 50% of these lesions are located in the lumbosacral region, 35% in the clival and cervical area, and the remainder are spread throughout the vertebral column. Chordomas are the most common primary neoplasms of the sacrococcygeal region and occur predominantly in the fifth and sixth decades of life. Neurological deficit in the form of bowel and bladder dysfunction may be present at the time of diagnosis. MRI is probably the radiographic modality of choice for total tumor evaluation, because of the ability to evaluate soft-tissue involvement. CT remains the modality of choice for imaging the extent of bony destruction (Fig. 19.3). Diagnosis is based upon CT or fluoroscopic-guided biopsy. Treatment is en-bloc resection, when feasible. Radiation is usually reserved for local recurrence and surgically inaccessible disease. There is considerable debate on pathological subtypes with respect to grade, recurrence and outcome. Age at presentation is probably the best prognostic indicator for disease-free survival following surgery, with younger patients having a better prognosis [1–4,6,10,11].

*Chondrosarcomas* are rare, malignant, cartilage-forming neoplasms, arising from cartilaginous elements. These tumors primarily affect the adult appendicular skeleton, with rare spinal involvement (6% of cases). Chondrosarcomas arise either primarily or from pre-existing solitary osteochondromas, hereditary multiple exostosis or Paget's disease. There is an even distribution of tumor involvement among cervical, thoracic and lumbosacral locations.

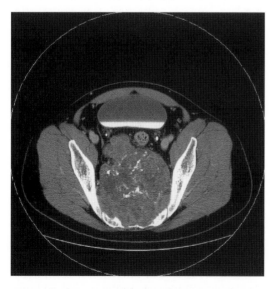

**Fig. 19.3.** Axial CT scan of a large sacrococcygeal chordoma. The patient is a 43-year-old male who presented with a 2–3-year period of progressive sacral pain. The patient went on to undergo an anterior L5/S1 discectomy, with bilateral sectioning of the sacroiliac ligaments, followed by posterior total sacrectomy, followed by L3 through iliac reconstruction.

Primary and secondary chondrosarcomas usually arise in middle-aged and older patients, and show a predilection for males. Diagnostic characteristics on MRI and CT radiographic imaging include bone destruction, associated soft-tissue mass and characteristic flocculent calcifications in the soft tissue mass. Definitive diagnosis is based upon biopsy of the tumor. Treatment is en-bloc resection, if feasible. Neither radiation therapy nor chemotherapy is of much benefit. Prognosis correlates with tumor extension and grade. Unresectable chondrosarcoma has a 5-year survival rate of only 20% [1–4,6,12].

*Osteogenic sarcomas* are primary malignant tumors of bone that are exceedingly rare in the axial skeleton. Only 2% of all osteogenic sarcomas arise in the spine. When they do involve the vertebral column, osteogenic sarcomas are more likely to be metastases than primary tumors. Osteogenic sarcomas may arise primarily or secondarily. The vertebral body is involved in over 95% of cases and these lesions are distributed evenly throughout the spine. The majority of cases of primary osteogenic sarcoma present in the first 20 years of life; secondary sarcomas arise in the fifth to sixth decades, as a result of irradiated bone or pre-existing Paget's disease. This neoplastic disease has a slight predilection for males. Radiologically, osteogenic sarcomas typically exhibit combined lytic and sclerotic lesions, with cortical destruction and ossification in the tumor mass. CT or fluoroscopic-guided biopsy will provide a diagnosis and guide pre-operative adjuvant therapy. Pre-operative embolization, chemotherapy and surgical extirpation with adjuvant radiotherapy are the current treatment modalities. Overall prognosis is poor, with a life expectancy of 10 months to 1.5 years, although there are a few long-term survivors [1–4,6].

*Ewing's sarcomas* are small, blue cell tumors of bone, whose cell of origin remains unclear (Fig. 19.6). Only 3–4% of Ewing's sarcomas arise within the axial skeleton, and Ewing's sarcomas only account for 6% of all primary malignant bone tumors, making these rare primary neoplasms of the spinal column. The incidence of spinal column involvement decreases from caudal to rostral, with more than 50% of Ewing's sarcomas arising within the sacrum. Vertebral body involvement is most common. Ewing's sarcoma is primarily a disease of the pediatric population, with over 85% of cases occurring during the first two decades of life. Males are affected more frequently than females, with a ratio of 2:1. Radiological imaging with MRI and CT will usually reveal a lytic lesion, with possibly a blastic component. Diagnosis is based upon biopsy of the tumor. Treatment involves a multidisciplinary approach that combines surgical extirpation, radiation and chemotherapeutic protocols. Younger patients tend to have a better prognosis. Survival at 5 years for younger patients approaches 75% [1–4,6,13].

*Multiple myelomas* (MMs) and solitary plasmacytomas are two manifestations on a continuum of B-cell lymphoproliferative diseases. Spinal involvement leading to extradural compression is a common finding in multiple myelomas. MMs are the most common malignant neoplasms of bone in adults and affect the spine in 30–50% of reported cases. The thoracic spine is affected most commonly, followed by the lumbar spine and, rarely, the cervical spine (less than 10%). The vertebral body is usually the site of tumor involvement. MM is primarily a disease of the fifth, sixth and seventh decades of life. There is an equal distribution for MM among males and females; however, approximately 75% of solitary plasmacytomas occur in males. Unlike the classic axial skeletal tumor presentation of pain with recumbency, MM lesions are sometimes relieved by rest and aggravated by mechanical agitation, mimicking other degenerative sources of pain. Diagnosis for MM is based upon characteristic serum protein abnormalities and radiological imaging. Plain radiographs and CT can be almost solely diagnostic because of the characteristic osteolytic picture without sclerotic edges involving the vertebral body and sparing the posterior elements. Treatment and prognosis vary greatly, depending on whether the diagnosis is a solitary plasmacytoma or the systemic MM. Both conditions are exquisitely radiosensitive, but with significantly longer survival rates for solitary plasmacytoma [1–4,6].

# Metastatic Spinal Disease

Cancer is a leading cause of death in the USA, claiming nearly half a million deaths each year. The vast majority of these patients will have some evidence of metastatic disease. In fact,

spinal metastases occur in virtually all types of systemic carcinomas. Although certain cancers are more likely to spread to the spine, surgical or autopsy studies have found that as high as 90% of patients with systemic carcinomas have spinal metastases. Between 5 and 20% of these patients will have epidural compression secondary to this, leading to neurological compromise [2,14–23].

Overall, metastatic lesions are equally spread throughout the thoracic and lumbosacral spine; however, the number of symptomatic thoracic metastases is greater. Epidural compression leading to neurological compromise is found in the thoracic region in roughly 70% of cases and in the lumbar region 20% of the time. Most series report symptomatic cervical lesions occurring in only 6–8% of patients. The axiom, however, that acute neck or back pain in a patient with a known malignancy is metastatic disease until proven otherwise remains a prudent guideline. The majority of patients have involvement at a single level, although 15–20% of patients have compression at two or more sites [2,14–23].

The vertebral body is involved most commonly (85%), with the posterior elements and epidural space involved less frequently (10–15% and less than 5%, respectively). The intervertebral disk is almost universally spared from metastatic disease, even when the vertebral body is completely destroyed. Two factors have been proposed to explain this distribution. First has been the high concentration of growth factors found in the rich medullary bone of the body to both attract tumor cells and promote their growth. Many of these factors, such as basic fibroblast growth factor (bFGF), hepatocyte growth factor (HGF) and tumor necrosis factor-( (TNF-(), are well known to facilitate angiogenesis and subsequent tumor growth. The second mechanism involves the draining of the venous plexus of the thoracic, abdominal and pelvic viscera, as described by Batson [2,14–23].

Most frequently, metastases result from hematogenous spread into the vertebral body. To establish a presence in the medullary bone, tumor cells must bypass the filters of the liver and lungs to reach the capillary system of the bone. This explains the fact that in a significant number of patients with spinal metastasis, additional lesions are found in those organs.

Another potential route is via direct flow from segmental arteries from the lungs or through Batson's para-vertebral venous plexus. A mechanism of retrograde flow though this plexus has been described with Valsalva's maneuvers, such as coughing or straining. This hypothetically allows for direct implantation of tumor cells into the spinal column. The final pathway is via direct extension into the bony column from the cancer's primary site. This is seen in lung cancer that extends into the thoracic spine and occasionally in rectal cancer that spreads into the sacrum [2,14–23].

The most common metastatic spinal column tumors are breast, lung and prostate malignancies. Additional cancers that also frequently metastasize to the spine include renal cell, thyroid cancer and multiple myeloma. Although there has been some argument between authors as to whether the latter lesions represent true metastasis or primary lesions of the medullary bone, we have included it in our section on primary bony malignancies [2,14–23].

A variety of studies have compared the results of radiation therapy and surgical management of metastatic disease. Many of these studies compared laminectomy to radiation therapy. Over the past 10 years, there has been a re-evaluation of the surgical approach to vertebral metastasis. The principal site of neural compression in metastatic spine disease is from an anterior or antero–lateral direction. Laminectomy further destabilizes an already compromised spinal column, resulting in progressive deformity and pathological fracture. Laminectomy also results (at best) in incomplete resection of the metastatic disease. Recent studies using aggressive anterior surgical approaches and current instrumentation techniques have shown very promising results in reducing pain, improving function with a relatively low complication rate [24] (Figs 30.4 and 30.5).

## Breast Carcinoma

By far the most prevalent of all metastatic tumors found in the spine, breast cancer has been cited to spread to the spinal column in 85% of all cases. However, the natural history of these tumors varies considerably. Some patients may present with a prolonged course of minimal symptoms, while others deteriorate

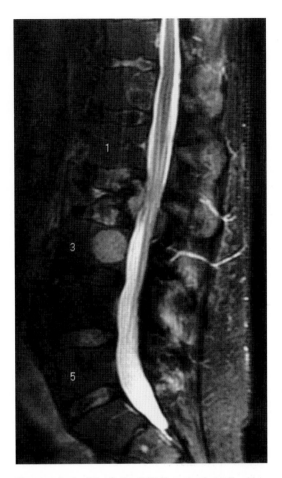

**Fig. 19.4.** Sagittal T2-wieghted MRI (for patient's details, please see Fig. 19.5).

rapidly. Local, radicular and referred pain are the most common symptoms seen in patients with metastatic breast cancer. This is reasonably tied to the biologic activity and, potentially, the hormonal sensitivity of the primary lesions. It is therefore useful to know the degree to which estrogen and progesterone receptors are present, as this can have a considerable impact on the modality of treatment that patients are offered. In such patients, hormonal manipulations via medical treatment are often used.

Often leading to osteolytic lesions, breast carcinomas are the primary cause of pathologic fractures due to metastatic disease. In certain series, breast carcinomas have been cited as being responsible for more than 50% of pathologic fractures.

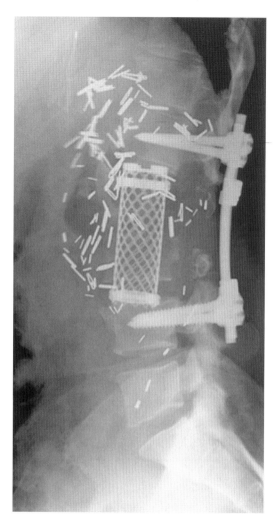

**Fig. 19.5.** Post-operative lumbar radiograph of a 42-year-old male with a history of metastatic renal cell carcinoma. The patient initially underwent radiation therapy but continued to have severe intractable pain and progressive neurological deficits. The patient went on to undergo a two-stage procedure, including L2 and L3 laminectomies, with L1–L4 posterior segmental instrumentation, followed by a right-sided retroperitoneal approach to the lumbar spine, followed by L2 and L3 corpectomies, with L1–L4 anterior reconstruction using a titanium cage. Prior to surgery, the patient underwent angiography and tumor embolization.

Many patients with previously diagnosed and treated breast cancer have undergone some form of radiotherapy. It is therefore important for the clinician to evaluate the patient's cardio–pulmonary function prior to considera-

tion of further therapy. Pulmonary function often can be significantly impaired in patients with parenchymal pathology, either from radiation to the chest wall or from primary lymphangitic spread of the breast cancer itself.

Most cases of breast carcinoma are fairly radiosensitive; therefore, radiation is the first-line treatment for spinal metastasis. Surgery is reserved for cases in which clear instability or neurological deficit is present, severe pain that is unresponsive to conservative measures, tumors that have not responded to radiation treatment or when previous irradiation fields overlap with areas of new disease, making further irradiation contraindicated [2,14–20].

## Prostate Carcinoma

Prostate cancer is second only to lung cancer as the leading cause of cancer-related deaths in men. Histological evidence of prostate cancer is directly related to increasing age. The incidence of occult disease has been shown to be as high as 30% in patients over the age of 50 years and over 70% in patients over the age of 80 years. The presence or absence of metastases primarily determines the prognosis of prostate cancer. The highest incidence of prostate metastases is found in bone, and lesions in the spine are felt to precede those in other areas of the body, such as the lung or liver. Kuban et al. found that spinal cord compression occurs in approximately 7% of all men with prostate cancer. Many argue for a backward venous spread of tumor to the spine. This is felt to account for the gradual decrease in spine involvement from the lumbar to the cervical spine (from 97 to 38%).

New onset of back pain in elderly men should be carefully evaluated for evidence of metastatic prostate cancer. For those patients with a known medical history of prostate cancer, back pain should also lead the clinician to entertain a diagnosis of recurrence, with metastases. In such patients, it is often helpful to routinely check the serum prostate-specific antigen (PSA) level. If the serum PSA level is greater than 100 ng/ml, then the positive predictive value for bony metastasis is 74%. Conversely, a level of less than 10 ng/ml indicates a negative predictive value of 98%. As the PSA level is a relative marker for extent of disease, it is useful to have prior levels and trends to compare current levels with.

Prostate cancer is distinct from other bony metastasis in that it produces mainly osteoblastic lesions. Whereas most cancers typically produce osteolytic lesions, this is true in only 5% of cases of metastatic prostate cancer. The proposed mechanism of this is related to the production of peptide growth factors, such as insulin-like growth factors (IGFs).

Most prostate metastases are fairly radiosensitive; thus, surgical management is generally reserved for those cases that have responded poorly to radiation or where spinal instability or pathological fracture is present. Surgery may also be indicated when a patient's prior prostate radiation fields preclude the use of additional radiation. The latter is not an uncommon event for lesions found in the lumbar spine, due to the close proximity to the prostate. Since most patients present later in life, the overall medical condition and medical co-morbidities which could complicate surgery must be carefully weighed against the patient's expectations from surgery [2,14–19,21].

## Lung Carcinoma

Metastasis to bone is the most frequent extra-pulmonary site of recurrence in patients with non-small cell lung carcinoma, accounting for as many as 43% of all distant recurrences. Of these, metastases to the spine are the most significant and potentially debilitating. Lung carcinoma may invade the spinal column, through direct extension or via hematogenous routes. Most frequently, metastases produce osteolytic lesions, which result from a variety of acid phosphatases, acid hydrolases and alkaline phosphatases. Lung carcinoma follows the typical pattern of spread, with the thoracic spine being most commonly involved, followed by the lumbar spine and finally the cervical spine.

The ultimate biologic activity of the subtypes of lung carcinoma is directly linked to their presumed cell of origin. Squamous cell carcinoma is thought to arise from the basal cell of the bronchial epithelium; adenocarcinoma from the CLARA cell of the bronchiole; bronchoalveolar carcinoma from the type II pneumocytes; and for small (oat) cell carcinoma, the neuroendocrine cells of the bronchoalveolar system are felt to be responsible. The cell of origin for large cell carcinoma is yet to be clearly defined. Of these, however, the spine surgeon rarely encounters those patients with disease other than non-small cell adenocarcinoma. This is due to the rarity of some lesions, such as large cell carcinoma, and to the exquisite sensitivity to radiation for small cell tumors. Patients with squamous cell disease typically have very aggressive disease that is widely disseminated in the lungs and liver, with overall survival looked at in terms of months.

Overall, the prognosis of patients with vertebral metastasis from lung carcinoma remains poor. With the exception of some patients with small cell carcinoma, in which significant responses or even remissions may be seen after chemotherapy and radiation, for the majority of patients with non-small cell disease, the goal of therapy is palliation and prevention of neurological deficits. Due to the relative radio-insensitivity of non-small cell carcinoma compared to breast or prostate cancer, patients may more frequently require surgical intervention to attain these goals [2,14,15,17–19,22].

## Renal Carcinoma

Although renal cell carcinoma (RCC) is relatively rare compared to lung, breast or prostate cancer, it is an aggressive malignancy that frequently metastasizes. The approximately 30,000 cases of renal cell carcinoma account for only 2.5% of all cancer patients. However, as many as 50% of these patients will have evidence of metastatic disease at the time of diagnosis [25]. Although metastatic renal cell carcinoma is found in multiple organs, there is a disproportionately high number of metastases to the spine, making it the fourth most common cancer to affect the spine, and the most common type to present with a neurological deficit as an initial presentation [25].

In contrast with breast and prostate cancer, however, the majority of RCCs are highly resistant to systemic chemotherapy and radiation therapy. In a minority of patients, immunotherapy such as interferon- or interleukin-2 will show a partial response. Therefore, at many institutions, surgery is considered to be the primary treatment option.

Surgery is most often indicated in patients with severe, medically intractable pain, neurological deficit or spinal instability. Classically, RCC is richly vascularized in comparison to other metastatic tumors of the spine. Therefore, many patients undergo pre-operative tumor angiography and embolization to minimize the degree of blood loss during surgery. Although the effectiveness of pre-operative embolization has been debated, it is typically performed prior to non-emergent surgery in patients with large tumors.

Due to the absence of effective systemic therapy, the prognosis of metastatic RCC remains poor, with less than 15% survival at 5 years. Surgical resection and stabilization can provide effective pain relief and neurological preservation or improvement, and the goal of therapy is palliation and prevention of neurological deficits, rather than increase in length of survival [2,14,15,17–19,25].

## Diagnosis

The first symptom of bony metastasis is often back pain. In fact, pain is the most common presenting symptom for tumors involving the axial skeleton and spinal cord. The hallmark of neoplastic lesions of the axial skeleton is localized spinal pain, associated with recumbency and night pain. Pain in the axial skeleton occurs in up to 85% of patients in the larger series of vertebral column tumors and usually begins well prior to any radicular pain or neurological deficit. However, ultimate diagnosis relies on a combination of laboratory investigation, radiographic studies and, potentially, tumor biopsy.

Diagnostic imaging is a cornerstone in the diagnosis of metastatic lesions of the spine. Typically, patients with known carcinoma are staged using multiple modalities of imaging, although, frequently, the spinal axis is not routinely screened unless symptoms are present.

The initial work-up for all patients should include plain radiographs of the spine. Anterior–posterior and lateral X-rays of the region in question can often give important information in the diagnosis of malignancy and can typically be done in an expedited fashion, with little cost to the medical system or patient. Pathologic compression fractures, the presence of a blastic lesion or destructive process within the vertebral bodies, or the destruction of the pedicle on AP views are often characteristic of spinal metastasis. Further, important information on sagittal alignment, including the presence of a kyphotic or scoliotic deformity, is best seen with plain X-rays. These caveats can be helpful in determining a requirement for stabilization or corrective procedures.

CT scanning of an involved area is also often warranted. The sensitivity of CT scanning is higher than that of plain films, although this modality is used most commonly to further define the degree of bony involvement and/or destruction. The detail of bony anatomy is useful in surgical planning, especially if instrumentation will be used for stabilizing the spine. Finally, in patients in which MRI is not an option, such as those with known metal fragments in their body or incompatible devices such as pacemakers, CT scanning with the administration of intrathecal contrast can help to define the degree of epidural extension

Recently, MRI has become the gold standard for radiological diagnosis of spinal metastasis. The ability of MRI to clearly visualize both the soft tissue, extradural and intradural contents in multiple planes makes this modality unique. Further, pending any contraindications to MRI, it enables the surgeon to evaluate the neural elements, with little or no risk to the patient. As MRI technology advances and as MRI-incompatible devices and hardware become less common, the utility of invasive tests such as myelography is sure to become more limited.

Another screening test that is commonly used in patients thought to have bony metastasis is isotope Tc99m bone scan. Often, bone scans are used as an adjuvant to standard screening examinations for patients with cancer. While these tests are useful in detecting bony lesions in patients with metastatic disease, the specificity of them is poor, as patients with degenerative processes or infectious processes can have lesions that are similarly bright on bone scan [2,14–23].

## Treatment

The primary goal in treating all of the above malignancies remains palliation rather than cure. Therefore, relief of pain and preservation of neurological function should be optimized. Treatment options for metastatic disease of the spine include medical therapy, radiation and surgical intervention. Operative intervention is palliative, with pain control and maintenance of function and stability as the goals.

Surgery is usually reserved for neurological compromise, pathological fracture, intractable pain, radiation failure, spinal instability or uncertain diagnosis. The patient's pre-operative functional status and level of activity directly correlate with the post-operative result. When neurological deficit is present, those patients who suffer progressive neurological deficits, occurring within a 24-hour period, have a higher chance of permanent paraplegia, while those with slowly evolving deficits are more likely to regain ambulatory function. Overall prognosis is directly related to neoplastic type, spinal location and extent of systemic involvement [2,14–23].

# Key Points

- *Tumors of the axial skeleton arise primarily from the bone or spread to the bone via hematogenous routes.*

- *Primary bone tumors can be benign or malignant; benign lesions are typically found in patients who are younger than 30 years of age and are more commonly found in the posterior elements; malignant lesions are typical in older patients and most commonly found within the vertebral body.*

- *The most frequent metastatic lesions to the spine arise from malignancy of the breast, prostate and lung.*

- *Diagnostic studies include physical examination, plain roentgenography, CT scanning and MRI, with the latter being the gold standard in imaging.*

- *Treatment for metastatic disease is primarily palliative; initial treatment is typically radiation therapy, with surgical treatment reserved for unclear diagnosis, intractable pain, spinal instability or neurological deficit.*

# References

1. Dreghorn CR, Newman RJ, Hardy GJ, Dickson RA. Primary tumors of the axial skeleton: experience of the Leeds Regional Bone Tumor Registry. Spine 1990;15: 137–40.
2. Boden SD, Laws ER. Tumors of the spine. In: Boden S, editor. The aging spine: essentials of pathophysiology,

3. diagnosis, and treatment. Philadelphia: WB Saunders, 1991; 221–52.
3. Boriani S, Weinstein JN. Differential diagnosis and surgical treatment of primary benign and malignant neoplasms. In: Frymoyer JW, editor. The adult spine: principles and practice. 2nd Edition. Philadelphia: Lippincott–Raven, 1997; 951–1014.
4. Ebersold MJ, Hitchon PW, Duff JM. Primary bony spinal lesions. In: Benzel EC, editor. Spine surgery: techniques, complication avoidance, and management. New York: Churchill Livingstone, 1999; 663–77.
5. Weinstein JN, McLain RF. Primary tumors of the spine. Spine 1987;12:843–51.
6. Weinstein JN. Tumors of the spine. In: Simeone FA, editor. The spine. 3rd Edition. Philadelphia: WB Saunders, 1992; 1279–319.
7. Gupta VK, Gupta SK, Khosla VK, Vashisth RK, Kak VK. Aneurysmal bone cysts of the spine. Surg Neurol 1994;42:428–32.
8. Faria SL, Schlupp WR, Chiminazzo H Jr. Radiotherapy in the treatment of vertebral hemangiomas. Int J Radiat Oncol Biol Phys 1985;11:387–90.
9. De Schepper AM, Ramon F, Van Marck E. MR imaging of eosinophilic granuloma: report of 11 cases. Skeletal Radiol 1993;22:163–6.
10. Bjornsson J, Wold LE, Ebersold MJ, Laws ER. Chordoma of the mobile spine: a clinicopathologic analysis of 40 patients. Cancer 1993;71:735–40.
11. O'Neill P, Bell BA, Miller JD, Jacobson I, Guthrie W. Fifty years of experience with chordomas in southeast Scotland. Neurosurgery 1985;16:166–70.
12. Slater G, Huckstep RL. Management of chondrosarcoma. Aust N Z J Surg 1993;63:587–9.
13. Sharafuddin MJ, Haddad FS, Hitchon PW, Haddad SF, el-Khoury GY. Treatment options in primary Ewing's sarcoma of the spine: report of seven cases and review of the literature. Neurosurgery 1992;30:610–18; discussion 618–19.
14. Gerszten PC, Welch WC. Current surgical management of metastatic spinal disease. Oncology (Huntingt) 2000;14:1013–24; discussion 1024, 1029–30.
15. Welch WC, Jacobs GB. Surgery for metastatic spinal disease. J Neurooncol 1995;23:163–70.
16. Benjamin R. Neurologic complications of prostate cancer. Am Fam Physician 2002;65:1834–40.
17. Healey JH, Brown HK. Complications of bone metastases: surgical management. Cancer 2000;88(Suppl.12): 2940–51.
18. Ratanatharathorn V, Powers WE. Epidural spinal cord compression from metastatic tumor: diagnosis and guidelines for management. Cancer Treat Rev 1991;18: 55–71.
19. Byrne TN. Spinal cord compression from epidural metastases. N Engl J Med 1992;327:614–19.
20. Landreneau FE, Landreneau RJ, Keenan RJ, Ferson PF. Diagnosis and management of spinal metastases from breast cancer. J Neurooncol 1995;23:121–34.
21. Osborn JL, Getzenberg RH, Trump DL. Spinal cord compression in prostate cancer. J Neurooncol 1995; 23:135–47.
22. Greenberger JS. The pathophysiology and management of spine metastasis from lung cancer. J Neurooncol 1995;23:109–20.

23. Jahroudi N, Greenberger JS. The role of endothelial cells in tumor invasion and metastasis. J Neurooncol 1995;23:99–108.

24. Gokaslan ZL, York JE, Walsh GL, McCutcheon IE, Lang FF, Putnam JB Jr et al. Transthoracic vertebrectomy for metastatic spinal tumors. J Neurosurg 1998;89: 599–609.

25. Jackson RJ, Loh SC, Gokaslan ZL. Metastatic renal cell carcinoma of the spine: surgical treatment and results. J Neurosurg 2001;94(Suppl.1):18–24.

# Index